INTRODUCTION TO
HEALTH CARE SERVICES

Parts I & II — 3110
Part III — 3113

INTRODUCTION TO HEALTH CARE SERVICES

FOUNDATIONS AND CHALLENGES

Bernard J. Healey
Tina Marie Evans

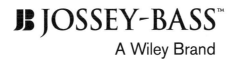

JB JOSSEY-BASS™

A Wiley Brand

Published by Jossey-Bass
A Wiley Brand
One Montgomery Street, Suite 1200, San Francisco, CA 94104-4594—www.josseybass.com

Jossey-Bass books and products are available through most bookstores. To contact Jossey-Bass directly call our Customer Care Department within the U.S. at 800-956-7739, outside the U.S. at 317-572-3986, or fax 317-572-4002.

Wiley publishes in a variety of print and electronic formats and by print-on-demand. Some material included with standard print versions of this book may not be included in e-books or in print-on-demand. If this book refers to media such as a CD or DVD that is not included in the version you purchased, you may download this material at **http://booksupport.wiley.com**. For more information about Wiley products, visit **www.wiley.com**.

Library of Congress Cataloging-in-Publication Data

Healey, Bernard J., 1947-

    Introduction to health care services : foundations and challenges / Bernard J. Healey, Tina M. Evans.
        pages cm
    Includes bibliographical references and index.
   ISBN 978-1-118-40793-6 (pbk.)
  1. Medical care–United States. 2. Health care reform–United States. 3. Public health administration—United States. 4. Medical economics–United States. I. Evans, Tina M., 1976- II. Title.
   RA395.A3H3845 2015
   368.38'2 — dc23

                                                    2014026473

Printed in the United States of America
FIRST EDITION

PB Printing   10 9 8 7 6 5 4 3 2 1

To Kathy, my wife of forty-two years, my two wonderful children, Alison and Bryan, and my five-year-old grandson, John.

Bernard J. Healey

To my grandfather and fishing buddy, Edward Evans Sr., who has taught me so much about working hard and making a difference in the lives of others.
I love you!

Tina Marie Evans

CONTENTS

Part Three: Challenges in Health Care Delivery   265

Chapter 11 The Pursuit of Quality Care 267
Tina Marie Evans

Chapter 12 The Chronic Disease Epidemic 299
Bernard J. Healey

Chapter 13 Leadership Solutions to Health Care Problems 323
Bernard J. Healey

ch. 11 - 15

FIGURES, TABLES, AND EXHIBITS

FIGURES

TABLES

EXHIBITS

INTRODUCTION

The health care industry in the United States is undergoing very rapid change in all sectors of health services delivery. This change will continue into the foreseeable future due to pressures from government, third-party payers, health care providers, and the consumers of health services. One of the most important catalysts of this change is the Patient Protection and Affordable Care Act. This federal legislation was signed into law on March 23, 2010, and it will result in numerous reforms in the way health care services are delivered and received by almost all Americans. The final result of this health care reform will be a completely restructured health care delivery system.

Everyone seems to agree that change in the health services sector of the U.S. economy is inevitable and long overdue, even though the prospect of this change seems to terrify everyone, especially the providers of health care services. This is why there have been numerous efforts to bring about health care reform over the last fifty years with very little success. In fact, a great deal of the change that has occurred over the years has only made our problems in delivering health care services worse.

The major problems found in our current health care system continue to be cost escalation, lack of access to care for a large number of Americans, and poor health for a large percentage of Americans. Of course, many of these problems will go away if more people remain healthy rather than becoming ill. The leading cause of morbidity and mortality in our country is no longer curable communicable diseases but rather incurable chronic diseases. This silent epidemic of chronic diseases cannot be treated, but it can be prevented if we as a nation are willing to invest the necessary resources in health education and health promotion programs designed to help people avoid acquiring these diseases in the first place.

Almost all the money spent on health care every year goes toward diagnosing curable disease and then working to cure it. The problem with this strategy is that once one acquires a chronic disease there is no cure; one can only manage the chronic disease in an attempt to prevent later complications from it. Fortunately, there is another strategy that can be used to deal with the epidemic of chronic diseases. This strategy will take a long time to develop, implement, evaluate, and improve, but given time and resources it will work. Our health care system must move a large amount of resources away from disease detection and attempted cure and direct those resources instead to health education designed to prevent disease. Health education is also a valuable strategy for preventing the complications that usually arise from having a chronic disease for a long period of time.

This text outlines many of the changes that are coming in the very near future to the American health care delivery system. It is divided into three sections: an overview of health care services delivery in the United States, a thorough survey of the major players in health care services, and a discussion of the challenges in health care delivery. In addition to the usual topics found in an introduction to health care services, it provides extensive coverage of the chronic disease epidemic, discussions about the community-centered health home model, and a thorough explanation of how leadership and the empowerment of health care workers can unleash the creativity and innovation that are so necessary if we are to solve our major health care problems. This book concludes with four case studies that demonstrate the kinds of innovations already occurring in the delivery of health care services.

An instructor's supplement is available at www.wiley.com/go /healeyevans. Additional materials such as videos, podcasts, and readings can be found at www.josseybasspublichealth.com. Comments about this book are invited and can be sent to publichealth@wiley.com.

ACKNOWLEDGMENTS

We would like to begin by acknowledging the dedicated individuals who work in the field of health care delivery on a daily basis with the goal of improving the health of those who become ill or are attempting to remain well. They are working during very difficult times as the American health care delivery system reorganizes the way it delivers health care.

During the process of gathering the research for this new text, we met many dedicated people who went out of their way to provide us with the vital information required to make this book accurate and to the point on the numerous topics covered. A number of individuals, to whom we are truly indebted, helped us with the writing of particular chapters. Several of the wonderful individuals who work at Prevention Institute, a nonprofit national center dedicated to improving community health and equity through effective primary prevention, wrote the chapter on the community-centered health home. They are Jeremy Cantor, Larry Cohen, Leslie Mikkelsen, Rea Pañares, Janani Srikantharajah, and Erica Valdovinos.

Two more individuals assisted us on two of the most important topics for a book designed to introduce students to the new world of health services delivery: hospitals and health insurance. Denise Yanchik contributed the comprehensive chapter about the historical development of hospitals and the many challenges these institutions are facing today in the United States. Jeffrey R. Helton contributed a great deal of up-to-date information as the coauthor of the chapter on health insurance in the United States.

In addition, Francis G. Belardi, Jeff Kile, Daniel J. Amorino, and Joseph J. Marrone contributed the case studies in health care administration that conclude this book. These case studies offer the reader a great deal of information about the enormous creativity and innovation going into the restructuring of the U.S. health care delivery system. Thanks to all of these generous individuals, we believe that this text captures the most important components of this country's new health care delivery system.

We would also like to thank reviewers Joy Renfro, Karoline Mortensen, Janice Frates, and Aaron G. Buseh, who provided thoughtful and constructive comments on the complete draft manuscript.

There are many wonderful people who gave of their time to help make our ideas better. We are very fortunate to have had the opportunity to write a book for a national publisher, and we are equally fortunate to have been able to work with such talent.

Bernard J. Healey is a professor of health care administration at King's College in Wilkes-Barre, Pennsylvania, and has been teaching college courses since 1974. He began his career in 1971 as an epidemiologist for the Pennsylvania Department of Health, retiring from that position in 1995. During his tenure with government he completed advanced degrees in business administration and public administration. He received his doctoral degree from the University of Pennsylvania in 1990. Healey has been teaching undergraduate and graduate courses in business, public health, and health care administration at several colleges for over thirty years.

The author of over one hundred published articles about public health; health policy, leadership, and marketing; and health care partnerships, Healey has also written and published four books on various topics in health care administration. He is a member of the Association of University Programs in Health Care Administration, a part-time consultant in epidemiology for the Wilkes-Barre City Health Department, and a consultant for numerous public health projects in Pennsylvania.

Tina Marie Evans is an associate professor and department head of applied health studies at the Pennsylvania College of Technology. She is a 1998 summa cum laude graduate of Marywood University with a bachelor's degree in sports medicine, and she completed her master's degree in health care administration at King's College in 1999. After teaching at King's College in the Department of Sports Medicine for five years, and serving as the interim director of sports medicine there, she then taught at Marywood University for two years, receiving her doctoral degree in 2004 from Marywood, with a specialization in health promotion. She is active in grant writing, publishing scholarly manuscripts, and presenting on various allied health topics on the local, regional, national, and international levels. She also engages in volunteer activities in her church and community. Outside of work, she enjoys the outdoors, swimming, golf, ballroom dancing, and spending time with her family.

Daniel J. Amorino is a quality improvement specialist in the Geisinger Quality Institute at Geisinger Health System. In this role he acts as a process improvement consultant and coach, using Lean/Six Sigma methodologies on various projects throughout the health system. His work varies from improving the patient experience by addressing throughput and clinic flow to helping teams that are struggling with performance measures in the inpatient setting. Previously, he worked at the Department of Veterans Affairs in New York City, first as an administrative Fellow and then as a process improvement specialist. He earned his BA degree in sociology from Brigham Young University-Idaho and his MHA degree from The Pennsylvania State University. He lives in northeast Pennsylvania with his wife, Jennifer, two daughters, Ellie and Evangeline, and twin boys, Calvin and Cooper.

Francis G. Belardi is currently president and CEO of the Guthrie Medical Group in Sayre, Pennsylvania. While serving as executive vice president of the Guthrie Clinic, he developed a physician leadership curriculum in conjunction with King's College. This program has trained forty-five Guthrie physicians in physician leadership over the past five years, and twelve of those physicians are pursuing the MHA degree to further enhance their leadership skills. He has served in many other leadership roles at the Guthrie Clinic, including program director for the family medicine residency, chairman of family medicine for Guthrie-Robert Packer Hospital, and designated institutional official for all Guthrie graduate medical education programs. He is a Fellow of the American Academy of Family Practice, and he has contributed several articles to the primary care medical literature over his forty-year career. Born and raised in Pearl River, New York, Belardi received his BS degree from Iona College and his MD degree from the Creighton University School of Medicine. He completed an internship at the Rhode Island Hospital–Brown University Program in Medicine in Providence, Rhode Island, a family medicine residency at the Ohio State University Affiliated Hospitals, and an academic teaching fellowship at the University of North Carolina School of Medicine. He has been married to his wife, Ann Marie, for forty-four years and has three children and three grandchildren.

Jeremy Cantor is a program manager at Prevention Institute. In addition to functioning as part of the organization's management team, he focuses on advancing the integration of clinical care and community prevention and creating healthy, safe, sustainable, and equitable communities in California. His recent projects include authoring a brief on sustainable resources for prevention (*How Do We Pay for a Healthy Population?*), functioning as lead consultant on the Eden Area Livability Initiative (an eighteen-month project to build community capacity and prioritize community needs in the unincorporated areas of Alameda County), and identifying opportunities and model practices for connecting clinical and community health data in order to inform prevention strategy. He has provided training and consultation to a variety of groups, including developing a health disparities training series for The California Endowment and training modules on the use of social determinant indicator data in communities for the Centers for Disease Control and Prevention. Prior to joining Prevention Institute, Cantor was the founding director of Destination: College, a University of California, Berkeley–based AmeriCorps program that trains and supervises undergraduate advisors placed in underresourced Bay Area schools. Cantor holds a BA degree in psychology from Haverford College and a master of public health degree from the University of California, Berkeley.

Larry Cohen is founder and executive director of Prevention Institute, a national nonprofit center that has helped to shape the way this country thinks about health and prevention—improving community conditions and taking action to build resilience and to prevent illness, injury, and violence before they occur. Prevention Institute has helped to advance a deeper understanding of how social and community factors and the design of communities shape health, and it works with communities to address health inequities. Prevention Institute has also helped to incorporate a focus on prevention into the national stimulus and health care reform legislation and has developed a framework for integrating prevention, public health, and clinical care. Cohen has created tools and frameworks for advancing comprehensive solutions through multidisciplinary collaboration—for example, for improving eating and activity environments in communities that are strongly affected by violence. Prior to founding Prevention Institute in 1997, he served as founding director of the Contra Costa County Prevention Program, where he engaged the American Cancer Society, American Heart Association, and American Lung Association in forming the first coalition in the United States for changing tobacco policy, an effort in which they advocated for passage of the nation's first multicity smoking ban.

Jeffrey R. Helton is an assistant professor of health care management at Metropolitan State University of Denver in Denver, Colorado, where he teaches health care finance, health informatics, and health economics. He is also an adjunct assistant professor at the University of Denver and at George Washington University. Helton is a certified management accountant, a certified fraud examiner, and a Fellow of the Healthcare Financial Management Association. He also serves on the board of examiners of that association. A former health system chief financial officer, he has over twenty years of experience in a variety of health care organizations across the United States. Helton earned his PhD degree from the University of Texas.

Jeff Kile is a pediatrician at Pediatric Associates of Kingston, where he has practiced for the last ten years, and an associate medical director for Blue Cross of Northeastern Pennsylvania, a position he has held since July 2010. A native of Wilkes-Barre, Pennsylvania, he graduated from the Drexel University (MCP/Hahnemann) School of Medicine in 1999, and completed his pediatric residency in 2002 at Rainbow Babies and Children's Hospital in Cleveland, Ohio, where he was elected to serve as chief resident for the 2002–2003 academic year. He was also a clinical faculty member in the department of pediatrics at Case Western Reserve University School of Medicine that same year. After returning to Wilkes-Barre as a general pediatrician, he completed an MHA degree at King's College in 2009, to attain skills in health care economics, organization, and management. Kile is actively involved in many sections of the American Academy of Pediatrics (AAP), especially the Section on Telehealth, serving on that section's nominating committee (as chair in 2008) and, since 2009, on its executive committee as the education chair. He was the activity director for the AAP's virtual grand rounds on telehealth, he has spoken on the topic of telehealth and reimbursement at the AAP National Conference and Exhibition, and he has published several peer-reviewed articles on reimbursement for telephone care and physician executive education, among other topics. He has volunteered for the United Way's Success by Six program, which promotes developmental milestone awareness among parents. He has served as an advisory board member for the Luzerne and Wyoming County Mental Health and Mental Retardation Program, and he also serves as a clinical instructor for the King's College physician's assistant program and as clinical faculty in pediatrics at Commonwealth Medical College.

Joseph J. Marrone currently works with Prudential Insurance in its Information Technology Department, working with a Windows server-client environment. These systems have ranged from Windows NT and Windows 95 up to the present-day Windows 2008 R2 and Windows 7 client. Previously, he was employed by Wang Laboratories, Inc., installing and maintaining various information systems, including telephony systems, mini and micro data systems, and office information systems. He has earned degrees in information technology along with an MBA degree from Excelsior College.

Leslie Mikkelsen is managing director at Prevention Institute, serving on the senior management team and supporting organizational operations and development to advance the practice of primary prevention. She directs the community-centered health systems team, with the goal of shifting the nation's health paradigm in order to elevate the critical need to address community determinants of health and thus to improve health equity and safety outcomes by marshaling the most effective community prevention strategies. The team is currently engaged in assessing how medical care organizations can institutionalize activities to address community determinants of health and is also researching and disseminating promising state and federal policies for supporting these efforts. Mikkelsen supports the Convergence Partnership—a consortium of national funders—with strategy development and implementation for promoting their vision of "healthy people, healthy places." She regularly serves as a technical assistance provider for a variety of foundations and community prevention collaborations at the state and local levels. Current efforts include investigating opportunities for advancing community-centered health homes for the Blue Cross Blue Shield of North Carolina Foundation and the Blue Shield of California Foundation. She also cofounded and served as project director for the Strategic Alliance for Healthy Food and Activity Environments, a California coalition that has successfully advanced a broad, multifaceted environmental change agenda that has influenced state legislation and was incorporated into the California Obesity Prevention Plan.

Rea Pañares is a senior advisor with Prevention Institute (PI), a national center dedicated to building momentum for community prevention. In this role she oversees projects related to health reform and advancing community prevention in health care settings, with a particular focus on supporting community health centers. Prior to her work with PI, she served as director of minority health initiatives at Families USA in Washington, DC, a national policy advocacy organization and a leading voice in the health reform debate. In this role she led efforts to strengthen health policies and programs, with an eye toward improving racial and ethnic minorities' access to care, and established Families USA's relationships with key stakeholders, including leading advocacy organizations, the media, and members of Congress and other elected officials. Before this she was a program associate at Grantmakers In Health (GIH), where she was responsible for leading GIH's work in the areas of racial and ethnic health disparities, which included language access, immigrant health, and the social determinants of health. She has also held positions at the National Business Group on Health and the Centers for Medicare & Medicaid Services. Pañares holds a master's degree in health policy and management from the Johns Hopkins Bloomberg School of Public Health and is a graduate of the University of California, Berkeley in molecular and cell biology.

Janani Srikantharajah is currently a student at the David Geffen School of Medicine at the University of California, Los Angeles. From 2006 to 2011, she worked as a program coordinator at Prevention Institute (PI), supporting that organization's research, advocacy, consulting, and administrative functions. She was involved in PI's national health reform efforts, health equity and injury prevention projects, and statewide efforts focused on the built environment. She earned her BA degree in molecular and cell biology, with a minor in conservation resource studies, from the University of California, Berkeley.

Erica Valdovinos is currently a medical student at the University of California, San Francisco. She was formerly a program assistant at Prevention Institute, where her work included analysis of the health reform process, building the economic case for community prevention, and researching better integration of clinical and community preventive services. She received her BA degree in English from the University of California, Berkeley in 2009.

Denice Yanchik is a senior director of clinical operations for Kindred Healthcare, Inc., Hospital Division, providing oversight to fourteen long-term acute care hospitals in Pennsylvania, New Jersey, Massachusetts, and Kentucky. She is a registered nurse with thirty-five years' experience in health care. Twenty-eight of those years were spent in short-term acute care, working for the Geisinger Health System in Pennsylvania. She has experience in critical care, diabetes education, performance improvement, leadership, and management. Yanchik started her nursing education at Luzerne County Community College in Nanticoke, Pennsylvania, received her bachelor's degree in nursing from College Misericordia in Dallas, Pennsylvania, and her master's degree in health care administration from King's College. She is a member of the American Nurses Association and the Pennsylvania Nurses Association.

INTRODUCTION TO
HEALTH CARE SERVICES

PART ONE

OVERVIEW OF HEALTH CARE SERVICE DELIVERY

CHAPTER 1

AN OVERVIEW OF HEALTH CARE DELIVERY IN THE UNITED STATES

Bernard J. Healey

What has happened to the health care delivery system in the United States, once considered the best system anywhere? This is a complicated question, and the answer you will hear depends on the biases of the group you are talking to. Physicians blame insurance providers, insurance providers blame employers, employees fault government regulation, and the consumers of health services blame everyone. This book is intended to help you better understand all of the important sectors of the U.S. health care system while developing an appreciation for all that needs to be done to improve health outcomes at a price those paying for health care can afford.

The health care delivery system in the United States is in a crisis situation that threatens its long-term survival. At the same time, this crisis offers tremendous opportunities for positive changes that will lead to a better system of care for all. The U.S. health care delivery system costs more than the system of any other industrialized country and yet delivers far fewer positive health outcomes to its population. Several indices of health care in America, such as infant mortality, fall below the results found in other industrialized countries, despite our extensive use of the newest and most expensive technology (Budrys, 2012).

According to Fuchs (1998) the major problems found in the U.S. health care system involve *costs, access,* and *health levels and outcomes.* There is also a serious problem with the *quality* of the health services received by many Americans. The *cost* of health care delivery has continued to rise for the last several years and was a leading reason why Congress recently passed the health care reform legislation titled the **Patient Protection and Affordable Care Act of 2010 (ACA).** The ACA is a federal statute designed

LEARNING OBJECTIVES

After reading this chapter you should be able to

- Describe the major problems found in the U.S. health care delivery system.

- Describe the need for reform of the present system of health care delivery in the United States.

- Discuss how health care services are financed in the United States.

- Explain the advantages of a focus on health outcomes rather than activities in the health care delivery system.

- Demonstrate the value of preventing disease rather than mostly attempting to cure disease.

Patient Protection and Affordable Care Act of 2010 (ACA)
Signed into law on March 23, 2010, the ACA seeks to increase the quality and availability of health care coverage for most Americans.

to increase the availability of health care coverage to most Americans and to improve the quality of that care. This new legislation attempts to solve the *access* problem for the millions of Americans who are without health insurance, and it should cause the number of uninsured people in the United States to drop dramatically in 2014. Unfortunately, this new legislation pays far less attention to *health levels and outcomes*, or wellness, in the U.S. population. We are currently dealing with an epidemic of chronic diseases, and these diseases and their complications are responsible for 80 percent of current health care costs.

Many health policy experts argue that the problems with costs, access, health levels, and quality are symptoms of a health care delivery system that is in immediate need of tremendous reform. This chapter will explore various aspects of these problems and their causes.

Health Care Costs

The cost of health care delivery has become one of the major problems confronting the United States as its health care system seeks to achieve reform. Forty years ago a typical American family spent approximately $450 per year on health care delivery, which at that time represented 8 percent of the gross domestic product (GDP) (Fuchs, 1998). In 2010, an average American family spent $8,402, representing over 17 percent of GDP. Carroll, Chapman, Dodd, Hollister, and Harrington (2013) argue that health care costs will continue to rise and, by the year 2020, will total $4.6 trillion, representing almost 20 percent of GDP. This cost escalation will occur despite the fact that the new health care reform law will have been fully implemented by 2020. In a recent article, Fuchs (2013) points out that even though the escalation in health care costs has slowed in the last few years, if it returns to its prior level, the United States will be spending over 30 percent of GDP on health care in 2040. Baumol (2012) calls such rapidly rising costs **cost disease**, an economic ailment that is forcing a crisis of public choice on how limited federal dollars are spent each year. Baumol argues that education, the performing arts, and health care all suffer from cost disease due to the fact that the quantity of labor required to produce these services is very difficult to reduce. In other industries, in contrast, productivity increases have occurred, allowing the costs of products to be lowered. Baumol also notes that the price increases for health care are "real price increases": that is, they are above the U.S. rate of inflation. This cost escalation is unsustainable and will result in this country being unable to deliver basic health care and many other goods and services in the near future unless we gain control over rising costs.

cost disease
The cost increase that occurs when the quantity of labor required by a product or service cannot be reduced, as in education, health care, and the performing arts, for example.

Table 1.1 shows expenditures for various components of the health care sector of the U.S. economy. It provides evidence of cost disease in action as we look at national health expenditures as a percentage of GDP from 1960 to 2011. It is again important to note that these price increases were real price increases; they were above the inflation rate for most of the years since 1960.

Conversely, there has been some recent good news regarding the costs of health care delivery. According to Lowrey (2012) health care spending rose only 3.9 percent in 2010, following a similarly low increase in health care costs in 2009. Also, the Centers for Medicare & Medicaid Services (2012) reports that consumers made fewer physician visits in 2010 than 2009, which resulted in very slow growth in the use and intensity of physician services. Unfortunately, this reduction in physician use was probably due to the loss of private insurance resulting from job loss and reduced personal income because of the recession of 2008.

Demographic and Population Change and Health Costs

Age, gender, ethnicity, and culture can be very useful in explaining health care concerns, along with providing the raw numbers to predict future health care problem areas. The population of the United States is aging, and there is usually a direct relationship between growing older and increasing expenditures for health care services. This may be a critical factor in the rising expenditures for health care services as the baby boom generation begins to receive Medicare benefits.

The first baby boomer reached age sixty-five on January 1, 2011, meaning that a very large cohort of Americans is now beginning to receive Medicare. In less than twenty years the Medicare rolls are expected to double.

Figure 1.1 reveals that in 2010 there were over 40 million Americans over age sixty-five in the United States, and this segment of the population is continuing to increase. In the last ten years, the overall American population increased by 9.7 percent while the number of those sixty-five years old and older grew 15.1 percent. The growth in this elderly segment of our population is going to pose tremendous challenges for our current health care delivery system, particularly in these two areas:

1. The already epidemic levels of chronic diseases and their complications will most likely become even greater in future years.

2. The difficult question of how to deal with end-of-life care that has low if any marginal value must be addressed.

Sultz and Young (2011) argue that the ramifications of treating chronic diseases are becoming a huge challenge for the U.S. health care

Table 1.1 National Health Care Expenditures: Aggregate and per Capita Amounts, Annual Percentage Change and Percentage Distribution: Selected Calendar Years 1960–2011

Item	1960	1970	1980	1990	2000	2001	2002	2003	2004	2005	2006	2007	2008	2009	2010	2011
Amount in Billions																
National health expenditures	$27.4	$74.9	$255.8	$724.3	$1,377.2	$1,493.3	$1,638.0	$1,775.4	$1,901.6	$2,030.5	$2,163.3	$2,298.33	$2,406.6	$2,501.2	$2,600.0	$2,700.7
Health consumption expenditures	24.8	67.1	235.7	675.6	1,289.6	1,402.1	1,535.9	1,665.5	1,784.2	1,904.0	2,032.4	2,154.6	2,252.8	2,355.1	2,450.8	2,547.2
Personal health care	23.4	63.1	217.2	616.8	1,165.4	1,265.3	1,371.9	1,480.2	1,589.4	1,697.1	1,804.4	1,914.1	2,010.4	2,111.6	2,190.0	2,279.3
Government administration and net cost of health insurance	1.1	2.6	12.0	38.8	81.2	90.0	111.9	131.8	141.0	150.9	165.7	171.8	169.8	167.9	181.5	188.9
Government public health activities	0.4	1.4	6.4	20.0	43.0	46.8	52.0	53.5	53.8	56.0	62.3	68.7	72.6	75.6	79.3	79.0
Investment	2.6	7.8	20.1	48.7	87.5	91.3	102.0	110.0	117.4	126.5	130.9	143.7	153.8	146.1	149.1	153.5
Millions																
U.S. population[1]	186	210	230	254	282	285	288	290	293	295	298	301	304	307	309	311
Amount in Billions																
Gross domestic product[2]	$526	$1,038	$2,788	$5,801	$9,952	$10,286	$10,642	$11,142	$11,853	$12,623	$13,377	$14,029	$14,292	$13,974	$14,499	$15,076
Per Capita Amount																
National health expenditures	$147	$356	$1,110	$2,854	$4,878	$5,240	$5,695	$6,121	$6,497	$6,875	$7,255	$7,636	$7,922	$8,163	$8,417	$8,680
Health consumption expenditures	133	319	1,023	2,662	4,568	4,919	5,340	5,742	6,096	6,447	6,816	7,158	7,416	7,686	7,934	8,187
Personal health care	125	300	943	2,430	4,128	4,439	4,770	5,103	5,430	5,746	6,051	6,360	6,618	6,891	7,090	7,326
Government administration and net cost of health insurance	6	12	52	153	288	316	389	454	482	511	556	571	559	548	588	607
Government public health activities	2	6	28	79	152	164	181	185	184	190	209	228	239	247	257	254

Investment	14	37	87	192	310	320	355	379	401	428	439	477	506	477	483	493

Average Annual Percentage Change from Previous Year Shown

National health expenditures		10.6%	13.1%	11.0%	6.6%	8.4%	9.7%	8.4%	7.1%	6.8%	6.5%	6.2%	4.7%	3.9%	3.9%	3.9%
Health consumption expenditures		10.5	13.4	11.1	6.7	8.7	9.5	8.4	7.1	6.7	6.7	6.0	4.6	4.5	4.1	3.9
Personal health care		10.4	13.2	11.0	6.6	8.6	8.4	7.9	7.4	6.8	6.3	6.1	5.0	5.0	3.7	4.1
Government administration and net cost of health insurance		9.4	16.4	12.4	7.7	10.8	24.4	17.7	7.0	7.0	9.8	3.7	−1.2	−1.1	8.1	4.1
Government public health activities		13.8	16.9	12.0	8.0	8.7	11.2	2.8	0.5	4.1	11.2	10.3	5.8	4.1	4.9	−0.5
Investment		11.7	10.0	9.2	6.0	4.3	11.8	7.8	6.8	7.8	3.5	9.7	7.1	−5.0	2.1	2.9
U.S. population[1]		1.2	0.9	1.0	1.1	1.0	0.9	0.8	0.9	0.9	1.0	0.9	0.9	0.9	0.8	0.7
Gross domestic product[2]		7.0	10.4	7.6	5.5	3.4	3.5	4.7	6.4	6.5	6.0	4.9	1.9	−2.2	3.8	4.0

Percentage Distribution

National health expenditures	100.0%	100.0%	100.0%	100.0%	100.0%	100.0%	100.0%	100.0%	100.0%	100.0%	100.0%	100.0%	100.0%	100.0%	100.0%	100.0%
Health consumption expenditures	90.6	89.6	92.1	93.3	93.6	93.9	93.8	93.8	93.8	93.9	93.7	93.6	94.2	94.3	94.3	
Personal health care	85.4	84.3	84.9	85.2	84.6	84.7	83.8	83.4	83.6	83.4	83.3	83.5	84.4	84.2	84.4	
Government administration and net cost of health insurance	3.9	3.5	4.7	5.4	5.9	6.0	6.8	7.4	7.4	7.7	7.5	7.1	6.7	7.0	7.0	
Government public health activities	1.4	1.8	2.5	2.8	3.1	3.1	3.2	3.0	2.8	2.9	3.0	3.0	3.0	3.1	2.9	

Table 1.1 *Continued*

Item	1960	1970	1980	1990	2000	2001	2002	2003	2004	2005	2006	2007	2008	2009	2010	2011
Investment	9.4	10.4	7.9	6.7	6.4	6.1	6.2	6.2	6.2	6.2	6.1	6.3	6.4	5.8	5.7	5.7
							Percentage									
National health expenditures as a percentage of gross domestic product	5.2%	7.2%	9.2%	12.5%	13.8%	14.5%	15.4%	15.9%	16.0%	16.1%	16.2%	16.4%	16.8%	17.9%	17.9%	17.9%

Note: Numbers and percentages may not add to totals because of rounding. Dollar amounts shown are in current dollars.
[1] Census resident-based information less armed forces overseas and population of outlying areas. *Source*: U.S. Bureau of the Census.
[2] U.S. Department of Commerce, Bureau of Economic Analysis.
Source: Centers for Medicare & Medicaid Services, n.d, tbl. 1. Data from Centers for Medicare & Medicaid Services, Office of the Actuary, National Health Statistics Group; U.S. Department of Commerce, Bureau of Economic Analysis; and U.S. Bureau of the Census.

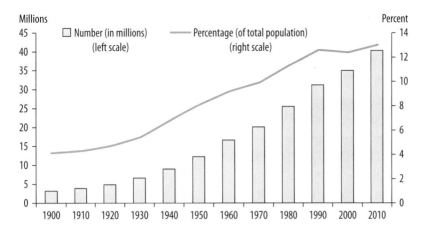

Figure 1.1   U.S. Population Aged Sixty-Five and Older, by Size and Percentage of Total Population, 1900–2010

Source: U.S. Census Bureau, 2011, fig. 2. Data from U.S. Census Bureau decennial census of population, 1900–2010.

delivery system, with very few solutions readily available. The cost burden of chronic diseases alone is causing many health policy experts to question whether the U.S. health care system can survive if costs continue to rise.

Examples of Other Health Care Systems

Every country is having difficulty dealing with cost escalation in health care services, but most countries are having greater success than the United States is with the issues of access to care and levels of health. It makes sense for us to look at how these countries have improved both access and health indices while not spending nearly as much as we do on health services delivery. There are many industrialized countries in the world that are achieving better health outcomes at a much lower cost than the United States currently is. Starr (2011) points out that during the last half of the last century, the United States became the only advanced society that did not provide universal health care. Yet, even without universal health insurance coverage, the United States spends two and a half times as much as other industrialized countries on providing health care just to its citizens who are able to access that care. The health care delivery systems in other industrialized countries have two things in common: extensive government involvement and limitations on the availability of many health care services. In many other countries, governments pay for health care services through higher taxes. In contrast, the United States has decided, for the time being, that it does not want to begin a single-payer system for health services that would be financed through higher taxes. Let's compare the U.S. health care system to the systems in three other industrialized countries: Germany, the United Kingdom, and Canada.

Health Care in Germany

The German system of health care delivery is one of the oldest in Europe. Started by Bismarck in 1883, it makes use of a number of *sickness funds* (insurance plans) and came into being through a law that provided funds to operate health clinics. "In 2008, Germany was spending $3,737 per person for health care services. The men were living to 76.7 and the women were living to 82 years of age" (Budrys, 2012, p. 132). These life expectancy figures are very close to the U.S. figures of 75.4 years for men and 80.4 years for women in 2007 (see Table 8.1 in Chapter Eight), but the cost of health care on a per capita basis in Germany is much lower than the nearly $8,000 per capita spent in the United States in 2008 (Table 1.1).

In Germany, enrollment in the government-financed social insurance programs is mandatory. In this system those who work must have health insurance that is financed by both the employer and employee. The insurance fees are collected and disbursed by the 240 sickness funds. According to Budrys (2012) the German government does not actually run the health care system but does oversee the health care market.

Health Care in the United Kingdom

In 1948, the National Health Service (NHS) was formed in Great Britain and was directed to provide health care services to all residents of the country. In 2005, the United Kingdom spent only $2,724 per capita on health care, representing 8.3 percent of the country's GDP (Linden, 2010). There are trade-offs for spending less on health care, and the National Health System restricts access to many parts of the system. Yet despite this fact, the World Health Organization (WHO) points out that the UK health care system ranks eighteenth among the systems of 191 countries in terms of health care performance (Linden, 2010).

The UK system offers residents relatively easy access to primary care, but specialty care is rationed through the use of waiting lists. Health services are paid for mostly through individual taxes, and physician payment is capitated, while physicians in hospitals mostly hold salaried positions. This payment mechanism has resulted in physician and nurse shortages along with limited availability of acute care beds in hospitals. Despite these shortages and the resultant rationing of care, life expectancy in the United Kingdom is as good if not better than that found in the United States.

Health Care in Canada

Many health policy experts in the United States look at the Canadian health care system as a model for the reform of the U.S. health care system. In fact this system was used as an example for the United States during the failed attempt at health care reform during the Clinton administration. Because Canada is similar to the United States in so many ways, it seems natural to look to its health care system for answers to many of the most pressing health care problems in the United States.

The Canadian health delivery system was started in 1947 and is sometimes referred to as medicare (not to be confused with the U.S. system of Medicare for the elderly). It is available to all residents from birth to death and is paid for through taxes, resulting in taxes higher than those in the United States. It is a single-payer system, allowing every citizen access to hospitals and medical care while not imposing any deductibles or copayments on patients. The costs of health care delivery are restrained through a series of rationing techniques that keep physician and hospital costs in line and restrict the development and use of technology through the government's large purchasing power.

According to Feldstein (2011) this system of health care delivery has improved life expectancy while lowering administrative costs, allowing health care in Canada to command a smaller percentage of GDP and lower spending per capita than health care in the United States. Administrative costs are lower in Canada than in the United States because third-party payers are eliminated when there is only one payer, the government. Despite this cost containment, Canada's health care system would be virtually impossible to duplicate in the United States due to many U.S. citizens' concerns over big government and the power of the special interest groups involved in the U.S. insurance market.

Lower health care costs in Canada also result from a restriction on technology development that is not present in the United States. Feldstein (2011) points out that because the Canadian government would have to pay for innovation in technology by raising taxes, there is a reluctance to invest in technology that may result in only limited benefits for the population overall.

According to Feldstein (2011) the Canadian plan has two major cost-saving features:

1. Reduced administrative costs, resulting in large part from the single-payer approach.

2. Imposed expenditure limits on providers of care.

Armstrong and Armstrong (2008) point out that the Canadian health care system has also achieved reasonable access to quality health services.

As reforms to the American health care delivery system proceed over the next several years, we need to adapt and implement the positive parts of these other systems. It is interesting that in Germany, the United Kingdom, and Canada, less testing and fewer medical procedures may be part of the reason that life expectancy in these countries quite often exceeds that in the United States. Fewer medical tests and procedures may result in fewer medical errors, reducing costs and mortality. All three of these systems of health care delivery focus on using large-scale purchasing power to keep health care costs low while making services available to the entire population. Physician fees, hospital charges, and the costs of purchasing and using expensive technology are kept low by restrictions imposed by the purchaser of the services. This results in restrictions of supply and some rationing but also the elimination of many unnecessary and wasteful expenditures of low marginal value.

Evidence-Based Medicine and Health Costs

In order to improve health outcomes while also reducing the cost of health services, we must use scarce health care resources wisely. According to Schimpff (2012) a large number of medical tests and procedures currently in use cost a great deal and offer little or no value. Evaluations supported by well-documented research need to be completed on numerous medical interventions in order to determine their true value.

Other countries deliver quality health services and produce better health outcomes while also spending less on health service delivery than the United States. They have accomplished this improvement in value while reducing costs by researching the value of almost every medical procedure and applying a cost-benefit analysis to reimbursement decisions for these procedures. One important way to improve health care delivery in the United States is to ask these same questions about the medical care being delivered here. This will help the United States determine how to achieve health outcomes similar to those in other developed nations while spending less.

evidence-based medicine (EBM)
The conscientious, explicit, and judicious use of current best evidence from relevant and valid research in making health care decisions.

Evidence-based medicine (EBM) is the conscientious, explicit, and judicious use of current best evidence in making decisions about the care of individual patients. According to Shi and Singh (2012), using evidence-based medicine can improve the value of medicine by curtailing the misuse and overuse of health care. It allows us to make informed choices concerning the use or nonuse of scarce health care resources. Sultz and Young (2011) point out that EBM offers the best available support for decisions in clinical practice, management, and health policy. EBM has the capacity to improve the health of the entire population by allowing those responsible for medical care to better understand what works and what does not work in patient health care delivery.

This approach to making medical decisions relies on results from randomized clinical trials involving large numbers of participants. These evaluations are necessary on both individual and population bases so we can better understand which health services provide a benefit that justifies their cost. The tools of EBM have been developed over time but still require more work in order to expand their potential for use in all areas of health services delivery. Having research that supports informed medical decisions is increasingly relevant for dealing with the complications produced by chronic diseases and, more important, for creating programs designed to prevent chronic diseases. In other words, we need to also evaluate the value of prevention programs and see how it compares to the value of current efforts focused on treatment and cures for disease.

The most promising solution to the problem of physicians ordering useless medical tests and procedures is the development and use of **comparative effectiveness research (CER)**. CER is designed to inform health care decisions by providing evidence on the effectiveness, benefits, and harms of different treatment options. The evidence is generated from research studies that compare drugs, medical devices, tests, surgeries, and other ways to deliver health care. Weinstein and Skinner (2010) argue that CER offers a potential solution to runaway health care costs in the United States because it will help us to cut medical waste without reducing the quality of health care services.

> **comparative effectiveness research (CER)**
> Research into the relative effectiveness, benefits, and harms of different treatment options.

Mushlin and Ghomrawi (2010) point out that the vast majority of countries that have reformed their health care systems are using some form of CER for deciding what should and should not be reimbursed in health services delivery. They are doing so to protect patients from potentially harmful medical tests and procedures while attempting to improve quality and tame health care costs. According to Nussbaum, Tirrell, Wechsler, and Randall (2010), the Patient Protection and Affordable Care Act includes an appropriation of an additional $500 million a year for this type of research. This research should reduce costs by identifying wasteful medical tests and procedures and could produce $700 billion in health care savings every year. CER will be discussed in more depth in Chapter Two.

Technology and Health Costs

Health care organizations must learn how to adapt if they are to remain relevant as providers of choice to consumers in the future. A truly adaptable business is able to change its behaviors, aspirations, and management systems. "Organizations lose their relevance when the rate of internal change lags the pace of external change" (Hamel, 2012, p. 95). There has been a rapid growth in technology in the United States, and this growth has moved into the area of health services delivery, increasing both productivity and costs at the same time. This rapid development and use of technology will continue, despite its extreme influence on cost escalation in health care delivery (Shi & Singh, 2012). It must be remembered that productivity is usually determined by two factors: efficiency in the use of inputs and the value that customers place on the outputs (McKinney, 2012). This applies to the improvement of health care services as there is great concern about the cost of delivery and the quality of the services received by the consumer. Improvements in productivity in health care delivery are welcomed, but the enormous escalation in the costs associated with this growth cannot be sustained in the long run.

According to Kaufman and Grube (2012), technology can help us reduce costs and improve the quality in health care if this technology is used correctly. The emergence of new technology will help to improve success rates along with producing cost reductions as it encourages the migration of health care delivery from the hospital to the outpatient clinic and ultimately to the home.

At the same time, we also have to be concerned with the effects of **moral hazard**, a concept from economics. It applies to health care because, as Budrys (2012) points out, many people are unable to resist the temptation to acquire goods and services like health care that they consider to be free to themselves, even when they do not actually need them and they know someone else will have to pay for them. This concept applies equally to the use of advanced technology, since quite often the patient does not actually see a bill for this type of purchase.

Seeking better technology will allow disruptive innovation to become the norm in how we deliver and improve health care in our country. **Disruptive innovation** occurs when resources are combined in the production process in new ways that usually allow greater value to be produced by the process. According to Christensen, Grossman, and Hwang (2009), disruptive innovation has worked well in lowering the cost and increasing the availability of products and services in the business world, and health care is ripe for this same type of innovation. The catalyst for disruptive innovation in health care could very well be public health agencies and the preventive strategies they have developed with a focus on wellness rather than illness. This is exactly what is required for our health care system to survive and deliver better quality services at lower prices. Responding to the opportunities presented by this disruption will require leadership in public health departments at the federal, state, and local levels, as the disruptive

moral hazard

A condition that exists when an individual is more likely to take risks because the costs associated with the risk are borne by another.

disruptive innovation

A new product or service that is capable of changing an existing market by improving convenience, access, and/or affordability.

innovations that are so needed in health care delivery have often been blocked by special interest groups, which tend to see change as detrimental to profits margins.

Health Care Access

The United States is the only developed country in the world that does not guarantee health care access to all its citizens. According to Starr (2011) the United States stands out among other rich nations for leaving large segments of its population without health care services, allowing the number of uninsured Americans to reach 50 million in 2010. Access to health care services in the United States has become a very complicated issue because different policymakers define access in different ways. While most politicians agree that some aspect of access is the most important issue facing our current health care system, many also believe that the provision of health insurance to the population will automatically improve the health of the population. This is clearly not the case, since there are many determinants of good health other than simply having insurance.

The question of who should receive health insurance coverage has been a controversial political issue for the last seventy years. With the passage of the Patient Protection and Affordable Care Act of 2010, most Americans will be able to get health insurance coverage as of January 1, 2014. But does the new legislation actually provide *access* to health care or simply insurance coverage for health care services? It must be emphasized again that the provision of insurance by itself does not guarantee good health. In fact it is well known that many individuals having health insurance never actually seek care from a health care provider until they become very ill. Therefore it is wrong to assume that merely providing health insurance will automatically improve the health of the country's population. Nevertheless, if more individuals have health insurance, then there is a greater opportunity to improve the health of the population. As Schimpff (2012) points out, good health care services become available only when individuals have access to those services, as they do when they have adequate health care insurance.

How should we define health care access? According to Shi and Singh (2013), *health care access* is "the ability to obtain needed, affordable, convenient, and effective personal health services in a timely manner." These authors point out that access to health care is one of the major determinants of good health. Other determinants are a person's environment, behavior, lifestyle, and heredity. To improve the health of the population it is necessary to look at all determinants of health, of which access to medical care is only one. In addition, there must also be access to health care providers and, importantly, health information.

When we talk about access, we have to define the goal. Are we talking about access to health insurance, to a physician, to primary care, or to the many other determinants of good health? If a person visits a physician only to find that the physician does not have time to provide a complete discussion of the many health issues facing that person, has that person experienced access or not? It is important to define access properly in order to discover solutions.

Fuchs (1998) introduced the concept of two main categories of access, which he labeled "general" and "special." On the one hand those individuals facing **general access issues** have the resources to pay for their health care but may have problems acquiring the care they want and need. They have health insurance but for a variety of reasons do not use their opportunity to seek medical care. For example, they may feel well and think that they don't require health care, or they may be frightened of actually entering the health care system. On the other hand, Fuchs argues, those facing **special access issues** are usually the poor or those living in rural areas of the United States. People with special issues may have insurance but be unable to find a provider due to their location or because their provider does not accept their type of insurance. Another problem often prevalent in both urban and rural America is poverty, which quite frequently means that individuals do not have health insurance or are underinsured.

In recent years there has been an improvement in the United States in many of the health indices considered important determinants of a country's overall health status. At the same time, a distinct group of Americans have seen their health regress. Owing to race, ethnicity, socioeconomic status, geography, gender, age, or disability status, people in this group have faced enormous problems in obtaining health insurance or finding a provider and, therefore, satisfactory health care. This group and also specific segments of it are commonly referred to as a **disparate population**. Cohen, Chavez, and Chehimi (2007) point out that the best definition of *health disparities* is provided by Margaret Whitehead, who defines these disparities as "differences in health that are not only avoidable and unnecessary but in addition unjust and unfair" (p. 31). Cohen et al. argue further that the only way to prevent health disparities is to utilize a holistic approach that pays particular attention to medical resources, quality care, and the environment where individuals live.

They also introduce the concept of the trajectory of health care disparities, diagrammed in Figure 1.2. This diagram is useful because it shows the three major determinants that contribute to the inequitable health outcomes found in a disparate population. These determinants are environmental factors, exposures and behavioral factors, and medical care factors. The environmental factors include things like discrimination and

general access issues
Problems in getting the type of care needed when it is needed.

special access issues
Problems faced by certain groups such as the poor and rural residents.

disparate population
A population with differences in health from other populations for reasons that are avoidable and unfair.

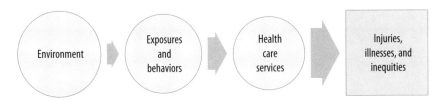

Figure 1.2   Trajectory of Health Disparities
Source: Cohen et al., 2007, p. 31.

poverty and also unemployment and restricted access to nutrition and to exercise, which quite often lead to behavioral factors such as poor diet, lack of exercise, and violence. The beauty of this diagram is that it tells policymakers and community leaders where to seek the root causes of health disparities. It also gives further credibility to the idea that access to health care alone is not usually sufficient to improve the health of the population.

Health Levels and Outcomes

Besides health care costs and access, another major concern is health levels and outcomes, including life expectancy and infant mortality, as compared to other countries. Despite the fact that the United States spends more on health care services than any other country in the world, the overall health levels of its population and the health outcomes produced by the delivery of its health services do not rank very high when compared with other countries. In fact the overall health levels of the U.S. population are at an all-time low, ranking twenty-seventh out of all industrialized countries, due to constant growth in the practice of high-risk health behaviors among all segments of the population. Although tobacco use is slowly dropping, the number of overweight and obese children and adults continues to escalate. The American diet of fast-food meals along with a preference for a sedentary lifestyle continues to provide ideal conditions for the development later in life of chronic diseases and the medical complications that typically follow them. For example, the United States is currently experiencing an epidemic of type 2 diabetes that is due primarily to poor diet, obesity, and lack of physical activity. Figure 1.3 shows the number of new cases of diabetes in the United States.

As with most chronic diseases, this epidemic of type 2 diabetes could be substantially reduced if the national system of health care focused more on diabetes prevention than on treatment of its complications. This is a clear example of how the improvement of health levels decreases the problems of cost escalation and access to health services. When people remain well, there is a lower demand for access.

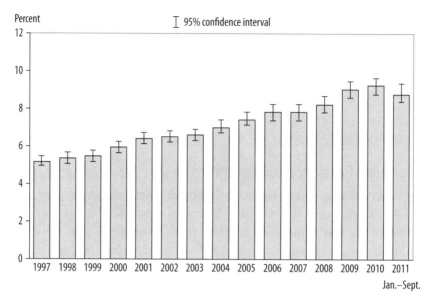

Figure 1.3   Prevalence of Diagnosed Diabetes Among U.S. Adults Aged Eighteen and Over, 1997–September 2011

Source: Centers for Disease Control and Prevention, 2013, fig. 14.1.

Numerous public health policy experts have concluded that the most important variables affecting individual health are personal behavior, social relations, the environment, economic well-being, and access to health care services (Schmitz, 2012). Unfortunately, these variables that are known to affect health seem to be ignored until an individual becomes ill. Making matters worse, once an individual becomes ill, he or she may have developed a chronic disease that cannot be cured but only treated with expensive therapies. Often as patients age and develop complications from chronic diseases, they become objects of referral from one medical specialist to another, thus increasing cost. Because there is little money to be made in preventing disease, the incentive for health care providers is to treat rather than prevent illness. As a result of disregarding the prevention of illness, we have created a fragmented system of medical care, one that begins with illness not wellness.

Champy and Greenspun (2010) point out that poor health outcomes and escalating health care costs are also a direct result of problems with efficiency and quality and that we require an effort in **reengineering** to improve how health care services are delivered. Reengineering entails disregarding previous ways of doing things in order to develop a new and process-oriented way of doing business. In health, reengineering will require looking at health care service delivery as interconnected processes designed to achieve one overall goal, good health for the population.

reengineering
Disregarding previous ways of doing things in order to develop a new and process-oriented way of doing business.

Unfortunately, special interest groups that profit from illness determine payment and reimbursement mechanisms and are reluctant to make such changes. To achieve this reengineering, we will have to determine health care outcomes based on whether or not predetermined goals of care were in fact achieved. It is reasonable to assume that most consumers are looking for good health as the most sought after outcome from the purchase of health care services.

Changing Patterns of Disease

The disease pattern in the United States has changed over the last few decades. There has been a remarkable shift in prevalence from communicable diseases to the even more dangerous and expensive chronic diseases and their complications. Table 1.2 shows the leading causes of death in the United States in 1900. The top three causes of death at that time were influenza, tuberculosis, and illnesses causing diarrhea, and all three quite frequently resulted in death because effective treatments were not available. These diseases have a short incubation period and are usually spread from person to person through close personal contact. These communicable diseases became less of a threat with the discovery and widespread use of antibiotics and vaccines along with the provision of a clean water supply.

Table 1.3 shows the leading causes of death in 2000. Chronic diseases such as heart disease, cancer, and stroke have replaced communicable diseases. These chronic diseases do not lend themselves to a cure or administration of a vaccine. They cause disability, early retirement, loss of

Table 1.2   Number of Deaths and Crude Mortality Rate for Leading Causes of Death in the United States in 1900

Cause of Death	Number of Deaths	Crude Mortality Rate per 100,000
Pneumonia and influenza	40,362	202.2
Tuberculosis	38,820	194.4
Diarrhea, enteritis, and other gastrointestinal problems	28,491	142.7
Heart disease	27,427	137.4
Stroke	21,353	106.9
Kidney disease	17,699	88.6
Unintentional injuries (accidents)	14,429	72.3
Cancer	12,769	64.0
Senility	10,015	50.2
Diphtheria	8,056	40.3

Source: Cohen et al., 2007, p. 31. Data from the National Center for Health Statistics.

Table 1.3   Number of Deaths and Crude Mortality Rate for Leading Causes of Death in the United States in 2000

Cause of Death	Number of Deaths	Crude Mortality Rate per 100,000
Heart disease	710,760	258.1
Cancer	553,091	200.9
Stroke	167,661	60.9
Chronic lower respiratory disease	122,009	44.3
Unintentional injuries (accidents)	97,900	35.6
Diabetes mellitus	69,301	25.2
Influenza and pneumonia	65,313	23.7
Alzheimer's disease	49,558	18.0
Kidney diseases	37,251	13.5
Specticemia	31,224	11.3

Source: Cohen et al., 2007, p. 31. Data from the National Center for Health Statistics.

quality of life, and premature death, along with an escalation in the costs of health care delivery. Moreover, according to the Centers for Disease Control and Prevention (CDC), seven out of ten deaths among Americans each year result from chronic diseases. Heart disease, cancer, and strokes account for more than 50 percent of all deaths each year (Kung, Hoyert, Xu, & Murphy, 2008). In 2005, 133 million Americans, or almost one out of every two adults, had at least one chronic illness (Wu & Green, 2005). Chronic diseases have become epidemic in the United States and show no signs of leveling off in the near future. Educational programs designed to prevent the development of poor health behaviors like tobacco use, improper diet, physical inactivity, and alcohol abuse could curb the onset of these diseases.

The Nation's Health, the monthly newspaper of the American Public Health Association, reports there is no question that our health care delivery system is facing a major challenge resulting from the obesity epidemic and the resultant monumental escalation in the prevalence of type 2 diabetes. According to the annual report titled *America's Health Rankings*, health levels in the United States are in serious trouble. The report for 2011 points out that although tobacco use is declining, it is still practiced by 17.3 percent of the population. The prevalence of obesity has increased 137 percent, rising from 11.6 percent of the population in 1990 to 27.5 percent of the population in 2011. The report also issues some frightening news concerning the epidemic of diabetes that is escalating every year. There are now over 20 million individuals with diabetes, representing 8.7 percent of the population in 2011 (Johnson, 2012). If this trend continues, the bill for this chronic disease alone will represent 10 percent of our entire budget for health care delivery. Those living with this disease face premature mortality as well.

Reversing the epidemic of chronic diseases is going to be the most difficult problem ever undertaken by our medical care system. The only way to prevent chronic diseases and their complications is through health education programs designed to prevent the high-risk health behaviors that predispose individuals to these diseases. These educational programs are not hard to develop, but there are tremendous challenges in making these programs available to large segments of the population at convenient times and a reasonable cost. In addition, because there is no profit to be gained in the prevention of chronic diseases, much of the funding for prevention programs will need to come from the government. Health education programs are a long-term investment that is expected to present large payoffs in terms of the improved health of the population in the future.

Involving Patients and Communities in Health Care

Patient involvement is a critical component of improved outcomes in health care. In the world of rapidly developing medical information, the patient must become an active participant in the medical decision-making process. The question, of course, is how to get normally passive patients to become active in their own health care decision making. The answer seems to involve a combination of incentives and the availability of relevant medical information that is easy to understand. Härter and Simon (2011) argue that shared decision making in medicine is a process where physicians and patients work together to make the best choice of medical interventions given the available medical information. Clinicians support their patients with the necessary medical information to allow them to make their preferences known to their medical team. This shared decision making has become an absolute necessity when dealing with complicated chronic diseases and their potentially deadly consequences. Thanks to information technology, including online medical information sources such as PubMed, this is currently possible but is still not the norm.

At the same time, there is a new wellness model of health care delivery that is moving away from the individual patient to the population and from illness to wellness, requiring a very different role for the providers of health care services. The need for prevention efforts that have a chance of success will require community leadership in order to improve the health of the population. For example, Aetna, a health insurer, offers a free blood pressure unit to its health plan members who have hypertension. The only requirement is to take your blood pressure every day and call the elevated readings into a nurse manager once each month for evaluation.

Several other health insurance companies are also using nurse educators to monitor and coach patients with elevated glucose readings. Members take their own glucose readings and then receive education about diet and exercise from the nurse educator.

If we are ever to reduce the current epidemic of chronic diseases, health care providers, especially hospitals, will require new relationships with the community. More than ever before these health care providers will be expected to deliver activities designed to improve the health of the population in their community. This will become a critical factor in sustainability for many hospitals aligned with their communities. In the past, public health departments and the U.S. medical care system have had tremendous successes in improving the health and life expectancy of most Americans. Now the medical community and health departments need to partner with Americans to face the health challenge found in the expanding epidemic of chronic diseases.

Improving Outcomes with Technology

Technology can help in the improvement of health, especially in the battle against the growing epidemic of chronic diseases. Technology is now available to improve the prevention of risky behaviors in large portions of the population. Public health departments have the information necessary to help individuals prevent chronic diseases from ever developing. The problem has been that the money budgeted for public health departments has never been sufficient to develop, implement, and evaluate a massive dissemination of chronic disease information to the entire population. This is not to say that there have not been chronic disease education efforts by health departments. Many successful programs have been developed and implemented in schools, workplaces, and communities to prevent chronic diseases and their complications. But these are limited efforts. Such educational efforts need to be expanded to larger populations.

There needs to be a greater use of technology to get more health information to the population on a consistent basis in innovative ways. Mukherjee (2009) argues that in a crisis there is a need to employ technologies that allow "intelligent adjustment to major environmental shifts." This recommendation rings true for public health departments. The chronic disease epidemic is an environmental shift that public health departments must address, and information technology must be employed in innovative ways to solve the crisis.

Mukherjee (2009) points out that the drivers of increased productivity and quality involve the transformation of systems and the nature of work, of worker skills, and of the structure of organizations. He is talking about the development of an adaptive business strategy. These kinds of transformation are also extremely important in the improvement of the health of the individual and the community. They need to become a functional part of the new world of the improvement of the health of the population. Goldstein, Groen, Ponkshe, and Wine (2007) argue that the current health care system with a focus on medical cure must change to a population-based disease prevention system supported by an advanced health informatics system. The drivers of innovation in our health care system today involve using information technology along with chronic disease connectors (the primary care doctors who coordinate patients' health care), finding ways to reduce medical errors, and developing sophisticated consumer self-care.

According to Turnock (2009), computers and electronic communications have improved our ability to gather, analyze, and disseminate large amounts of disease surveillance data. This technological approach will need to be expanded to provide a continuous stream of information about chronic diseases, their effects on health, and prevention techniques to the entire population. Examples of doing this successfully with innovative uses of technology already exist, such as the CDC's Epi-X and eCards. Epi-X (Epidemic Information Exchange) is a system that offers web-based communications for public health professionals. This system was created to provide public health officials with current information and alerts involving the health of the public. State and local health departments and poison control centers are able to access and share preliminary health surveillance information with large numbers of health care professionals. This system supports postings of up-to-date medical information and discussions about disease outbreaks and other public health events that involve many parts of the nation and the world. Epi-X provides rapid communications whenever they are needed, and its staff are available twenty-four hours a day, seven days a week to provide consultation. The system's primary goal is to inform health officials about important events that can affect the public's health and to help them respond to public health emergencies. This type of system would be excellent for the rapid sharing of chronic disease information with the population. All that would be required is that individuals sign up for prevention messages from the CDC. They would then receive a daily email with tips on the prevention of chronic diseases and their complications.

The CDC also currently has available over one hundred free Health-e-Cards (electronic greeting cards). These cards are colorful greetings that encourage healthy living, promote safety, and can even celebrate a health- or safety-related event. This concept could also be expanded to include information about the prevention of chronic diseases along with ways of preventing the complications that can develop later in life as a result of practicing the unhealthy behaviors that lead to chronic diseases.

A unique use of technology in health care is found in the emergence of digital games as a new tool for increasing healthy exercise. *The Nation's Health* (Krisberg, 2012) reports that a school district in Alabama is one of a number of districts using the Nintendo video game Wii Fit, which requires children to move around to earn points. The children use the game two to three times each week in their physical education period. According to teacher Audrey Gillis, the children don't even realize that they are exercising, and she reports that some younger children actually began to cry when they found out that it was not their Wii day.

The Nation's Health (Krisberg, 2012) reports that this type of gaming technology is also being used to deal with many other health issues, including tobacco cessation, mass vaccination, physical inactivity, health promotion, and chronic disease management and rehabilitation. "Games can influence everything from your attitudes about health to your perception of risk to your belief in your capability to take care of your own health, which is critical," said Debra Lieberman, director of the Health Games Research program at the University of California, Santa Barbara (Krisberg, 2012, p. 10).

Health Care Quality

The last major health care problem that requires immediate attention is the quality of health services received by many Americans. According to Schimpff (2012), although we spend 50 percent more on health care services than the next closest developed country, the quality of our health care is subpar and medical errors are epidemic. Torinus (2010) argues that there is no proven relationship between the price of health care services and the quality of those health services. In fact the opposite often seems to be the case, with lower price quite often indicating efficiency in production along with improved quality. That is, by producing large quantities of goods and services, a company or institution not only achieves economies of scale allowing it to lower prices, but it also becomes more productive in its processes, which allows it to actually improve quality.

Torinus (2010) further argues that although quality in health care is not what it should be in the United States, it can be improved if the country is willing to put in the necessary time and effort. Quality improvement can reduce costs, improve access, and improve health outcomes.

Another key indicator of diminished quality in the delivery of health care services is the rate of medical errors, errors that have become epidemic in the United States over the last decade. The Institute of Medicine (IOM) defines a **medical error** as "the failure of a planned action to be completed as intended or the use of a wrong plan to achieve an aim." Medical errors typically occur in operating rooms, emergency departments, and intensive care units. There is mounting evidence that entering the medical care system at any location increases a person's risk of adverse drug events, errors in care delivery, and the development of hospital-acquired infections. Such errors are increasing the cost of health care delivery, requiring longer hospital stays, and causing disability, death, and a loss of trust in medical care. In fact the CDC now classifies medical errors as the eighth leading cause of death in the United States.

medical error
The failure of a planned action to be completed as intended or the use of a wrong plan to achieve an aim.

In 1999, the IOM released a study revealing that as many as 98,000 of the 33 million individuals hospitalized each year die and many more hospitalized patients receive secondary infections or incur other problems because of poor quality health care while hospitalized. According to Black and Miller (2008), the percentage of hospital admissions experiencing injury or death is between 2.9 and 3.7 percent. Ironically, many of the costs associated with medical errors are actually reimbursed by patients' insurance companies.

Health care services are produced and delivered by people, and the improvement process must begin and end with these people. According to Black and Miller (2008), the solution to problems in delivering health care services will be found in the skills and ideas of the people who do the work of delivering health care services to patients. These service providers control the creative power so necessary for success in problem resolution. Unfortunately, health care institutions often pay little attention to these individuals. This lack of attention to medical errors will need to change as the health care system undergoes reform.

Because health care services are produced as needed rather than ahead of demand, they need to be produced error free each time. This makes medical error a *systems problem.* When a mistake is made in the delivery of a service, it is too late to correct the faulty delivery. It is very important, therefore, that systems be designed to prevent errors in the delivery of health care services before they are delivered. When mistakes are made, they must be evaluated and corrected immediately in order to prevent future occurrences. The results of this evaluation then need to be shared with all employees in order to prevent future problems.

In order to deal with these new demands, health care providers are beginning to realize that they are obligated to spend time focusing on delivering quality care and providing exceptional service to their customers. This will require employees who understand that it is the consumer who ultimately determines their success or failure as health care providers and also the success or failure of the health care system. Baldoni (2012) also points out that the key to pleasing the consumer is for employees to understand their purpose. This means that health care employees must be in tune with the wants and needs of their consumers.

SUMMARY

The health care delivery system that was once the best in the world is in a crisis situation that threatens its very survival. The major health care problems causing this crisis revolve around escalating costs for health care services and poor access to and outcomes from the very services that are supposed to improve our health. The entire system of health care found in the United States is in need of tremendous reform. Our health care system seems to be plagued with high costs, access problems for many, and health levels lower than those in many other industrialized countries. Making matters worse, the United States is facing an epidemic of incurable chronic diseases and an epidemic of preventable medical errors.

Several countries offer all their citizens health care services that are less expensive than services in the United States and that result in improved health indices for these countries' entire populations. The critics of these health systems argue that they ration health care and that is why their costs are so much lower than costs in the United States. If that is the case, perhaps rationing some care may make sense if it improves health at the same time. As the United States moves through health care reform, it is very important that we look at how these countries deliver their health care and determine whether some of their approaches can be helpful to the United States.

Health care services delivery in the United States is going to change in a dramatic way in the next several years. This change is going to involve every health care organization and every person who works in the field of health services delivery. The new health care system that evolves from the change process is going to focus on health outcomes that can be produced at a price that everyone involved can afford.

KEY TERMS

comparative effectiveness
   research (CER)

cost disease

disparate population

disruptive innovation

evidence-based medicine (EBM)

general access issues

medical error

moral hazard

Patient Protection and Affordable
  Care Act of 2010 (ACA)

reengineering

special access issues

DISCUSSION QUESTIONS

1. Name the major problems in the health care industry as outlined by Victor Fuchs. What are some of the reasons for these problems? Are the problems Fuchs identifies the largest problems, or are they symptoms of even bigger problems?

2. How do other industrialized countries deal with cost escalation in health care delivery?

3. What are the reasons for the *cost disease* in the health services sector of the U.S. economy?

4. How is the development of new technology expected to help in the reduction of future health care costs?

REFERENCES

Armstrong, P., & Armstrong, H. (2008). *About Canada: Health care.* Nova Scotia, Canada: Fernwood.

Baldoni, J. (2012). *Lead with purpose: Giving your organization a reason to believe in itself*. New York, NY: American Management Association.

Baumol, W. J. (2012). *The cost disease: Why computers get cheaper and healthcare doesn't.* New Haven, CT: Yale University Press.

Black, J., & Miller, D. (2008). *The Toyota way to healthcare excellence: Increase efficiency and improve quality with Lean.* Chicago, IL: Health Administration Press.

Budrys, G. (2012). *Our unsystematic health care system* (3rd ed.). New York, NY: Rowman & Littlefield.

Carroll, L. E., Chapman, S. A., Dodd, C., Hollister, B., & Harrington, C. (2013). *Health policy: Crisis and reform* (6th ed.). Burlington, MA: Jones & Bartlett Learning.

Centers for Disease Control and Prevention. (2013). *Early release of selected estimates based on data from the January–September 2012 National Health Interview Survey.* Retrieved from http://www.cdc.gov/nchs/data/nhis/early release/earlyrelease201303_14.pdf

Centers for Medicare & Medicaid Services. (2012). *National health expenditure data: Historical* (Highlights). Retrieved from www.cms.gov/NationalHealth ExpendData/02_NationalHealthAccountsHistorical.asp

Champy, J., & Greenspun, H. (2010). *Reengineering health care: A manifesto for radically rethinking health care delivery*. Upper Saddle River, NJ: Pearson Education.

Christensen, C., Grossman, J., & Hwang, J. (2009). *The innovator's prescription: A disruptive solution for health care*. New York, NY: McGraw-Hill.

Cohen, L., Chavez, V., & Chehimi, S. (2007). *Prevention is primary: Strategies for community well-being*. San Francisco, CA: Jossey-Bass.

Feldstein, P. J. (2011). *Health policy issues: An economic perspective* (5th ed.). Chicago, IL: Health Administration Press.

Fuchs, V. R. (1998). *Who shall live? Health, economics, and social choice* (2nd exp. ed.). Hackensack, NJ: World Scientific.

Fuchs, V. R. (2013). The gross domestic product and health care spending. *New England Journal of Medicine, 368*(12), 107–109.

Goldstein, D., Groen, D., Ponkshe, S., & Wine, M. (2007). *Medical informatics 20/20*. Sudbury, MA: Jones & Bartlett Learning.

Hamel, G. (2012). *What matters now: How to win in a world of relentless change, ferocious competition, and unstoppable innovation*. San Francisco, CA: Jossey-Bass.

Härter, M., & Simon, D. (2011). Do patients want shared decision making and how is it measured? In G. Gigerenzer & J. A. Muir Gray (Eds.), *Better doctors, better patients, better decisions: Envisioning health care 2020*. Cambridge, MA: MIT Press.

Institute of Medicine. (1999). *To err is human*. Washington, DC: National Academies Press.

Johnson, T. D. (2012, February). Nation's overall health not improving, assessment finds: Obesity, diabetes stalling U.S. progress. *The Nation's Health, 1*, 18.

Kaufman, K., & Grube, M. E. (2012). The transformation of America's hospitals: Economics drives a new business model. In *Futurescan 2012: Healthcare trends and implications 2012–2017*. Chicago, IL: Health Administration Press.

Krisberg, K. (2012, March). Digital games emerge as new tool to foster health, exercise. *The Nation's Health, 1*, 10.

Kung, H.-C., Hoyert, D. L., Xu, J. Q., & Murphy, S. L. (2008). Deaths: Final data for 2005. *National Vital Statistics Reports, 56*(10). Retrieved from http://www.cdc.gov/nchs/data/nvsr/nvsr56/nvsr56_10.pdf

Linden, R. A. (2010). *The rise and fall of the American medical empire*. North Branch, MN: Sunrise River Press.

Lowrey, A. (2012, May 1). In hopeful sign, health spending is flattening out. *New York Times*. Retrieved from http://blog.targethealth.com/?p=22153

McKinney, P. (2012). *Beyond the obvious: Killer questions that spark game-changing innovation*. New York, NY: Hyperion.

Mukherjee, A. S. (2009). *The spider's strategy: Creating networks to avert crisis, create change, and really get ahead*. Upper Saddle River, NJ: Pearson.

Mushlin, A. I., & Ghomrawi, H. (2010). Health care reform and the need for comparative effectiveness research [Perspective]. *New England Journal of Medicine, 10*(1058), 1–3.

Nussbaum, A., Tirrell, M., Wechsler, P., & Randall, T. (2010, April 5). Obamacare's cost scalpel. *BusinessWeek*, 64–66.

Schimpff, S. C. (2012). *The future of health-care delivery: Why it must change and how it will affect you.* Washington, DC: Potomac Books.

Schmitz, P. (2012). *Everyone leads: Building leadership from the community up.* San Francisco, CA: Jossey-Bass.

Shi, L., & Singh, D. A. (2012). *Delivering health care in America: A systems approach* (5th ed.). Sudbury, MA: Jones & Bartlett Learning.

Shi, L., & Singh, D. (2013). *Essentials of the U.S. health care system* (3rd ed.). Burlington, MA: Jones & Bartlett Learning.

Starr, P. (2011). *Remedy and reaction: The peculiar American struggle over health care reform.* New Haven, CT: Yale University Press.

Sultz, H. A., & Young, K. M. (2011). *Health care USA: Understanding its organization and delivery* (7th ed.). Sudbury, MA: Jones & Bartlett Learning.

Torinus, J. (2010). *The company that solved health care.* Dallas, TX: BenBella Books.

Turnock, B. (2009). *Public health: What it is and how it works* (4th ed.). Sudbury, MA: Jones & Bartlett Learning.

U.S. Census Bureau. (2011, November). *The older population: 2010* (2010 Census Briefs). Retrieved from http://www.census.gov/prod/cen2010/briefs/c2010br-09.pdf

Weinstein, M. C., & Skinner, J. A. (2010). Comparative effectiveness and health care spending—implications for reform. *New England Journal of Medicine, 362*(5), 460–465.

Wu, S. Y., & Green, A. (2005). *Projection of chronic illness prevalence and cost inflation.* Santa Monica, CA: RAND Health.

CHAPTER 2

THE FORCES OF CHANGE IN HEALTH CARE

Bernard J. Healey

Tremendous changes are rapidly engulfing the entire health care sector of the U.S. economy. These changes are a direct result of a very strong effort by the federal government to gain control of escalating costs in the delivery of health care to Americans. These cost increases, on an annual basis, are far above the inflation rate in the American economy. Policymakers have finally come to the full realization that cost escalation in health care has become a drag on the economy, has bankrupted many hard-working Americans, and is no longer sustainable. Americans need a health care system with decreased costs for increased quality of care.

There are many who believe that the United States has the greatest health care system in the world. However, this belief is not supported by the majority of health care indices, which reveal that the United States ranks quite low when compared to other countries on many important measures, including individual life expectancy and infant mortality rate. The World Health Organization (WHO) (2013) points out that the United States spends much more than any other country on health care services but is only thirty-seventh out of 191 countries in the WHO's ranking of health care delivery systems, based on a range of measures. It is reported that the United States spends twice as much as other industrialized countries on health care delivery, yet all this spending results in inferior health outcomes for its population. To be sure, in many ways the U.S. system of health care offers a superior array of advanced and expensive curative medical care. Unfortunately, this medical care system does a very poor job of keeping people from becoming ill in the first place. This is the reason why the winds of change directed at the U.S. system of health care are so strong. Changes to the U.S. system will require a united

LEARNING OBJECTIVES

After reading this chapter you should be able to

- Understand the need for real change in the way health care services are produced and delivered to consumers.

- Be aware of the changes in health care that will result from passage of the Patient Protection and Affordable Care Act of 2010.

- Understand the value of using concepts from economics to determine the value of various medical procedures.

- Describe why better use of technology would improve health care delivery.

effort by government, the providers of health care services, employers, and even consumers to develop a new system that concentrates scarce resources on good health outcomes, rather than on wasteful, unproductive activities of low marginal value.

Schimpff (2012) argues that several medical megatrends are emerging that will result in changes in the practice of medicine over the next few years. All told, they will create five shifts in medicine:

1. An increase in custom-tailored medicine

2. A greater emphasis on prevention

3. An improvement in the ability to repair, restore function to, or replace organs, tissues, or cells

4. Fully digitized medical records available instantly, anytime or any place

5. An enhanced level of safety and quality of care (p. 42)

This chapter will consider the effects of shifts 2, 4, and 5, focusing especially on the chronic disease epidemic, cost-effectiveness analysis, and health promotion and disease prevention as the factors most likely to foster real change in the near future.

Consequences of Forty Years of Health Care Cost Escalation

U.S. health care costs have increased from 4.6 percent of gross domestic product (GDP) in 1950 to greater than 17 percent of GDP in 2010. This cost escalation, which is projected to reach over 20 percent of GDP in the next few years, is simply not sustainable. If the health care sector continues to consume an ever-larger portion of the GDP, then the United States will have progressively less to spend on other public services such as education and national defense. As the appetite for more and more expensive health care services continues to grow, the costs of this growth will place ever-greater limitations on both public and private expenditures for everything else produced by the economy. This in turn affects international competitiveness, take-home pay from employment, and most important, the availability of health care services for a large part of the population.

According to Fuchs (2012) the growth of health care expenditures in the last several decades is affecting the viability of the U.S. government and is also a primary cause of the stagnation of wages in the vast majority of American industries. The continual increase in health care expenditures, especially in recent years, is one of the greatest challenges to ever face the United States. Fuchs (2012) also argues that the real cause of health care cost escalation over the last several years has been the development and use of new technology and the increased labor specialization that results from this technology. Often new technology adds costs to health care delivery while offering very little benefit. The key is to use cost-benefit analyses before adopting any new technology; however, there is little that can be done to slow the growth of technology in health care, even if that were what was wanted. The good news is that much of the new technology being developed should improve health outcomes and, in the long run, result in lower health care costs, as long as we make certain that the costs are equal to the benefits and we are not wasting scarce resources.

The availability of health insurance from employers has also been a major cause of cost escalation in health care. Until recent years it was the norm for health insurance premiums to be part of an employee's benefit package. The government subsidized this benefit by allowing businesses to claim these health insurance costs as a tax deduction and by ruling that employees do not have to treat the value of their health insurance as income. Since there was thus little cost to the company or the employee for a better insurance package, individuals and their unions could periodically demand and receive better health insurance packages from their employers. Insurance companies, moreover, have been reluctant to invest in any change that increases costs in the short term, even when a change could produce benefits, including lower costs, in the long term. A good example of this is that insurance companies often refuse to pay physicians to return patient phone calls or emails, even though this practice might result in fewer emergency room visits. There is also a reluctance by many health insurance plans to pay physicians for providing health education to patients, yet such education is a necessary component of preventing chronic diseases.

Medicare and Medicaid

As health care costs have continued to rise over the last several decades so has the amount the U.S. government spends on this sector of the economy. Fuchs (2012) calculates that the government pays for about half of health care spending in the United States and that this percentage is continuing to increase.

The middle of the 1960s marked the beginning of federal government involvement in health care in a large way with the passage of the legislation creating Medicare and Medicaid. The **Medicare** program was established in 1965 as part of Title XVIII of the Social Security Act Amendments. It is focused on providing health insurance that covers many health care costs to Americans sixty five years of age and older and also to younger individuals with disabilities or end-stage renal disease. The **Medicaid** program was also established in 1965, through Title XIX of the Social Security Act

Medicare
A government program that provides health insurance to Americans sixty-five and over and younger individuals with disabilities or end-stage renal disease.

Medicaid
A government program that provides health insurance to many low-income individuals and families.

Amendments. This program is limited to providing insurance that covers health care costs for certain categories of individuals with low incomes, and it is now the largest health care payer for these individuals. Both programs are run by the Centers for Medicare & Medicaid Services (CMS). These two entitlement programs brought increased government money and regulation to the health care industry. Both the dollars and the regulation would grow and become more complicated over the ensuing decades.

Figure 2.1 reveals the major problem underlying the Medicare program. As the population ages, the number of Medicare recipients increases while the number of workers who are paying taxes to support this government-financed program diminishes. One does not have to be an economist to figure out that before the program goes broke, benefits must be reduced, reimbursements for health services must be lowered, or workers must pay higher payroll taxes, or a combination of all three.

The cost of the Medicare program is paid out of the federal government's general revenues (42%), by payroll taxes (37%), and by premium payments by beneficiaries (13%). Owing to population growth among the elderly and expected increases in the cost of health care services for this group, the cost of this entitlement program is projected to go from $555 billion in 2011 to $903 billion in 2020. The Medicaid program is a mandatory, joint federal and state program. An additional program, the **State Children's Health Insurance Program (SCHIP or CHIP)** was enacted in 1997 by Congress (as part of the Balanced Budget Act of 1997) and is designed to provide coverage to uninsured, low-income children who are not eligible for the Medicaid program. SCHIP provides federal matching funds to states to provide this coverage. The Kaiser Commission on Medicaid

State Children's Health Insurance Program (SCHIP or CHIP)

A joint federal and state government program that provides health insurance to uninsured, low-income children not eligible for Medicaid.

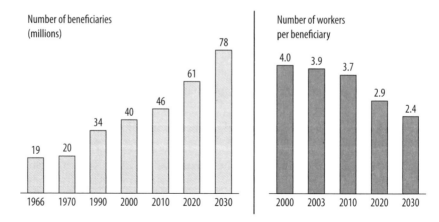

Figure 2.1   The Medicare Population Is Growing, but Fewer Workers Will Support This Population in the Future

Source: Henry J. Kaiser Family Foundation, 2005b, fig. 7.6. Data from 2001 and 2005 annual reports of the board of trustees of the Federal Hospital Insurance and Federal Supplementary Medical Insurance trust funds.

and the Uninsured (2013) points out that "Medicaid covers over 62 million Americans, . . . more than 1 in 3 children and over 40 percent of births. . . . More than 60 percent of people living in nursing homes are covered by Medicaid" (p. 1). Figure 2.2 shows the groups whose members may be eligible for Medicaid and the percentages of these groups that actually receive Medicaid funds for health care services. This figure clearly shows that decisions have to be made concerning the reimbursement of costs for nursing home care and the poor, especially pregnant women and low-income children.

The U.S. government is heavily involved in financing and regulating health care services and certainly shares the blame for the cost escalation and reduction in outcomes being experienced in the American health care system. The government has not done a good job of controlling the costs associated with entitlement programs, as can be seen by the fact that the three largest government programs—Social Security, Medicare, and Medicaid—are all approaching bankruptcy.

Longman (2012) argues that if we could affect the practice patterns in higher-spending hospitals and bring them in line with the patterns in lower-spending hospitals, we could retain or improve the quality of care and reduce the costs of Medicare by 30 percent. The higher-spending hospitals use more resources per patient than the lower-spending hospitals. If Medicare would use its financial muscle to accomplish this task, this program could

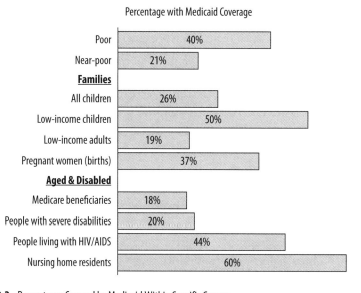

Figure 2.2　Percentages Covered by Medicaid Within Specific Groups

Note: "Poor" is defined as living below the federal poverty level—$14,680 for a family of three in 2003.
Source: Henry J. Kaiser Family Foundation, 2005a. Data from Kaiser Commission on Medicaid and the Uninsured, Kaiser Family Foundation, and Urban Institute estimates; Birth data: National Governors Association, Maternal and Child Health Update.

be preserved into the far distant future. Medicare and Medicaid will be discussed in depth in Chapter Six.

The Chronic Disease Epidemic

As discussed in Chapter One (Table 1.2), in 1900, the leading causes of death in the United States were communicable diseases such as influenza, pneumonia, and tuberculosis, which usually resulted in death at a very young age because there were no effective treatments for these diseases. That all changed with the discovery of antibiotics in the mid-1930s and their subsequent widespread use. Many public health measures also came into play in the early 1900s, including better hygiene, greater access to clean water, and better food-handling techniques, lowering the chances of contracting a communicable disease. Communicable diseases have a short **incubation period**, the amount of time between exposure to the cause of a disease and the development of the symptoms of that disease. When a communicable disease occurs in large numbers of people, there is an immediate response by health providers and public health departments in order to discover the cause, treat the ill, and implement control measures in order to prevent the epidemic from spreading.

incubation period
The amount of time between exposure to the cause of a disease and the development of disease symptoms.

This type of response does not work very well against chronic diseases, for various reasons. As we have been discussing, the leading causes of death in the United States today have become chronic diseases such as heart disease, cancer, stroke, and diabetes. These diseases have long incubation periods, have multiple causes, and usually cannot be cured. Often complications arise from their presence over long periods of time. Health providers and public health departments do not have to look for an immediate cause because their causes are long term and they are not infectious; also, they cannot be thoroughly treated because there is no cure. Another major difference between communicable and chronic diseases is that people often cause their chronic diseases through their practice of high-risk health behaviors.

For example, according to the Centers for Disease Control and Prevention (2011), during the period from 2005 to 2008, approximately 35 percent of the U.S. population aged twenty years or older had prediabetes and 26.9 percent of the population sixty-five years or older had diabetes. This epidemic has continued to grow, and diabetes is now the leading cause of kidney failure, nontraumatic lower limb amputation, and new cases of blindness in the United States. Over 90 percent of individuals with diabetes have type 2 diabetes, which is largely a result of poor personal health behaviors like overeating, poor diet, and lack of physical activity. Unfortunately, these high-risk health behaviors not only lead to diabetes but also usually lead to the serious health complications mentioned earlier as people age.

The chronic disease epidemic must be better understood by providers of care and health policymakers before it becomes the most dangerous and expensive epidemic ever to be faced by the U.S. system of health care delivery. It is dangerous and expensive because these incurable diseases usually result in disability and quite often in premature death as well. Morewitz (2006) reports that individuals with chronic diseases are often unable to work, experience a decrease in quality of life, and incur significant medical costs as they grow older and experience the many complications typical of these diseases.

Figure 2.3 outlines the path of a typical disease such as heart disease, cancer, or diabetes. The patient quite often is the first to recognize symptoms of disease and usually then begins to seek information from friends, family, and now the Internet. The patient then proceeds to visit the family physician, who begins examinations and testing to determine the medical problem and give it a name. This primary care physician will then begin referring the patient to a number of specialists in an attempt to verify a diagnosis and begin a series of attempts at treating the disease once the stage of illness is determined. When a chronic disease is determined as the cause of illness, the process of referral to specialists may be never-ending, and the patient may have increasing numbers of drugs to take each day. He or she also has the constant worry of complications that may result from the disease.

Chronic diseases thus usually require an approach much different from the one the medical system is currently designed to provide. Because there is usually no complete cure available, these diseases require more numerous episodes of care than communicable diseases do. Another major problem with chronic diseases is that often an individual has more than one of them, requiring **coordination of care** (typically by the primary care physician) among multiple specialists and medications. Chronic diseases are going to require the adoption of new methods of treatment in which patients are more active participants in order to improve the quality of care while also reducing the costs of treatment. Some very important innovations in the care of these diseases are coming from other countries. Richman, Udayakumar, Mitchell, and Schulman (2008) argue that health

coordination of care
Having one person responsible for organizing all of a patient's care to avoid errors and duplication and ensure the right treatment at the right time.

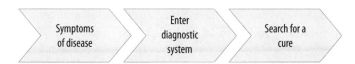

Figure 2.3 The Disease Path

care found in some other countries is capable of achieving outcomes similar to those of the United States, but at 10 percent of the cost. For example, these authors found open-heart surgery similar in quality to that found in the United States being performed at Fortis hospital in India for $6,000, compared to $100,000 in the United States. The major reasons for lower costs in India involve scale and organizational efficiency along with better coordination among providers, which is lacking in the United States. Encouraged by health care executives, many of whom are physician leaders, and their managers, medical team members in India encourage continuous innovation in the way health care services are delivered to their customers. This is a demonstration that quality and lower costs are compatible in all industry segments, including health care.

In brief, chronic diseases currently affect over half of the U.S. population, cost over a trillion dollars a year, and are for the most part the result of individuals' own high-risk health behaviors. The number of Americans suffering from chronic diseases is certainly going to rise in an aging population, and the costs of these diseases will continue to rise into the distant future. The increased aging of the U.S. population is only going to make this chronic disease epidemic larger and cause it to consume a greater percentage of the resources devoted to health care. Because a vast number of individuals with chronic diseases and their complications are over age sixty-five, this epidemic will place further strains on the Medicare program. Fineberg (2012) points out that in 2001, 5 percent of Medicare recipients accounted for 43 percent of the program's expenditures, and 75 percent of these individuals had one or more chronic diseases. It seems obvious that the answer to controlling health care costs while improving the overall health status in this country is to be found in the control of chronic diseases. This new epidemic of chronic diseases is going to require an entirely different approach in which resources are focused more on the prevention of disease through health education than on the management of disease. More will be said about the chronic disease epidemic in Chapter Twelve.

Health Care Reform

When discussing health care reform, politicians usually concentrate on increasing access for a greater portion of Americans as one of the goals, with finding sustainable ways to finance that access being the second goal. In the last few decades there have been numerous attempts at reforming the American health care system, with very little, if any, success.

Starr (2011) points out that several presidents and members of Congress have actively supported some form of national health insurance or universal coverage for all Americans over the last fifty or so years, with very little to show for their efforts. The most ambitious attempt at national health insurance, made by President Bill Clinton, was soundly defeated in 1993; the campaign against it was funded by massive outlays of money from physician groups and third-party health insurers. The desire for health reform became a major issue in the 2008 presidential campaign, contributing to a win for President Obama and the Democrats. This victory brought forth the latest attempt at health care reform, the **Patient Protection and Affordable Care Act,** which is better known as the Affordable Care Act (ACA) and which was passed by Congress in 2010. This new law is attempting to make major changes in health care delivery that will ultimately affect all health care organizations and consumers of health care services in the United States.

Patient Protection and Affordable Care Act (ACA)
Signed into law on March 23, 2010, the ACA seeks to increase the quality and availability of health care coverage for most Americans.

The Congressional Budget Office (2011) points out that this new law should provide insurance for most Americans while reducing the federal deficit over the next ten years. The law currently contains nine titles, and each one addresses a key piece of health care reform. Critics argue that the new law is nothing more than government-run health care that will cause the government deficit to explode while doing very little to improve the health of most Americans. Supporters of the health care reform effort point out that the new law requires insurers to cover preventive services and immunizations and to provide continued coverage for dependent children up to age twenty-six, eliminates lifetime annual limits on benefits, and extends coverage to those who are uninsured because of a preexisting condition.

As Koh and Sebelius (2010) show, the Affordable Care Act offers a whole array of prevention initiatives, including funding through Title IV of the act. These initiatives deal with the prevention of chronic diseases by improving access to clinical preventive services. However, Starr (2011) points out that although the Affordable Care Act does require major changes in how health insurance works, it does little to change how medical care is organized and will not accomplish long-term reductions in the cost escalations of health care delivery. Wennberg (2010) argues that true reform of our system of health care will require a movement from delegated decision making by the physician to shared decision making with the patient. It will also require a movement to an organized system of care delivery that begins to eliminate wasteful testing and procedures that may place the patient at extreme risk while offering the patient very little in the way of medical value.

According to Schimpff (2012), "The first step in any set of decisions about the future of health care is to envision the care system, then the payment system. Most efforts to date begin with the payment system and ignore the care system" (p. 29). This suggests real problems for health care reform because, historically, we have never been able to get beyond costs and into the improved health care outcomes made possible through a redesigned health care system. Christensen, Grossman, and Hwang (2009) argue that the practice of medicine needs to move from intuitive medicine to empirical medicine, finally emerging as precision medicine. According to Christensen et al. (2009), intuitive medicine involves diagnosis and treatment of disease-based symptoms with treatment that is uncertain. In contrast, precision medicine involves accurate diagnoses of the diseases underlying the symptoms along with treatments that are predictably effective. In order to move from intuitive medicine to precision medicine, providers need the results of cost-effectiveness analyses that can identify the medical interventions that actually improve health, and at what cost. According to Fuchs (2007), health care reform is inevitable in the United States simply because current escalations in costs are not sustainable. In order for health care reform to be successful, it must improve cost-effective care by providing the physician with information about appropriate care and incentives to change the way health care is delivered.

Agus (2011) agrees that two very important components of health care reform are the growing database of empirical medical information being supplied by information technology and the addition of provider and consumer incentives to the health care delivery process. Medical information can be mined and converted to knowledge made available to the physician as evidence-based recommendations and then shared with the consumer in the form of medical care customized to his or her needs.

Cost-Benefit Analysis and Comparative Effectiveness Research

In the real world of economic rules and limitations, markets of supply and demand distribute resources that utilize the price system to make allocation decisions. In many cases the price system in our economy acts as a rationing force to exclude lower-income individuals from many high-price purchases. This rationing function should also serve as a regulating mechanism to force consumers to make rational choices for products and services due to a limited budget. Price can also provide incentives for individuals to work harder if they want to achieve the income level required to purchase higher-priced items in the economy. Markets for goods and services, along with a price system, allow a capitalist system to deliver superior output at reasonable prices to those who can afford the purchase. The regulating mechanism that discourages waste and inefficiency is the price system. Unfortunately, this price system usually favors those with higher incomes, allowing them to receive larger amounts of the goods and services available in an economy.

Phelps (2010) observes that the health care sector of the U.S. economy shares many characteristics with the rest of the economy but also exhibits many differences. These differences involve government reimbursement of some health care; uncertainty about the availability of care, which may depend on where you live and whether providers will accept your insurance plan; and the large difference between the provider of health care and the consumer of this care in their knowledge of medicine. In many ways the health care sector has defied normal market reactions to high prices and poor quality services. These market differences have made it difficult to apply economic analysis to the health care sector in an attempt to improve its performance.

One of the economic evaluation procedures used by many economists is the **cost-benefit analysis (CBA)**, which compares both costs and benefits in dollar terms to estimate the strengths and weaknesses of alternative choices. (The costs and benefits are adjusted to their present value through a process called discounting that accounts for the passage of time.) Thus, if a program demonstrates a net benefit, it is considered to provide good economic value and, other things being equal, should be continued or perhaps even expanded. It must be mentioned that rational individuals also practice cost-benefit analysis every day when purchasing most things other than health care. Whenever they shop for a product or service they usually compare price with value before making a purchase decision. The free-market economy usually allocates resources based on information that becomes available through the price system. Nas (1996) argues that the impact of CBA grew significantly in the 1960s because the federal Office of Management and Budget made such analyses a principal tool in the evaluation of government programs. The CDC has been using CBA for years to evaluate the costs and potential benefits of prevention programs (CDC Evaluation Working Group, 1999). In order to compare different prevention strategies, researchers need reliable and consistent cost and effectiveness data.

Table 2.1 offers an overview of the various types of economic analysis used by both for-profit and not-for-profit organizations when they make decisions. Among government agencies the most commonly used forms of economic analysis are cost-benefit analysis and cost-effectiveness analysis. **Cost-effectiveness analysis** compares the cost of an intervention to its effectiveness as measured in health outcomes, such as the number of years of life saved, whereas cost-benefit analysis assigns a dollar value to the outcomes.

cost-benefit analysis (CBA)
A way to estimate (in dollar terms) the strengths and weaknesses of alternative choices in terms of benefits, time, and costs.

cost-effectiveness analysis
A method of comparing the cost of an intervention to its effectiveness as measured in health outcomes.

Table 2.1   Overview of Economic Evaluation Methods

Economic Evaluation Method	Purpose of Method	How Health Effects Are Measured	How Results Are Expressed
Cost analysis	Used to compare net costs of different programs, for planning and assessment	In dollars	Net cost; cost of illness
Cost-effectiveness analysis	Used to compare interventions that produce a common health effect	In natural units	Cost-effectiveness ratio; cost per case averted; cost per life year saved
Cost-utility analysis	Used to compare interventions in terms of morbidity and mortality outcomes	In years of life, adjusted for quality of life	Cost per quality-adjusted life year (QALY)
Cost-benefit analysis	Used to compare programs with varied units of outcomes (health and nonhealth)	In dollars	Net benefit or cost; benefit-cost ratio

comparative effectiveness research (CER)

Research into the relative effectiveness, benefits, and harms of different treatment options.

Many of these principles have been carried over for use in **comparative effectiveness research (CER)**, which is designed to inform health care decision makers by providing evidence on the effectiveness, benefits, and harms of different treatment options. It involves studying two or more existing health care interventions to determine which ones work best for which patients and which offer the greatest benefits or pose the greatest detriments (Jacobson, 2007). This economic analysis usually addresses both effectiveness and costs, asking whether a given medical treatment or procedure actually works and, if so, whether its medical value is sufficient to justify its cost. According to Weinstein and Skinner (2010), the use of CER by government agencies resulted from the government's overriding concern with runaway health care costs.

There is widespread agreement among health economists that a large number of medical tests and procedures will prove to be wasteful when subjected to rigorous analysis of their benefits, let alone their large costs. This issue becomes even more significant when we realize that many medical procedures are very dangerous for the patient while providing little if any medical benefit. According to the Congressional Budget Office, (2011), there is very little evidence currently available to tell us which treatments work best for individuals, despite the fact that many of the newer treatments cost a great deal more than previous ones. Unfortunately, the U.S. health care system tends to rapidly adopt expensive new technology and treatments in health care delivery without any real evaluation of their true value or cost. This is where CER comes into play, because it gathers evidence that compares different medical interventions in terms of costs and patient value.

CER has become the latest version of economic decision making related to the use of scarce health care resources. It can help us to determine what medical interventions work best so we can target our resource use and improve health outcomes. Mushlin and Ghomrawi (2010) point out that there is a lack of understanding among health policy experts about how CER works and what it attempts to accomplish. They also argue that fears exist that CER threatens the autonomy of the physician, and a concern that health care will be rationed for some Americans even though they have health insurance. Emanuel, Fuchs, and Garber (2007) comment that it is important that both cost and effectiveness information be communicated to all the stakeholders involved in medical decision making. Everyone needs to become aware of the results of reliable, trustworthy, and legitimate CER results so that wasteful, dangerous, and expensive medical tests and procedures can be eliminated.

This increase in economic analysis of medical tests and procedures is starting to gain support from unlikely sources. Rabin (2012) states that nine medical specialty boards have recently recommended that forty-five common medical tests and procedures be used less frequently. These boards also recommended that patients begin to question their physicians about the need for many routine tests and procedures that are regularly ordered. This represents a monumental change in the attitude of the medical profession, which is finally acknowledging that many profitable tests in medicine are not necessary and may actually produce harm for the patient. Some of the medical procedures that are no longer recommended are EKGs done during routine physicals, MRIs to diagnose back pain, and antibiotics to treat mild sinusitis. In the past these have been routine recommendations made by many physicians. It is thought by many health policy researchers that unnecessary treatment may account for as much as one-third of all medical spending annually in the United States. Brody (2012), for example, argues that we now know that one-third of health care costs could be eliminated without depriving the patient of necessary tests and medical procedures. He believes that the elimination of wasteful testing and unnecessary medical procedures is not rationing but sound practice of medicine. In fact it may also represent protecting the patient from tests that are not only wasteful but that may expose the patient to such dire consequences as excess radiation, medical errors, adverse drug reactions, and several hospital-acquired infections.

CER has become a major factor in the government's ongoing effort to reform the health care sector of our economy. Weinstein and Skinner

(2010) argue that CER offers the opportunity to substitute cost-effective medical interventions with high-quality health outcomes for those medical approaches that are more expensive and usually result in poorer health outcomes. This is exactly what is required to save the U.S. medical care system from bankruptcy and focus all its limited resources on producing the best health outcomes at an affordable price.

CER offers the opportunity to discover the evidence that is so necessary if clinicians, payers, and consumers are to make good decisions concerning medical choices. Mushlin and Ghomrawi (2010) state that the "final result should be that important medical decisions will be guided and influenced by the scientific community, not solely the capricious nature of the marketplace" (p. 152). They also note that the vast majority of Western countries that have reformed their health care systems have used some form of CER. The countries using this form of economic analysis hope to better inform consumers, clinicians, and purchasers of health care services so that they can make decisions based on good evidence that will ultimately improve individual and population health. These decisions will help eliminate wasteful spending, lower costs, and ultimately improve the quality of health care services.

electronic medical record (EMR)

A systematic gathering of all medical information concerning a given patient in a digital format.

electronic health record (EHR)

A record of a patient's health information generated over time across various health care delivery settings and providers and available at any time and any place.

Electronic Medical Records

An **electronic medical record (EMR)** is nothing more than an electronic replacement of the paper chart that would be generated by one particular provider. Physicians purchase EMR systems to use in their offices. An **electronic health record (EHR)** is a record of a patient's health information generated over time across the various health care delivery settings and providers used by the patient. The EHR connects these various clinical settings and providers and also includes such information as patient demographics, progress notes, medications, past medical history, immunizations, laboratory data, and radiology reports. The important aspect of this record is that it becomes a virtual medical file that can be made available to the patient and all providers of care at any time and any place. Christensen et al. (2009) point out that the EHR allows data that were once available only to the physician and the hospital to become a tool that shifts control of the medical record to the patient. In addition, Fallon, Begun, and Riley (2013) point out that the adoption of the EHR for both inpatient and outpatient care can go a long way toward improving the quality and safety of patient care.

According to Sultz and Young (2011), as we move into the future of health care delivery, physicians and nurses will rely more on computer-based decision-support systems accompanied by electronic programs that outline best practices in health care delivery. EHRs focus on the total health of the patient—going beyond the standard clinical data collected in the provider's office to achieve a broader view of a patient's care. EHRs are designed to reach out *beyond* the health organization that originally collects and compiles the information. They are built to share information with other health care providers, such as laboratories and specialists, so they contain information from *all the clinicians involved in the patient's care.* Health information technology, especially EMRs and EHRs, will become a much greater part of medical decision making by both the health care provider and the consumer of health care services. This technology should result in better health outcomes, improved quality of service delivery, and ultimately, lower costs for health care services. Fuchs (2012) believes that if the system of health care is well organized, there will be tremendous advantages for patients and providers in the widespread use of EHRs. According to Kenney (2008) it currently takes far too long for new scientific knowledge to reach physicians. The rapidly accumulating, evidence-based medical information on medical procedures that have a positive value and on best practices needs to be disseminated to physicians in a more timely fashion. He believes that evidence-based care can work best when supported by EHRs, along with treatment guidelines that include various treatment options.

Halvorson (2009) argues that EHRs need to be patient focused, having all of a patient's medical records linked together with a full complement of computer tools that allow all doctors to use the same data for attainment of desired patient care. Halvorson believes that electronic records need to support the business model found in other industries that rewards successful outcomes and goal achievement.

One of the best EHRs, VistA, has been developed and used by the Veterans Administration (VA) for years. According to Longman (2012) employees of the VA, working mostly on their own initiative rather than under managerial direction, developed this EHR many years ago and have been improving its capabilities ever since. **VistA (Veterans Health Information Systems and Technology Architecture)** uses an open source software program that has been made available to everyone. Longman offers several examples of the advantages of this software in his book *Best Care Anywhere: Why VA Health Care Would Work Better for Everyone* (2012). One example of its successful use is found in the fact that all VA patients and all their nurses wear ID bracelets with bar codes. This allows computer verification that the right nurse is with the right patient with the right medication to be administered. If a mistake is about to be made, a computer-generated warning is administered. This has allowed the VA to eliminate prescription drug errors while these errors still persist in other U.S. hospital systems.

VistA (Veterans Health Information Systems and Technology Architecture)
An electronic health record system that operates throughout the VA medical system.

My HealtheVet
A program that gives veterans, military personnel, and their dependents electronic access to their medical records.

Another example of successful technology use cited by Longman is found in a new program called **My HealtheVet**. This program allows an enrolled individual to access his or her own complete medical record and to share this record with family members. Having this virtual record allows patients at one VA facility to visit other VA centers and know that their medical records will be available to staff there.

Health Promotion and Disease Prevention

According to Koh and Sebelius (2010), the poor health of a large number of individuals in the United States is due to preventable conditions. Americans are receiving only about half of the preventive services recommended to them, demonstrating the need for a greater role for health promotion in our current health care system. The Affordable Care Act attempts to rectify this problem by offering a wide array of prevention services along with the funding to pay for these services. Maciosek, Coffield, Flottemesch, Edwards, and Solberg (2010) argue that preventive services are an excellent investment because they offer a good value for the system of payment and the patient. According to Schimpff (2012) the greatest opportunity to improve health outcomes among the U.S. population is found in behavioral change; such change could affect over 40 percent of our current mortality in the United States by postponing the development of chronic diseases and their complications. Personal behaviors like tobacco use, poor diet, physical inactivity, and alcohol abuse are proven contributors to many of the major chronic diseases and their subsequent complications. The National Institutes of Health (Moolgavkar et al., 2012) reports that tobacco control programs have been responsible for preventing more than 795,000 lung cancer deaths in our country from 1975 through 2000. The report goes on to say that if all cigarette smoking had ceased following the release of the first U.S. surgeon general's report on smoking and health in 1964, a total of 2.5 million people would have been spared death due to lung cancer. (This report deals only with lives saved and with not health care expenses averted.) This is only one of many examples of the value of well-developed, implemented, and evaluated health promotion programs, a value that can be achieved at very low cost. At the same time, the *Nation's Health* (Johnson, 2012) reports that "after years of progress, declines in preventing America's teens and young adults from using tobacco products have stalled, according to a new U.S. surgeon general's report on preventing tobacco use among youth" (p. 10). Indeed, tobacco use among youth is at epidemic status, with 3.6 million U.S. teens smoking cigarettes. This indicates a continuing need for tobacco control programs.

There has always been an interest among many people in the United States in the prevention of health problems. This interest is evident when we look at the strong support for the elimination of childhood diseases through the funding of vaccine development and the distribution of vaccines by public health departments. Unfortunately, there has been a reluctance to move past children and young adults with well-developed disease prevention programs for the rest of the population. The problem is that all the incentives in medicine favor a focus on illness rather than wellness. In order for wellness programs to work, they must be made as profitable as programs for treating illness. In other words, the U.S. health care system needs to begin offering incentives for wellness program initiatives.

According to physician David Agus (2011) we need to discover the value of making informed health choices. In his new book titled *The End of Illness*, Agus offers insight into the requirements necessary to lead a long life free of illness. Wellness is a gift most of us are given at birth, but many of us allow it to be taken away by poor health decisions as we age. These decisions result in our using tobacco, consuming a poor diet, and leading a sedentary life. Any good intentions we have tend to be frustrated by the multitude of negative health influencers that we encounter every day and the relative lack of countervailing influences that promote wellness. It has become very clear that incentives to remain healthy are weak or nonexistent. If we really want to improve population health in America, we need to provide incentives for the development of healthy lifestyles. Money devoted to wellness programs must be looked at as an investment that pays dividends over the long run. These dividends come in the form of a reduction in the chronic disease epidemic leading to fewer hospitalizations, fewer medications, decreased sick days, and increased productivity at work.

The federal government, through the Department of Health and Human Services and the Centers for Disease Control and Prevention, has put forth numerous programs to help Americans develop a healthy lifestyle, most notably the Healthy People initiative. The Healthy People initiative began in 1979 as the result of the publication of *The Surgeon General's Report on Health Promotion and Disease Prevention*. This report started a national discussion on the relationship of personal behaviors to the development of many serious diseases and injuries. This eventually led to the development of Healthy People objectives, which were first stated in a 1990 report, followed by similar reports in 2000 and 2010. Each science-based report lists the general health *topics* to be addressed over the next ten years to improve the health of all Americans, and then breaks those topics down into *goals* and then *objectives*. Every ten years a new Healthy People report outlines accomplishments along with additional topics, goals, and objectives for the health of the nation for the next ten years.

As Koh (2010) notes, **Healthy People 2020** builds on past achievements and adds new, important goals that include promoting quality of life, encouraging healthy development and healthy behaviors across life stages, and creating social and physical environments that promote good health. Here are the continuing topics from 2010 and the new topics for 2020 (U.S. Department of Health and Human Services, 2014). Among other issues the new topics address the importance of understanding that individual health is directly related to the health of the community where the individual lives. Healthy People 2020 offers a vision of healthy people in healthy communities.

Topic Areas for Healthy People 2010 and 2020 Goals

* Access to health services
* Arthritis, osteoporosis, and chronic back conditions
* Cancer
* Chronic kidney disease
* Diabetes
* Disability and health
* Educational and community-based programs
* Environmental health
* Family planning
* Food safety
* Health communication and health information technology
* Hearing and other sensory or communication disorders
* Heart disease and stroke
* HIV
* Immunization and infectious diseases
* Injury and violence prevention
* Maternal, infant, and child health
* Medical product safety
* Mental health and mental disorders
* Nutrition and weight status
* Occupational safety and health
* Oral health
* Physical activity

- Public health infrastructure
- Respiratory diseases
- Sexually transmitted diseases
- Substance abuse
- Tobacco use
- Vision

New Topic Areas for Healthy People 2020 Goals

- Adolescent health
- Blood disorders and blood safety
- Dementias, including Alzheimer's disease
- Early and middle childhood
- Genomics
- Global health
- Health care–associated infections
- Health-related quality of life and well-being
- Lesbian, gay, bisexual, and transgender health
- Older adults
- Preparedness
- Sleep health
- Social determinants of health

SUMMARY

The winds of change are blowing through the entire U.S. health care delivery system and are growing in intensity. The current system of health care delivery has seen escalating costs over the last forty years while health outcomes and quality of care have diminished. The cost escalation in the health care sector is not sustainable because it is resulting in less money being available for other sectors of our economy, such as education and national defense.

There is a demand from the consumers and many providers of health care services for the creation of a new system of care that produces better health outcomes at a price that does not bankrupt those who use it. These demands for reform resulted in passage of the Affordable Care Act, which was signed into law by the president in 2010. This new health law changes the requirements for what health insurance needs to cover, increases access to that insurance, and improves access to care and the offering of preventive care services. Some of the highlights of the law are an attempt to improve the availability of preventive care, the elimination of lifetime and annual limits on health care benefits, and as of 2014, a requirement that insurers cannot discriminate against individuals with preexisting conditions by refusing coverage or charging them more than other individuals.

Unfortunately, this health care reform act does little to reform our system of health care delivery, which is the real cause of health care cost escalation. Although access to health care services is important, this access alone does not improve the overall health of the individual or the population. The major change that is required to lower costs and improve health outcomes involves reducing the number of Americans with chronic diseases by improving their health behaviors. This will require a focus on prevention throughout the health care system and more participation by individuals in their own health care. One of the tools that can help us achieve both these goals is better use of technology. As Shi and Singh (2013) argue, many Internet and e-health applications, including electronic health records, are capable of providing vital health information on demand to entire populations to help people make better health care decisions. The ability to have online visits with providers of care would also help people to get timely medical information and prevent illnesses from getting worse. Another essential tool is analysis of medical approaches and treatments to determine how to achieve the best outcomes at a manageable cost.

KEY TERMS

comparative effectiveness research (CER)

coordination of care

cost-benefit analysis (CBA)

cost-effectiveness analysis

electronic health record (EHR)

electronic medical record (EMR)

Healthy People 2020

incubation period

Medicaid

Medicare

My HealtheVet

Patient Protection and Affordable Care Act of 2010 (ACA)

State Children's Health Insurance Program (SCHIP or CHIP)

VistA (Veterans Health Information Systems and Technology Architecture)

DISCUSSION QUESTIONS

1. Name several reasons for the cost escalation in health care services over the last forty years. What are the main reasons for these cost increases?

2. Why has our health care delivery system been designed to focus on activities rather than outcomes?

3. Describe the history of health care reform in the United States. What are the reasons why these reform efforts have failed?

4. What is comparative effectiveness research? How can it be used to improve health outcomes?

REFERENCES

Agus, D. B. (2011). *The end of illness*. New York, NY: Free Press.

Brody, H. (2012). Medicine's ethical responsibility for health care reform—the top five list. *New England Journal of Medicine, 362*(4), 283–285.

CDC Evaluation Working Group. (1999). Framework for program evaluation in public health. *Morbidity and Mortality Weekly Report, 48*(RR-11). Retrieved August 28, 2006, from ftp://ftp.cdc.gov/pub/Publications/mmwr/rr/rr4811.pdf

Centers for Disease Control and Prevention. (2011). *National diabetes fact sheet*, 2011. Retrieved from http://www.cdc.gov/diabetes/pubs/pdf/ndfs_2011.pdf

Christensen, C. M., Grossman, J. H., & Hwang, J. (2009). *The innovator's prescription: A disruptive solution for health care*. New York, NY: McGraw-Hill.

Congressional Budget Office. (2011). *CBO's analysis of the major health care legislation enacted in March 2010* (Statement of Douglas W. Elmendorf, Director, before the Subcommittee on Health, Committee on Energy and Commerce, U.S. House of Representatives). Retrieved from http://www.cbo.gov/sites/default/files/cbofiles/ftpdocs/121xx/doc12119/03-30-healthcarelegislation.pdf

Emanuel, E., Fuchs, V., & Garber, A. (2007). Essential elements of a technology and outcomes assessment initiative. *Journal of the American Medical Association, 298*(11), 1323–1325.

Fallon, L. F., Begun, J. W., & Riley, W. (2013). *Managing health organizations for quality and performance*. Sudbury, MA: Jones & Bartlett Learning.

Fineberg, H. V. (2012). A successful and sustainable health system—how to get there from here. *New England Journal of Medicine, 366*(11), 1020–1027. doi: 10.1056/NEJMsa1114777

Fuchs, V. R. (2007). What are the prospects for enduring comprehensive health care reform? *Health Affairs, 26*(6), 1542–1544.

Fuchs, V. R. (2012). Major trends in the U.S. health economy since 1950. *New England Journal of Medicine, 366*(11), 973–977. doi: 10.1056/NEJMp 1200478

Halvorson, G. C. (2009). *Health care will not reform itself: A user's guide to refocusing and reforming American health care.* New York, NY: CRC Press.

Henry J. Kaiser Family Foundation. (2005a). *Key Medicare and Medicaid statistics.* Menlo Park, CA: Author.

Henry J. Kaiser Family Foundation. (2005b). *Medicare chartbook* (3rd ed.). Retrieved from http://www.nahc.org/assets/1/7/MedicareChartbook05.pdf

Jacobson, G. A. (2007). *Comparative clinical effectiveness and cost-effectiveness research: Background, history, and overview* (CRS Report for Congress). Retrieved from http://assets.opencrs.com/rpts/RL34208_20071015.pdf

Johnson, T. D. (2012, May/June). Youth tobacco use an epidemic, surgeon general report warns: New tobacco ads share hard-hitting stories. *The Nation's Health, 1,* 20.

Kaiser Commission on Medicaid and the Uninsured. (2013). *Medicaid: A primer: Key information on the nation's health coverage program for low income people.* Retrieved from http://kaiserfamilyfoundation.files.wordpress .com/2010/06/7334-05.pdf

Kenney, C. (2008). *The best practice: How the new quality movement is transforming medicine.* New York, NY: Public Affairs.

Koh, H. K. (2010). A 2020 vision for Healthy People. *New England Journal of Medicine, 362*(18), 1653–1656.

Koh, H. K., & Sebelius, K. G. (2010). Promoting prevention through the Affordable Care Act. *New England Journal of Medicine, 363*(14), 1296–1299.

Longman, P. (2012). *Best care anywhere: Why VA health care would work better for everyone* (3rd ed.). San Francisco, CA: Berrett-Koehler.

Maciosek, M. V., Coffield, A. B., Flottemesch, T. J., Edwards, N. M., & Solberg, L. I. (2010). Greater use of preventive services in U.S. health care could save lives at little or no cost. *Health Affairs, 29*(9), 1656–1660.

Moolgavkar, S. H., Holford, T. R., Levy, D. T., Kong, C. Y., Foy, M., Clarke, L., . . . Feuer, E. J. (2012). Impact of reduced tobacco smoking on lung cancer mortality in the United States during 1975–2000. *Journal of the National Cancer Institute, 104*(7), 541–548. doi: 10.1093/jnci/djs136

Morewitz, S. J. (2006). *Chronic diseases and health care.* New York, NY: Springer.

Mushlin, A. I., & Ghomrawi, H. M. (2010). Comparative effectiveness research: A cornerstone of healthcare reform. *Transactions of the American Clinical and Climatological Association, 121,* 141–145.

Nas, T. (1996). *Cost-benefit analysis: Theory and applications.* Thousand Oaks, CA: Sage.

Phelps, C. E. (2010). *Health economics* (4th ed.). New York, NY: Addison-Wesley.

Rabin, R. C. (2012, April 4). Doctor panels recommend fewer tests for patients. *New York Times.* Retrieved from http://www.nytimes.com/2012/04 /04/health/doctor-panels-urge-fewer-routine-tests.html

Richman, B. D., Udayakumar, K., Mitchell, W., & Schulman, K. A. (2008). Lessons from India in organizational innovation: A tale of two heart hospitals. *Health Affairs, 27*(5), 1260–1270.

Schimpff, S. C. (2012). *The future of health-care delivery: Why it must change and how it will affect you.* Washington, DC: Potomac Books.

Shi, L., & Singh, D. A. (2013). *Essentials of the U.S. health care system* (3rd ed.). Burlington, MA: Jones & Bartlett Learning.

Starr, P. (2011). *Remedy and reaction: The peculiar American struggle over health care reform.* New Haven, CT: Yale University Press.

Sultz, H. A., & Young, K. M. (2011). *Health care USA: Understanding its organization and delivery* (7th ed.). Sudbury, MA: Jones & Bartlett Learning.

U.S. Department of Health and Human Services. (2014). *Healthy People 2020: Topics and objectives.* Retrieved from http://www.healthypeople.gov/2020/topicsobjectives2020

Weinstein, M. C., & Skinner, J. A. (2010). Comparative effectiveness and health care spending—implications for reform. *New England Journal of Medicine, 362*(5), 460–465.

Wennberg, J. E. (2010). *Tracking medicine: A researcher's quest to understand health care.* New York, NY: Oxford University Press.

World Health Organization. (2013). *World health statistics: 2013.* Retrieved from http://apps.who.int/iris/bitstream/10665/81965/1/9789241564588_eng.pdf?ua=1

PART TWO

THE MAJOR PLAYERS IN HEALTH CARE SERVICES

CHAPTER 3

PROVIDERS OF HEALTH CARE SERVICES

Tina Marie Evans

Today's health care environment comprises a wide variety of educated individuals with many different skills who must work together to provide quality medical care services for the individuals who seek their care. Regardless of the particular setting, the provision of health care in the United States is a team effort, with each individual care provider contributing his or her own knowledge and skills toward the success of the team as a whole. To function well in either clinical medicine or administrative work, it is essential to have an understanding of the various categories of health care providers, their education and scope of practice, and the ways they interact as they work.

To help you achieve that understanding, this chapter introduces some of the more prevalent categories of health care workers and offers foundational background information about the training, specialization, and duties of each group. It then explains the necessity of collaboration in the current health care environment in order to keep the critical patient-centered focus. Finally, this chapter discusses the job outlook for health care providers and health care managers, as this is a common question and concern for students studying in the allied health professions as well as health care administration.

LEARNING OBJECTIVES

After reading this chapter you should be able to

- Understand the common categories of health care providers.

- Articulate the similarities and differences between a medical doctor and a doctor of osteopathic medicine.

- Explain the similarities and differences between a psychologist and a psychiatrist.

- Contrast the duties performed by the three levels of nurses.

- Summarize the various types of rehabilitation professionals and the duties of their specialties of care.

- Differentiate the responsibilities of radiologic and imaging professionals.

- Value the importance of collaboration among health care providers within or across specialties.

- Describe the projected job outlook for the various health care occupations.

Primary Care Physicians and Primary Care Assistants

The primary care provider is a cornerstone of the American health care system. These physicians, physician assistants, and nurse practitioners are the usual first point of contact for a patient entering the health care system. The physicians are often referred to as generalists, as they specialize in family practice or internal medicine and address a wide range of conditions and illnesses.

Primary Care Physicians

According to the World Health Organization (2013), primary care physicians, along with other *generalist medical practitioners*, "diagnose, treat and prevent illness, disease, injury, and other physical and mental impairments and maintain general health in humans through application of the principles and procedures of modern medicine" (p. 1). The **primary care physician** is responsible for planning, supervising, and evaluating the overall care plan of a patient, and will frequently counsel individuals on dietary practices, hygiene, and preventive health care. In addition, he or she will refer people to specialty care providers, who offer expert services in particular medical areas, and then he or she will help to coordinate the care offered by these other providers (most of whom are discussed in the following pages). A primary care physician often sees the same patients on a regular basis over time for both preventive care and also for illnesses and injuries. He or she may treat multiple members of families. For the most part these doctors emphasize a well-rounded and comprehensive plan of health care for patients of any age as well as for families (Stanfield, Cross, & Hui, 2009). Recent advances in medical technology have greatly expanded the scope of practice for these physicians, as new technologies replace older, outdated approaches and open up entirely new areas of medical practice (Field, 2007; Stanfield et al., 2009).

There are two types of licensed physicians: the **doctor of medicine (MD)** and the **doctor of osteopathic medicine (DO)**. MDs are also sometimes referred to as allopathic physicians. Both types of physicians are licensed by state boards, and both have a wide array of diagnostic and therapeutic interventions that they may perform and prescribe. They may use all accepted methods of medical treatment (including medications and surgery); however, DOs place a special emphasis on the alignment and health of the body's musculoskeletal system, preventive medical care, and holistic patient care. Approximately one-third of MDs and over half of DOs are primary care physicians. Both MDs and DOs may choose the general practice setting or (after additional training) a specialty. Many students enter medical schools already interested in a particular area of medicine, but they are also exposed to the various specialties during their training. In the final year of study, medical students decide which area of practice is the one that interests them the most and that they will choose for their career (Sugar-Webb, 2005). Although DOs are more likely to choose the primary care setting than are MDs, they can be found in all specialties, especially emergency medicine, anesthesiology, obstetrics and

primary care physician
The physician who is the first point of contact for a patient; general practitioner.

doctor of medicine (MD)
A medical professional who has earned a doctor of medicine (MD) degree.

doctor of osteopathic medicine (DO)
A medical professional who has earned a doctor of osteopathic medicine (DO) degree.

gynecology, psychiatry, and surgery. MDs who choose the general practice setting typically serve as primary care physicians in a family practice, pediatric, geriatric, or internal medicine setting.

Primary Care Physician Assistants

In current primary care settings, it is common for physicians, who are often working on tight time schedules, to delegate some of the patient care responsibilities. This has led to rising employment of the **physician assistant (PA)** and the **nurse practitioner (NP)** as adjunct care providers to assist in the day-to-day process of patient care. PAs are becoming a necessary part of primary care, as they are trained to perform many of the routine, time-consuming tasks that physicians face. PAs always work under the supervision of a physician and are skilled at taking medical histories, performing physical examinations, ordering routine laboratory testing, and providing care for minor injuries. They are midlevel health care providers who attain a skill level beyond that of a registered nurse but short of that of a licensed physician (Stanfield et al., 2009). In some areas of specialty care, the duties of a PA may be more specific to the needs of the particular care setting (Field, 2007). The specific training requirements for PAs are set by the respective states, but most include the completion of a bachelor's or master's degree program, followed by state board examinations. Some PAs choose to pursue postgraduate training in a specialty of interest as well.

Nurse practitioners are advanced-level nursing professionals who carry out many of the same duties that a PA does. Like PAs, NPs are allowed to provide primary care services as well as perform many of the routine clinical tasks in a medical office. This frees the physicians to focus on the more critical medical duties, such as the more seriously ill patients and the more complex cases. Although the training of a PA and an NP is similar, NPs have greater autonomy. In some states, NPs may practice independently and also prescribe medications and rehabilitation care such as physical therapy (Wischnitzer & Wischnitzer, 2011).

physician assistant (PA)
A clinician who provides health care services under the direction and supervision of an MD or a DO.

nurse practitioner (NP)
An advanced-level nursing professional who provides health care services.

Specialty Care Providers

After completing their schooling, some medical professionals decide to refine their skills and pursue an area of medical specialty rather than stay in general practice. These specialty care providers can choose to concentrate in one or more of a wide variety of disease categories, certain types of patients, or particular methods of treatment. They may also seek out teaching positions in medical education settings and undertake research activities in their chosen areas of specialization. Becoming skilled in a particular area of care requires the "completion of a university-level degree in basic medical education plus postgraduate clinical training in a medical specialization or equivalent" (World Health Organization, 2013, p. 2). Although specialists must spend quite a bit more time being educated than generalists do, the work of a specialist is rewarding in many ways. Here are some of the most common specialty care areas:

Areas of Specialty Care

- Allergy and immunology
- Anesthesiology
- Cardiology
- Chiropractic
- Dermatology
- Endocrinology
- Gastroenterology
- General surgery
- Geriatrics
- Hematology
- Immunology
- Infectious disease
- Medical genetics
- Nephrology
- Neurology
- Neurosurgery
- Obstetrics and gynecology
- Oncology
- Ophthalmology
- Orthopedics
- Otorhinolaryngology (ear, nose, and throat specialists)
- Pathology
- Pediatrics
- Physiatry
- Plastic surgery
- Podiatry
- Pulmonary
- Radiology

- Rheumatology
- Urology

Dentists, Dental Hygienists, and Dental Assistants

Dentists, registered dental hygienists, and dental assistants provide care and treatment to promote and restore oral health, which is a vital component of a person's overall health status.

Dentists

A **dentist** (this term includes oral and maxillofacial surgeons) diagnoses, treats, and prevents diseases, injuries, and abnormalities of the teeth, mouth, and jaws. Dentists make use of a wide range of specialized diagnostic, surgical, pharmacological, and other approaches either to promote or to restore oral health (World Health Organization, 2013). The majority of dentists work in a general practice, handling both routine and emergency dental cases. Others, however, choose to specialize within dentistry and to work primarily in pediatric care, periodontics (gum and jaw diseases), prosthodontics (bridges, crowns, dentures), or endodontics (root canal treatment). Each of these professionals is highly trained to provide preventive and restorative care, with the overarching goal of promoting good oral hygiene (Quan, 2007).

dentist
A specialist in the diagnosis, treatment, and prevention of injuries to and diseases of the teeth, mouth, and jaws.

Dental Hygienists

The **dental hygienist** is an important member of the dental health care team. Working closely with dentists, hygienists have duties that go well beyond the cleaning of teeth, as they also conduct assessments and examinations of patients for oral diseases such as oral cancers and gingivitis. In some states (the allowable duties vary by state), dental hygienists are allowed to provide some types of dental services, take impressions, place temporary fillings, take X-rays, and apply fluorides and sealants, and they may also be certified to administer local anesthesia prior to further care being performed by the dentist. They are a critical link in the overall patient care process, and they often take the lead in patient education, sharing their knowledge regarding ways to improve and maintain high levels of oral health (Bureau of Labor Statistics [BLS], 2013a).

dental hygienist
A health care professional who provides preventive dental care and patient education.

Dental Assistants

The **dental assistant** is also a vital member of the dental care team. These individuals assist dentists with patient care; however, they cannot perform teeth cleaning or most of the other duties of the dental hygienists. They

dental assistant
A member of the dental care team who assists the dentist in providing services.

also take care of many laboratory and day-to-day general office tasks, which keeps the facility running smoothly and ensures that it is organized, clean, and well stocked with needed supplies. In many states dental assistants can retrieve records, prepare, and set out the instruments the dentists will need for each patient, and clean and sterilize various types of equipment, as well as hand instruments to the dentist during a procedure. Other common duties of the dental assistant are to make and confirm appointments, to organize dental records, to inventory supplies, and (in some cases) to send out bills and assist in the processing of payments (Quan, 2007).

Mental Health Care Providers

The mental health care system in the United States employs a large variety of skilled providers who have a wonderful array of pharmacological and nonpharmacological therapies that can be tailored specifically to the person being treated. The category of mental health care providers comprises many types of professionals: psychiatrists, psychologists, mental health clinical nurses, psychiatric nurse practitioners, and social workers. These professionals offer their services to improve or maintain a patient's level of mental health on either a short-term or a long-term basis. Each of these professionals often works to provide care for the many different mental illnesses that patients present with; however, their scopes of practice, education, and training differ.

Psychiatrists

psychiatrist
A medical professional who is trained in the diagnosis and treatment of mental illness.

A **psychiatrist** is a professional who is fundamental in the management of mental illnesses, offering diagnostic services, treatment, and social support to those suffering from mental illness. Psychiatrists, like all medical doctors, first earn a bachelor's degree and then attend four years of medical school. To specialize in psychiatry, they complete one year of general residency and a period of specialty residency as well (Raffel & Barsukiewicz, 2002). Psychiatrists are licensed by the state that they practice in, and many receive certification from the American Board of Psychiatry and Neurology (ABPN), a process that requires testing and evaluation. The ABPN certifies psychiatrists for a period of ten years, after which time the certification can be renewed. Ten subspecialties are currently available to psychiatrists: addiction psychiatry, brain injury medicine, child and adolescent psychiatry, clinical neurophysiology, forensic psychiatry, geriatric psychiatry, hospice and palliative medicine, pain medicine, psychosomatic medicine, and sleep medicine (ABPN, 2013).

Most commonly, psychiatrists treat conditions involving psychoses, nonpsychoses, mood disorders, substance abuse, adjustment reactions, developmental disabilities, and sexual dysfunctions. They may evaluate and treat patients on either a short-term or long-term basis as well as order laboratory tests, prescribe medications, and provide various methods of psychotherapy. They may treat one person as an individual, or consult with and provide care to an entire family as a group if that family is dealing with a serious situation or a period of great stress. At times, psychiatrists will also offer their services as consultants to primary care physicians or to other health care professionals such as psychologists, social workers, and nurses (ABPN, 2013). Depending on their chosen subspecialty, they may use in-depth psychotherapy or medication therapy or a combination of both. Psychiatrists commonly provide outpatient services in the community and may also have admitting privileges for one or more hospitals or be employed by a hospital. It is common for individuals with mental illness to receive care from a team of professionals, often led by a psychiatrist, who as a medical doctor has the ability to prescribe medication and write diagnostic orders (Varcarolis & Halter, 2010).

Psychologists

In contrast to a psychiatrist, a **psychologist** earns an academic doctoral degree such as a PhD, EdD, or PsyD degree. Psychologists must be licensed by their respective state board to practice independently, a process that requires a review of a candidate's educational background and training. Although licensing requirements vary from state to state, a doctoral degree from an accredited institution and at least two years of supervised professional experience are necessary (American Psychological Association, 2013). Licensing is now required in all fifty states (Raffel & Barsukiewicz, 2002).

psychologist
An academic professional who is trained in the interactions among brain function, environment, and behaviors.

Psychologists universally study the interaction between a person's brain function and his or her behaviors, as well as between the environment and the person's behaviors. Using a variety of scientific methods, careful observation, creative experimentation, and thorough analysis, psychologists gather the information that allows them to diagnose and properly treat their patients. They study both normal and abnormal behaviors as they relate to human functioning, offering psychological testing and consultations and encouraging behaviors that help people develop physical and emotional wellness and increase their level of emotional resistance. Many psychologists are educators and researchers as well (American Psychological Association, 2013).

For the past few decades, the American Psychological Association and some state psychological associations have lobbied aggressively to earn psychologists the right to legally prescribe medication—a request that is passionately opposed by the American Psychiatric Association and some other physician organizations. Psychologists have already won the right to legally prescribe medication in New Mexico and Louisiana, with several other states currently considering this legislation. This heated legal battle between the organizations representing psychologists and psychiatrists will likely continue for years to come, as neither side is willing to back down from this legislative battle (Richard & Huprich, 2009). The lobbying efforts have contributed to an increase in tension between psychologists and psychiatrists, as the groups of professionals remain in disagreement over increasing the treatment privileges of psychologists.

Mental Health Clinical Nurses

registered nurse–psychiatric mental health (RN-PMH)
An RN who is clinically competent in mental health nursing.

advanced practice registered nurse–psychiatric mental health (APRN-PMH)
An RN who has passed the certification exam in psychiatric–mental health nursing.

Two levels of psychiatric mental health nurses are currently recognized in the United States: the **registered nurse–psychiatric mental health (RN-PMH)** and the **advanced practice registered nurse–psychiatric mental health (APRN-PMH)**. The RN-PMH has earned an associate's degree or a bachelor's degree in nursing. Registered nurses with a bachelor of science degree in nursing (BSN) are eligible to take the basic certification exam in psychiatric–mental health nursing of the American Nurses Credentialing Center to show that they are clinically competent and knowledgeable in mental health nursing. Employers in some states require this certification because of reimbursement requirements, and the certification additionally serves to distinguish a nurse as a competent clinician in this setting. At this basic level of training, RN-PMHs work in supervised settings and often handle multiple responsibilities, such as those of a staff nurse, a case manager, or a home care nurse. They may assess symptoms of mental illness, track responses to interventional care, coordinate interdisciplinary patient care, participate in counseling, hand out prescribed medications, and educate patients. It is estimated that 4 percent of the overall population of registered nurses choose to work in the mental health care setting (Varcarolis & Halter, 2010).

The next level of educational preparation for mental health clinical nurses is the APRN-PMH. These professionals are registered nurses who have earned either a master of science degree in nursing (MSN) or a doctor of nursing practice (DNP) degree focusing on psychiatric–mental health nursing. Certification through the American Nurses Credentialing Center is also available at this level of nursing, and there are currently four types of certification examinations available to the APRN-PMH. Almost 10 percent of these nurses choose to earn credentials in psychiatric mental health nursing, allowing them to function autonomously in this setting. These nurses are educated and skilled in diagnosing mental illnesses, prescribing psychotropic medications, and conducting psychotherapy. They frequently work in case management, consulting services, patient education, and research within psychiatric settings. Currently, there is great demand for both RN-PMHs and APRN-PMHs, making the future very bright for this group of knowledgeable and valuable professionals (Varcarolis & Halter, 2010).

Psychiatric Nurse Practitioners

The **psychiatric mental health nurse practitioner (PMH-NP)** is a health care professional who has earned a four-year bachelor's degree in nursing (BSN) and has completed an MSN or DNP degree in psychiatric-mental health nursing, inclusive of at least 600 clinical hours. PMH-NPs are qualified to provide psychiatric services to adults, children, adolescents, and families. They may practice autonomously in a great range of settings, and commonly work in primary care settings, ambulatory mental health clinics, psychiatric emergency or crisis centers, hospitals, community health centers, and private psychiatric practices. PMH-NPs are licensed to perform psychosocial and physical assessments, make diagnoses, conduct therapy sessions, formulate treatment plans, and dispense prescription medications. In other words, they can fully manage a wide range of patient care services. The legally permitted functions and licensing requirements for PMH-NPs currently vary from state to state. In almost half of the states, PMH-NPs may open and operate their own mental health care practices, but the remaining states require that they practice collaboratively with physicians (American College of Nurse Practitioners, 2012).

psychiatric mental health nurse practitioner (PMH-NP)
A nurse practitioner who provides a wide range of mental health patient care services.

Social Workers

A **social worker** is a professional who has earned either a bachelor's or a master's degree in social work. Social workers are essential support personnel who work in a variety of settings including community mental health programs, hospitals and skilled nursing facilities, private psychiatric practices, military and veterans' centers, schools, and rehabilitation centers. They are often the coordinators of basic mental health services in employee assistance programs and disaster relief programs.

social worker
A professional who helps to improve individuals' quality of life through the coordination of available programs and services.

One of the strengths of social workers is in case management, as they are skilled in arranging for various services that maintain or improve quality of life while meeting patients' psychosocial needs. Often they assist individuals in securing housing, employment, general medical care, and other necessary services based on the needs of each case. In addition, they are valuable consultants to other health care providers in helping people prepare and develop a support system that will facilitate good mental health upon their discharge from an inpatient facility. Licensing requirements for social workers vary among the states; up-to-date information on specific state requirements is provided on the licensing board website for each state (Varcarolis & Halter, 2010; Williams & Torrens, 2008).

Nurses

Nurses are a critical portion of the health care workforce in the United States, as they provide treatment, support, and care services for the ill, injured, and aged. In many cases, they help to plan and manage the care of patients with physical and mental illnesses. Nurses are also skilled in the practical application of many preventive and curative services, and can deploy these skills in either clinical or community settings (World Health Organization, 2013, p. 3).

Registered Nurses

registered nurse (RN)
A health care professional who helps to treat patients, coordinate patient care, and provide patient education.

A **registered nurse (RN)** is a highly educated individual who helps to treat patients, coordinate patient care, and provide patient education to individual patients, families, and the public about a variety of health conditions. They also serve to give advice and emotional support to patients and family members during stressful and difficult times. RNs are skilled in recording medical history data, assisting with diagnostic testing, and administering treatments and medications as ordered by a physician, as well as assisting with the follow-up process to ensure a good continuum of care. RNs can specialize in one or more areas of care, and find employment in a large number of health care settings. Some choose to specialize in critical care, diabetes education, orthopedics, forensics, HIV/AIDS, geriatrics, wound care, hospice care, or oncology; the number of specialty fields for nurses goes far beyond this short, illustrative listing. They work in a variety of settings, including hospitals, physicians' offices, ambulatory care facilities, home health care outreach services, and inpatient nursing care facilities. They work in correctional facilities, schools and universities, summer camps, and social assistance agencies, and they also find employment with the government and the military (BLS, 2013c; Stanfield et al., 2009).

Licensed Practical Nurses

licensed practical nurse (LPN)
A midlevel nursing care provider who supports day-to-day functions in the health care setting.

A **licensed practical nurse (LPN)** works under the direction of physicians and RNs, providing basic nursing care services to the sick, injured, convalescent, or disabled. LPNs are integral midlevel nursing care providers, supporting individuals' day-to-day functions in many settings, including nursing homes, extended care facilities, hospitals, physicians' offices, and home health care settings. The nature of their work varies by the scope of practice allowed by their respective state; however, most LPNs frequently provide bedside care. They measure and record vital signs, prepare injections, dress wounds, assist with personal care and hygiene, feed patients who need assistance, reposition patients, and help with ambulation and transferring. Many LPNs are trained to collect samples for laboratory testing, to clean and monitor medical equipment, to watch for and report adverse reactions to medications and treatments, and to teach family members or caregivers how to assist in caring for the patient. LPNs are often generalists, working in all areas of health care rather than specializing as RNs may do (BLS, 2013b; Stanfield et al., 2009).

Certified Nursing Assistants

The **certified nursing assistant (CNA)** is a hard-working professional who often carries the heaviest burden in terms of hands-on, routine patient care services. Working in the same settings as LPNs, CNAs are usually hired on an hourly basis to answer patient call lights, take vital signs, bathe patients, make beds, assist with dressing and other hygiene activities, feed patients, provide basic wound care, and also help with ambulation or transfer. They do not assess, interpret, make decisions, or delegate duties. They do, however, act as primary caregivers in settings such as nursing homes, often being the main point of social contact for patients who have little family or few visitors. These workers are the facilities' watchful eyes, as they know to report any changes in a patient's condition (and any other concerns) to the supervising RN (Quan, 2007).

certified nursing assistant (CNA)
A basic-level nursing care provider who provides routine patient care and personal assistance services.

Radiologic and Imaging Professionals

Most people are familiar with the basic practices of radiologic medicine, such as the taking of X-rays to diagnose bone fractures. This remains a popular procedure; however, the medical uses of radiation and other forms of imaging extend far beyond that. Radiation is used not only to provide images of the inside of a patient's body but also as a form of treatment for various diseases. Moreover, it is now possible to view and examine not only bones but also organs, tissues, vessels, and all systems of the body. This area of medicine employs a rapidly growing group of health care workers, comprising radiologic technicians, diagnostic medical sonographers, nuclear medicine technologists, and radiation therapists, and makes use of computerized equipment to produce sharp and clear images (Stanfield et al., 2009).

Radiologic Technicians

radiologic technician (RT)
An imaging professional who takes radiographs using a variety of equipment.

A **radiologic technician (RT)** is an imaging professional who takes radiographs using a variety of equipment. He or she will have earned either an associate's or bachelor's degree and will also have received specialized training. RTs help to prepare a patient for a prescribed test or procedure, answer questions, check that the patient is not wearing accessories that will obstruct the images, and then correctly position the patient for the test or procedure. The areas of the patient's body that are sensitive to radiation are shielded with lead-containing covers to minimize risk. Then the technician focuses the X-ray source at the correct height and angle for the body part to be examined, and sets the controls for the appropriate density, detail, and contrast (Wischnitzer & Wischnitzer, 2011). It is also common for RTs to assist with maintenance of the radiologic equipment and to keep patient records.

Some RTs, after more extensive training, choose to become certified in additional radiation modalities such as MRI (magnetic resonance imaging), CT (computed tomography), or mammography. These workers perform more complex levels of imaging procedures and can advance their careers by becoming able to perform a wider variety of tests. They commonly work in hospitals as members of the radiology department, but may also work in private practice settings, clinics, ambulatory care centers, and educational settings.

Diagnostic Medical Sonographers

diagnostic medical sonographer
A technician skilled in using sound waves to assess and diagnose a variety of conditions.

A **diagnostic medical sonographer** will have a two- or four-year degree and specialized training in this field. These technicians use specialized imaging equipment that directs nonionizing, high-frequency sound waves into a patient's body to help assess and diagnose various medical conditions. These technicians operate the equipment that collects the echoes of the sound waves and translates them into useful images that can then be saved as videotapes or photographs or transmitted directly to a physician for interpretation and diagnosis. As RTs do, they prepare the patient, answer questions, and take a variety of images. Once the images are recorded, they review them and carefully select the ones that are most clear and useful for the physicians' diagnostic purposes. Diagnostic medical sonographers may specialize in particular areas or systems of the body, such as obstetric and gynecological, abdominal, vascular, cardiac, or breast sonography or neurosonography (Stanfield et al., 2009).

nuclear medicine technologist
A professional who uses radioactive nuclides to diagnose and treat diseases.

Nuclear Medicine Technologists

A **nuclear medicine technologist** uses radioactive nuclides (unstable atoms that spontaneously emit radiation) to diagnose and treat diseases.

The radioactive nuclides are purified and then compounded to form radio-pharmaceuticals, which the nuclear medicine technologist administers to patients. Once the patient ingests the prescribed drug, the technologist monitors the characteristics and level of function of the tissues and organs that take up the drug. He or she watches the computer screen carefully for tissues that show higher than expected or lower than expected concentrations of the ingested drug, as these indicate abnormalities in those tissues. Testing using radiopharmaceuticals is thus different from the previously mentioned radiographic techniques in that it determines the presence of disease on the basis of metabolic changes rather than by changes in the tissue structures themselves (Stanfield et al., 2009).

Radiation Therapists

A **radiation therapist** is a member of a medical oncology team who is skilled in using a linear accelerator to administer radiation treatments to treat cancer and other diseases. Images from diagnostic X-ray, MRI, or CT exams are used to pinpoint the location of a patient's cancer or condition needing treatment. Sometimes, radiation therapy is provided with a curative intent (meaning that the treatment is given in the hope that it will cure a cancer either by destroying a tumor or preventing cancer recurrence, or both). In that case radiation therapy is provided either alone or in combination with surgery or chemotherapy, or with both. In other cases radiation therapy is provided with a palliative intent, meaning that the therapy is not expected to be a cure but rather is intended to relieve symptoms and reduce the amount of suffering caused by the cancer or other condition. The radiation used in this type of therapy can be produced by a machine outside the body (external-beam radiation therapy) or by radioactive material that is skillfully placed inside the body near tumors or cancer cells (internal radiation therapy, more commonly called brachytherapy).

radiation therapist
A member of a medical oncology team who is skilled in treating cancer and other diseases.

Radiation therapists also oversee systemic radiation therapy, in which the patient is given a radioactive substance, either by mouth or by injection into a vein, which then travels in the bloodstream to tissues throughout the body (National Cancer Institute, 2013). The radiation therapist monitors this type of treatment, watching diligently for any side effects while maintaining a positive attitude and providing any necessary emotional support along the way. Most patients will make appointments to see their radiation therapist on a daily basis (five days per week) for two to nine weeks, so a friendly patient–care provider relationship is often built in this setting.

Most radiation therapists work full-time in hospitals or cancer centers. In this particular job setting a considerable amount of physical work is performed, since many cancer patients require assistance getting on and off the treatment tables and transferring from chairs. Working with cancer patients as one's primary patient base can be stressful and at times emotionally taxing; however, many radiation therapists find their work to be both satisfying and rewarding (Stanfield et al., 2009).

It is interesting to note that the future generations of computer-assisted radiographic equipment are certain to be even more sophisticated and more capable of producing images of amazing clarity than the machines we have today. This will allow physicians to receive ever more accurate information to confirm or monitor the progress of a diagnosis. Treatments are becoming more and more focused on the exact location of the problem in the body, which is likely to continue to improve outcomes. It is expected that future patients will undergo their tests and treatments even more safely than they do today and with less risk or discomfort. Taken altogether, these benefits will likely lead to a more extensive use of radiologic procedures in the upcoming years (Stanfield et al., 2009).

Allied Health Rehabilitation Professionals

Practitioners of rehabilitation care are valuable health care workers who provide care and treatment for the purpose of enhancing and restoring a disabled or impaired patient's functional abilities as well as preserving his or her quality of life. Rehabilitation therapists use their skills to help patients with physical, mental, or social impairments to regain their strength and quality of independent life to the greatest extent possible. If a return to full function is not possible, these workers use their training and some creative thinking to teach patients ways to modify their environments or approaches to life activities to make the most of their lives after an illness or injury.

physical therapist
A clinician skilled in the assessment and treatment of physical injuries.

occupational therapist
A clinician who assists individuals with physical and/or emotional disabilities by teaching daily living or other related life skills.

There are many types of highly skilled rehabilitation professionals working in one or more specialty care settings. In a specialty care setting, these therapists often receive referrals from medical professionals of patients who have suffered an injury or illness that has affected the patient's ability to function. They often work collaboratively with physicians and others to create a detailed care plan with stated goals that can be measured and reassessed as the patient moves through the rehabilitation program over time. For example, some of these therapists work in a corrective environment, such as a physical therapy, occupational therapy, or athletic training setting. These workers use a range of techniques to assess and implement individualized plans of care to address specific deficits caused by trauma, strokes, illnesses, or birth defects. A **physical therapist** commonly uses heat, cold, exercise, electromodalities, ultrasound, and aquatic therapy to improve the deficits as much as possible. An **occupational therapist** assists individuals with physical and/or emotional disabilities by teaching daily living or activity skills or other related life skills. Occupational therapists are creative, out-of-the-box thinkers whose innovations lead to helpful ways to modify life and recreational activities to make necessary functions possible. A **certified athletic trainer** works primarily with physically active populations, caring for injuries and also taking steps to prevent injuries among those involved in school-related, amateur, and professional athletics. They use modalities similar to those of occupational therapists and, in addition, are well respected for their emergency care and assessment skills.

Patients who have lost all or a portion of a limb owing to trauma, disease, or a birth defect can benefit from the skills of an **orthotist** or **prosthetist**, an individual who is highly skilled in fitting patients for braces, supports, and artificial limbs. These individuals take the time to assess each patient's needs and limitations to ensure that the correct device is chosen, built, and properly fitted, and they then help to educate the patient on the use and proper care of the device for the best possible outcome over time.

A **speech-language pathologist** works with both children and adults who are diagnosed with speech or language impairments. Whether the impairments are the result of a brain injury, birth defect, developmental delay, Parkinson's disease, or Alzheimer's disease, these therapists see patients of all ages who suffer from a wide range of impairments from the very mild to those that are severely limiting. They are also helpful to those with voice disorders and swallowing difficulties, especially patients who are dealing with the aftereffects of some types of stroke and cancer. An **audiologist** is a doctoral-level trained professional who works with both children and adults with hearing impairments, from a variety of causes, evaluating their hearing and fitting hearing aids when needed. They may also work with people with balance problems. This growing profession is likely to expand even further in future years due to the aging of the population, since hearing loss tends to increase as people age.

Additionally, **art, dance, and music therapists** rely on creativity—applying both artistic and therapeutic skills to assist patients with mental and physical impairments. Because these art and dance and, to some extent, music therapies involve nonverbal communication, they may be particularly useful for patients with certain physical, mental, and social issues.

A **horticultural therapist** uses gardening as his or her main therapeutic technique. It has the advantage of being a relaxing, social, and enjoyable activity as well as a means of assessing a patient's capabilities in performing certain types of tasks (Stanfield et al., 2009). There are many more therapeutic specialties, as the following list shows.

Rehabilitation Professionals and Therapists

- Aroma therapists
- Art therapists

certified athletic trainer
A health care professional who specializes in preventing, assessing, and treating musculoskeletal injuries and illnesses.

orthotist
A clinician who measures, designs, fabricates, or fits an orthosis for a patient.

prosthetist
A clinician who measures, designs, fabricates, or fits a prosthesis for a patient.

speech-language pathologist
A clinician who helps children and adults who have been diagnosed with speech or language impairments.

audiologist
A health care professional who works with children and adults who have hearing impairments.

art, dance, and music therapists
Professionals who are highly skilled in using their respective creative medium to enhance the therapeutic process.

horticultural therapist
A therapist who uses gardening as a therapeutic technique.

- Audiologists
- Behavioral therapists
- Biofeedback therapists
- Certified athletic trainers
- Child life specialists
- Dance therapists
- Grief therapists
- Horticultural therapists
- Hypnotherapists
- Kinesiotherapists
- Massage therapists
- Music therapists
- Myotherapists
- Occupational therapists
- Occupational therapy assistants and aides
- Orientation and mobility specialists
- Orthotists
- Physical therapists
- Physical therapy assistants
- Prosthetists
- Recreation therapists
- Respiratory therapists and technicians
- Speech-language pathologists
- Substance abuse counselors

Rehabilitation and therapy is a diverse and rewarding field, with a broad spectrum of settings of care as well as opportunities for career exploration. Therapists may work in hospitals, clinics, or long-term care facilities, or travel to the homes of patients, and there is a type of therapist for almost every type of physical, mental, or emotional disability. As the population in the United States continues to age and live longer than previous generations, these professionals will become all the more critical for supporting those needing care as they either return to full function or learn to modify and adapt their functions after illness or injury.

Collaboration in Health Care

Regardless of the specialty or subspecialty of care in which one chooses to practice, collaboration and communication are critical to the success of the overall operation of the health care system, especially in an age of frugality in resources and high expectations for accountability. The current U.S. health care system involves numerous interfaces and patient handoffs among many health care providers, each with a particular educational preparation and level of training. In some cases patients who spend four to five days in the hospital will encounter approximately fifty different health care providers—including primary care physicians, specialists, various levels of nurses, technicians, and other assistants. Any breakdown in the chain of communication raises the risk of error, which has potentially devastating or deadly consequences for the patient. Each error caused by a lack of understanding of other professionals' work, scope of practice, and/or communication regarding the patient at hand creates situations where patient harm is likely to occur.

Especially since the Institute of Medicine released its landmark reports in 1999 and 2001, a clear call has been made for an increase in team collaboration by all types of health care providers in all settings. Without team collaboration, patient safety is at risk for many reasons, especially when critical information is not shared in a timely and complete way, information is misinterpreted, phone or written orders are unclear, and changes in patient status are overlooked or not properly brought to the attention of a supervising care provider. These types of medical errors, especially those caused by a failure of health care providers to work actively together to communicate well, are a pervasive problem in most current health care systems. In addition to causing medical errors, lack of communication is also associated with a reduction in quality of care as well as a higher cost for the care provided.

In fact The Joint Commission (formerly known as the Joint Commission on Accreditation of Health Care Organizations, or JCAHO) notes that if medical errors appeared on the National Center for Health Statistics list of the top ten causes of death in the United States, they would rank number 5. This would place medical errors ahead of accidents, diabetes, and Alzheimer's disease, as well as AIDS, breast cancer, and gunshot wounds. Even more upsetting is the fact that The Joint Commission cites communication errors among health care providers as the primary cause for medication errors, delays in treatment, and wrong-site surgeries, as well as the second most frequently cited cause for operative and postoperative events and falls leading to patient death (O'Daniel & Rosenstein, 2008).

There is an awareness that the current training of health care professionals involves "little cross-training or interaction with other professional groups with which a professional discipline must eventually work. There is also little transition or flow between and among the professional groups; the majority of training time during health care providers' education is spent in developing the unique skills necessary for one particular professional role. This results in health care providers who are highly competent in the specifics of their own field and, at the same time, are virtually unaware of the specifics of others" (Freshman, Rubino, & Chassiakos, 2010, p. 6). This disintegration and isolation of professional trainings leads to care providers who are well prepared in their particular discipline but poorly prepared to be members of health care–providing teams and collaborative patient care groups (Freshman et al., 2010).

So how can we work to increase cross-specialty collaboration among health care providers? First, educational institutions must work to identify the collaborative skills needed to increase communication among health care professionals and thereby reduce medical errors. It is also necessary for all health care providers to personally take active steps to become familiar with the work of the other providers around them, so that an understanding of cultures, methods of care, and values can be instilled. With a clear recognition of the needs of each group of care providers, an environment of support for the maximum effectiveness of each provider will begin to grow.

Health care organizations can further support this communication and collaboration by creating an environment with specific guidelines that support teamwork. Over time, following these guidelines for cross-communication will become more natural for health care providers, and errors are likely to decrease as communication increases. All types of patient care involve some degree of communication and collaboration among care providers, so teamwork must be emphasized from day one of both education and employment and must be reinforced on a consistent basis thereafter.

Employment Trends in the Health Care Sector

The job outlook and employment trends in the U.S. health care system remain extremely promising and strong. Nearly every person will have some type of contact with the health care system in their lives, from the time of birth in a delivery room, to incidental emergency room needs as a child, to preventive primary care services as an adult, to the last days of life that are sometimes spent in a nursing home or inpatient hospice facility.

According to the Bureau of Labor Statistics (2013a), health care is the fastest-growing sector of the U.S. economy, currently employing over 18 million workers. Of this 18 million, women represent nearly 80 percent of the overall health care workforce. Although a health care career has many opportunities for employment and financial reward, it also takes place in a setting where workers face several on-the-job hazards, including needlestick injuries, back injuries, latex allergies, patient-on-provider violence, fatigue, and stress. Facilities have already taken many steps to prevent or reduce health care workers' exposure to these hazards; nevertheless, many health care workers continue to experience injuries and illnesses in the workplace (Centers for Disease Control and Prevention, 2013).

In terms of wages, physicians and surgeons rank among the highest of all occupations. In 2012, physicians who practice in the primary care setting received total median annual compensation of \$220,942, while physicians who practice in medical specialties received total median annual compensation of \$396,233. The overall employment of physicians and surgeons is expected to increase by 18 percent from the year 2012 to the year 2022, a growth rate predicted to be faster than the average for all occupations. The job prospects are also very promising for primary care and specialist physicians who are willing to set up their practices in either rural or low-income areas, because these areas typically have difficulties in attracting physicians (BLS, 2014).

Many health care providers will continue to see a promising job outlook (Figure 3.1). The health care occupations with the largest projected employment increases include RNs, personal and home care aides, home health aides, nurse's aides, medical assistants, and LPNs. Nurses, in particular, will enjoy a high employment rate into the future years, both within and outside the traditional health care settings. With 2.5 million nurses already employed, even more nurses, as well as aides and support personnel, are necessary to support the continued needs of the health care system (BLS, 2013d).

Overall, the employment trend in the health care professions is expected to continue to be positive in the upcoming years (Figure 3.2). This strong and steady growth in employment is expected to be driven by the many technological advances in patient care that will allow a greater number of injuries and illnesses to be treated, which will lessen both morbidity and mortality rates. An increase in the emphasis placed on primary care drives these expected employment numbers up as well, as the number of professionals now needed to support the primary care setting has increased in recent years. In addition, advances in technology and innovations in pharmaceuticals are allowing people to live longer than ever before.

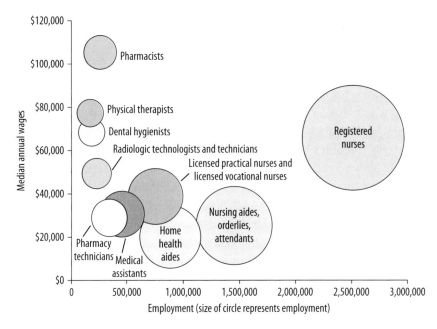

Figure 3.1   Employment and Earnings in Selected Health Care Practitioner and Health Care Support Occupations

Source: Bureau of Labor Statistics, 2013d.

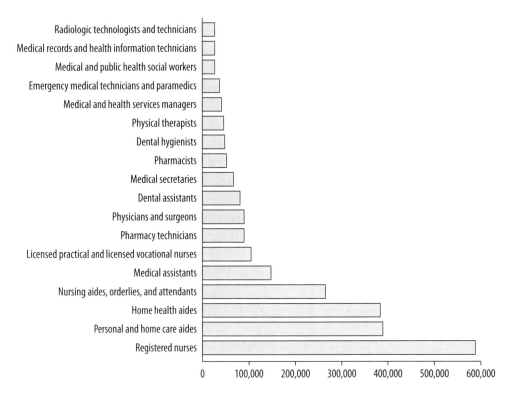

Figure 3.2   Projected Change in Total Employment, Selected Health Care Occupations

Source: Bureau of Labor Statistics, 2013d.

The aging of the baby boomer generation comes into play here, as it causes the need for a variety of health care personnel in both the generalist and the specialty care areas. The numbers of people needing nursing care and therapies is also greater than ever before, which translates to a positive job trend for health care professionals all across the disciplines.

SUMMARY

The current health care environment involves the work of many types of skilled individuals, knowledgeable in their particular disciplines and (optimally) working together in teams to fulfill the needs of each patient as an individual. Given the diversity of education, skills, and scope of practice among these health care providers, it is imperative that they work collaboratively in treating a patient. Each health care professional is a link in the overall chain of care and is to be valued for the knowledge and contributions he or she provides.

It is to be hoped that current and future health care workers are enlightened over time to realize that today's health care professions depend for success on a patient-centered team environment where the training and experiences of each team member have an additive effect, to the overall benefit of the patients who are seeking care. The importance of collaboration and communication among health care providers at all levels cannot be emphasized enough, as this has been identified as a critical point in preventing medical errors that cause both patient harm and patient deaths. The job outlook for providers of health care continues to be promising in all fields; those who are or will be employed in the fields presented in this chapter will enjoy a wide variety of settings and opportunities for utilizing their education and skills.

KEY TERMS

advanced practice registered nurse– psychiatric mental health (APRN-PMH)

art, dance, and music therapists

audiologist

certified athletic trainer

certified nursing assistant (CNA)

dental assistant

dental hygienist

dentist

diagnostic medical sonographer

doctor of medicine (MD)

doctor of osteopathic medicine (DO)

horticultural therapist

licensed practical nurse (LPN)

nuclear medicine technologist

nurse practitioner (NP)

occupational therapist

orthotist

physical therapist

physician assistant (PA)

primary care physician

prosthetist

psychiatric mental health nurse
    practitioner (PMH-NP)

psychiatrist

psychologist

radiation therapist

radiologic technician (RT)

registered nurse (RN)

registered nurse–psychiatric mental
    health (RN-PMH)

social worker

speech-language pathologist

DISCUSSION QUESTIONS

1. How would you describe the differences between MDs and DOs?

2. What are some of the specific differences in the duties of the three levels of nurses?

3. What are some of the specific differences between psychiatrists and psychologists?

4. What are the differences in the clinical functions of the three levels of mental health nurses?

5. In what ways are tests and treatments provided by radiologic and imaging professionals important in the overall chain of health care?

6. As the population ages and lives longer, why are the various rehabilitation professionals and therapists an important part of the future of health care?

7. What are some of the ways in which communication breakdown leads to medical errors?

REFERENCES

American Board of Psychiatry and Neurology. (2013). ABPN certification resources. Retrieved from http://www.abpn.com/what_is_abpn.html

American College of Nurse Practitioners. (2012). What is a nurse practitioner? Retrieved from http://www.acnpweb.org/i4a/pages/index.cfm?pageid =3479

American Psychological Association. (2013). What is psychology? Retrieved from http://www.apa.org/careers/resources/guides/careers.aspx?item=1

Bureau of Labor Statistics. (2013a). Dental hygienists. In *Occupational outlook handbook*. Retrieved from http://www.bls.gov/ooh/healthcare/dental -hygienists.htm

Bureau of Labor Statistics. (2013b). Licensed practical nurses. In *Occupational outlook handbook*. Retrieved from http://www.bls.gov/ooh/healthcare /licensed-practical-and-licensed-vocational-nurses.htm

Bureau of Labor Statistics. (2013c). Registered nurses. In *Occupational outlook handbook*. Retrieved from http://www.bls.gov/ooh/healthcare/registered -nurses.htm

Bureau of Labor Statistics. (2013d). Spotlight on statistics: Health care. Retrieved from http://www.bls.gov/spotlight/2009/health_care

Bureau of Labor Statistics. (2014). Physicians and surgeons. In *Occupational outlook handbook*. Retrieved from http://www.bls.gov/ooh/healthcare/physicians-and -surgeons.htm

Centers for Disease Control and Prevention. (2013). Healthcare workers. Retrieved from http://www.cdc.gov/niosh/topics/healthcare

Field, S. (2007). *Career opportunities in health care* (3rd ed.). New York, NY: Ferguson.

Freshman, B., Rubino, L., & Chassiakos, Y. R. (2010). *Collaboration across the disciplines in health care*. Sudbury, MA: Jones & Bartlett.

National Cancer Institute. (2013). *Radiation therapy for cancer* [Fact sheet]. Retrieved from http://www.cancer.gov/cancertopics/factsheet/Therapy /radiation

O'Daniel, M., & Rosenstein, A. H. (2008). Professional communication and team collaboration. In R. G. Hughes (Ed.), *Patient quality and safety: An evidence-based handbook for nurses*. Rockville, MD: Agency for Healthcare Research and Quality. Retrieved from http://www.ahrq.gov/professionals/clinicians providers/resources/nursing/resources/nurseshdbk/index.html

Quan, K. (2007). *The everything guide to careers in health care*. Avon, MA: Adams Media.

Raffel, M. W., & Barsukiewicz, C. K. (2002). *The U.S. health system: Origins and functions* (5th ed.). Albany, NY: Delmar.

Richard, D. C., & Huprich, S. K. (2009). *Clinical psychology: Assessment, treatment and research*. Burlington, MA: Elsevier Academic Press.

Stanfield, P. S., Cross, N., & Hui, Y. H. (2009). *Introduction to the health professions* (5th ed.). Sudbury, MA: Jones & Bartlett.

Sugar-Webb, J. (2005). *Opportunities in physician careers*. New York: McGraw-Hill.

Varcarolis, E. M., & Halter, M .J. (2010). *Foundations of psychiatric mental health nursing: A clinical approach* (6th ed.). St. Louis, MO: Saunders Elsevier.

Williams, S. J., & Torrens, P. R. (2008). *Introduction to health services* (7th ed.). Clifton Park, NY: Delmar/Cengage Learning.

Wischnitzer, S., & Wischnitzer, E. (2011). *Top 100 health careers* (3rd ed.). Indianapolis, IN: JIST.

World Health Organization. (2013). *Classifying health workers: Mapping occupations to the international standard classification*. Retrieved from http:// www.who.int/hrh/statistics/Health_workers_classification.pdf

CHAPTER 4

HOSPITALS

Denice Yanchik

The hospital. This is the place we go to be healed when we are sick. It is the place where many of us come into this world and where many of us will leave this world. But what do most people really know about this mysterious place with its high-tech, state-of-the art machines, staffs of diverse disciplines that speak a language known only unto them, and a billing and payment system that is as complex and mysterious as the federal tax code? The answer is probably not much. When asked, most people will tell you which hospital in their community gives the best care in their opinion, and whether they like the doctors and nurses there. But how did these institutions come into being? How are they paid? Who regulates them? How are they staffed and governed? Who monitors their quality? What does the future hold for hospitals?

LEARNING OBJECTIVES

After reading this chapter you should be able to

- Explain both horizontal integration and vertical integration of hospitals and the effect of this integration on the health care market.

- Explain the responsibilities of the hospital governing board.

- Describe how modern hospitals evolved.

- Describe the complexities of staffing a hospital.

- Describe a culture of safety.

History of Hospitals

Hospitals have their roots in early religious communities. It was in the early convents and monasteries of Europe that the sick and infirm sought comfort and healing. Unfortunately, the nuns and monks could offer little more than spiritual consolation, as the treatments and therapies that we take for granted were still hundreds of years away. In the eighteenth century, as medical education began to spread, the notion that recovery from disease was possible began to take hold (Wall, 2012). Prior to this time, medicine could cure little and surgical interventions many times served only to hasten the patient's demise (Goldin, 1984). Early American hospitals have their roots in charitable organizations. According to an article in the *California State Journal of Medicine*, Pennsylvania Hospital in Philadelphia was the first hospital in the United States. It was initially established as an institution to care for the "insane and indigent sick." The hospital charter was granted in May 1751 and the hospital was completed in December 1762 (Cutter, 1922). It's hard to imagine that Bellevue Hospital in New York City, which today is an 838-bed hospital with over 125,000 emergency room visits per year, 4,298 employees, and an operating budget of $726 million per year, was originally a 6-bed ward on the second floor of an almshouse founded in 1736 for the poor and infirm (City of New York, 2013).

During the 1800s and the early 1900s, most Americans never visited a hospital. The United States was largely rural at that time, and most medical care was provided at home, ranging from childbirth to, at times, surgery. Usually it was the poor or those needing to be isolated from others who were cared for in hospitals. The upper classes cared for their sick and infirm at home (Wall, 2012). The modern hospital began to emerge around the time of the Civil War. It was at this time that medicine and surgical procedures were beginning to advance. With these advances, physicians began to staff hospitals and nursing was becoming recognized as a profession. In 1859, Florence Nightingale established the first school of nursing at St. Thomas's hospital in London. This had a tremendous influence on the training of nurses in the United States as well.

Early hospitals were not-for-profit institutions and relied largely on charitable contributions. Patients were expected to pay out of pocket for the care and services they received. In the 1920s, as hospitals began to offer hope to many that they could be cured of their illnesses, many hospitals also began to shed their charitable focus on the poorer classes in favor of taking care of the upper-middle class (America's Essential Hospitals, n.d.). By the mid-1920s, hospitals were using new technologies such as X-rays, laboratory testing, and aseptic techniques for surgical procedures. With these advances it was becoming more difficult to justify taking care of people at home. Hospitals were becoming much safer than in the past, and it was also much easier to take care of individuals in the hospital than in their homes. It was at this time that many hospitals developed their own nurse training programs. It was the student nurses who provided most of the patient care in hospitals at this time, thus affording hospitals an almost free labor force (Domrose, 2012).

The demand for increased hospital capacity and services increased greatly following World War II. With this increased demand came increased government involvement. In 1946, Congress passed the Hospital Survey and Construction Act, commonly known as the **Hill-Burton Act**, a federal law that allocated funds to build, expand, and modernize community hospitals, nursing homes, and other health care facilities (Health Resources and Services Administration [HRSA], 2012). Moreover, any facility that accepted loans or grants associated with the Hill-Burton Act had to agree

Hill-Burton Act
A federal law that allocated funds to build, expand, and modernize community hospitals, nursing homes, and other health care facilities.

to provide a reasonable volume of services to those who were unable to pay and to make its services available to all people living in the facility's area. The Hill-Burton program ceased to provide funding in 1997, but as of 2012, approximately 170 health care facilities that previously accepted such funding were still obligated to provide free or reduced-cost care to people who qualified. It is estimated that since 1980, more than $6 billion in uncompensated services has been provided to eligible patients (HRSA, 2012).

One of the largest government programs to influence health care was introduced in 1965. **Medicare** was signed into law on July 30, 1965, as title XVIII of the Social Security Act Amendments. The goal of Medicare was to provide health insurance to all citizens aged sixty-five or older and also to younger individuals with disabilities or end-stage renal disease. Prior to the enactment of Medicare, almost 50 percent of the elderly population in the United States had either inadequate or no health insurance coverage. Medicare coverage was designed to reflect the commercial health care plans of the time, primarily Blue Cross and Blue Shield. This coverage was divided into two parts. Hospital insurance (Part A) covered hospital stays and related expenses. Supplemental medical insurance (Part B) covered such things as physician fees and costs of outpatient hospital care, laboratory tests, X-rays, therapy, medical equipment used at home, and home health not covered by Part A (National Bipartisan Commission on the Future of Medicare, 2012). For those who were not of retirement age, the expanding business sector provided health insurance for its employees. But this still left those who were poor and not of retirement age with no health insurance coverage. This was the population that the federal **Medicaid** program was developed to serve. The Medicaid program was passed by Congress at the same time as Medicare, as Title XIX of the Social Security Act Amendments of 1965. The Medicaid program, while funded by the federal government, is administered by the individual states (Moore & Smith, 2005–2006).

The Medicare and Medicaid programs ensured health care coverage for many of those in need, but with this came increased government oversight. Medicare and Medicaid program authority rests with the **Centers for Medicare & Medicaid Services (CMS)**. The CMS is a federal agency within the U.S. Department of Health and Human Services (HHS) that administers the Medicare program and also works in partnership with state governments to administer Medicaid, the State Children's Health Insurance Program (SCHIP), and health insurance standards. CMS has developed **conditions of participation (CoPs)** and **conditions for coverage (CfCs)** that health care organizations must meet in order to participate in the Medicare and Medicaid programs (CMS, 2013; to look up specific CoPs and CfCs, see Electronic Code of Federal Regulations

Medicare
A government program that provides health insurance to Americans sixty-five and over and to younger individuals with disabilities or end-stage renal disease.

Medicaid
A government program that provides health insurance to many low-income individuals and families.

Centers for Medicare & Medicaid Services (CMS)
The federal agency that administers the Medicare program and (with state governments) the Medicaid and SCHIP programs.

conditions of participation (CoPs)
Rules governing the eligibility of an organization to participate in Medicare and Medicaid programs.

conditions for coverage (CfCs)
Health and safety standards that organizations serving Medicare and Medicaid patients must meet.

[e-CFR], 2014). In other words, if an organization accepts money from CMS for caring for patients enrolled in either Medicare or Medicaid, it must adhere to the CMS CoPs and CfCs for *all* patients, not just those enrolled in these programs. These conditions set health and safety standards that are the foundation for improving quality and protecting the health and safety of beneficiaries. CMS also ensures that the standards of accrediting organizations recognized by CMS (through a process called *deeming*) meet or exceed the standards set forth in the CoPs and CfCs.

It was in the 1970s that community hospitals saw their greatest growth, due to funding from the government. In the period from 1960 to 1970, the number of beds in community hospitals increased by 32.7 percent (Wall, 2012). By this time hospitals were offering very complex and comprehensive services. With the increasing sophistication of medical technology came rapidly increasing costs for inpatient services. In the 1980s, Medicare introduced the **diagnosis related group (DRG)** payment system, a system under which a predetermined amount of money was paid to a hospital for treating a patient with a specific diagnosis, identified by a specific DRG. Gone were the days of fee-for-service payments. Linking payments to DRGs meant, for example, that if a patient were admitted for routine gallbladder surgery, the payment the hospital would receive would be the same no matter how long the hospital stay. This payment system forced hospitals to look at how they were providing care and to develop ways of working more efficiently.

Hospitals may be not-for-profit or for-profit. Community hospitals operate as **not-for-profit organizations**. This means that any profits they generate from operations are invested back into the hospital. Regardless of which classification it falls under, a hospital must turn a profit or it will not be in business for long. Profit must be realized in order to give raises to employees, upgrade equipment, and expand services. The 1980s saw a growth in for-profit organizations and the formation of larger hospital organizations, or systems (Wall, 2012).

The years of the late twentieth century and early twenty-first century have been difficult for hospitals. Many smaller community hospitals have closed their doors or been swallowed by larger organizations. With the changes in payment schedules and advances in technology, more treatments, procedures, and surgeries are now completed on an outpatient basis. This means that the patients who are actually admitted to the hospital, the inpatients, are more acutely ill than previously. However, inpatients are also released from the hospital more quickly than they used to be, leading to a host of new difficulties and challenges for hospitals, which will be discussed later in the chapter.

diagnosis related group (DRG)
A classification system, based on ICD diagnoses and procedures, for paying specific amounts for treatment of specific diagnoses.

not-for-profit organizations
Organizations that conduct business for the good of the general public, without shareholders or a profit motive.

Management of Hospitals

"The hospital must have an effective governing body legally responsible for the conduct of the hospital as an institution" (CoP 482.12). The **governing board** is the ultimate overseer of the hospital. The membership of the governing board may vary depending on the affiliation of the hospital. Typically the board will include influential members of the community, or members of the clergy if the hospital has a religious affiliation. If the hospital is connected to a university, the university board of trustees may oversee the hospital as well. A multihospital system will have one governing board that oversees all the hospitals in the system (Feigenbaum, 2012). Requirements about how often the board must meet vary from state to state, ranging from quarterly to biannually.

governing board
The supervising body of a health care organization.

The primary responsibilities of the governing board are regulated by the Medicare conditions of participation for hospitals. It is the governing board that is ultimately responsible for ensuring that each patient receives safe and quality care; it must also develop an operating budget, which is reviewed and updated annually. The operating budget must be prepared according to generally accepted accounting principles, include all anticipated income and expenses, and provide for capital expenditures for a period of at least three years. The governing board is also responsible for all contracted services that are provided (CoP 482.12[d]). This means ensuring that contracted service providers are in compliance with regulatory bodies, and monitoring providers' quality indicators. Contracted services may include services ranging from hemodialysis to housekeeping to security.

Each hospital is also required by law to have an organized medical staff and a **medical executive committee (MEC)**, which represents and acts on behalf of the medical staff. The MEC is made up of members of the medical staff and must meet a set number of times per year, as determined by the medical staff bylaws. The governing board is also required to "assure that the medical staff have bylaws and that they comply with state and federal law and requirements of the Medicare hospital conditions of participation (CoPs)." The **medical staff bylaws** govern the medical staff of the hospital and set forth in writing what authority the MEC has and also how that authority is delegated and removed (American Medical Association, 2009). The medical staff members are usually represented on the MEC by their department directors (medicine, surgery, orthopedics, etc.). The MEC is customarily chaired by the chief or president of the medical staff. The MEC also includes representation from nursing administration (typically the chief nursing officer), quality, finance, and other ancillary departments as needed. All policies and procedures must come through and be approved

medical executive committee (MEC)
A body that represents and acts on behalf of the medical staff.

medical staff bylaws
Rules for self-governance of the medical staff.

by the MEC. Once a year, the MEC is required to have a special meeting, generally referred to as the **committee of the whole**, and every member of the medical staff is invited to attend this meeting.

committee of the whole
A meeting of all the medical staff.

The hospital must have a chief executive officer (CEO) who oversees the running of the hospital on a day-to-day basis. The CEO reports directly to the board of directors and is wholly accountable to them. Other executives the organization may have include a chief administrative officer (CAO), chief medical officer (CMO), chief nursing officer (CNO), and a chief financial officer (CFO).

The nursing department is required to have a nurse executive who also reports to the CEO. The nurse executive must be a registered nurse (CoP 482.23[a]). The nurse executive may have the title of chief nursing officer, vice president or associate vice president of nursing, or chief clinical officer, depending on the organizational structure. Reporting to the nurse executive will be the nursing patient care managers of the various departments in the hospital. It is the responsibility of the nurse executive to ensure that the policies and procedures of the nursing department are adhered to, that the various levels of licensed nursing personnel practice within their scope of practice, and most important, that patients are cared for safely and attain the best possible outcomes. The patient care managers are usually department specific, although one manager may oversee multiple departments, depending on their size and areas of specialization. The **patient care department managers** oversee the staff that provide direct patient care. It is their responsibility to ensure that the policies and procedures of the hospital are carried out and followed appropriately. They are responsible for day-to-day operations, quality initiatives, scheduling, handling employee and patient complaints, and developing department budgets.

patient care department managers
Individuals who provide clinical and operational oversight to departments providing direct patient care.

If the organization is large, there may also be department directors who have specific oversight of medical or operational activities. For example, a large hospital may have department directors for pediatrics, obstetrics, orthopedics, surgery, and other patient care areas. In addition, it may have directors for operational departments that do not provide patient care but are important to the day-to-day operations of the hospital, such as food services, maintenance, housekeeping, supply, and security.

The nursing department is the largest department in a hospital (American Association of Colleges of Nursing, 2011). Nursing departments have traditionally used a top-down, hierarchal model of management, but in recent years, with the push for facilities to obtain the Magnet recognition designation (discussed later in the chapter), more and more nursing departments are adopting a shared governance model. Shared governance embraces practices such as employee autonomy, empowerment, involvement, and participation in decision making (Anthony, 2004). Shared governance first became popular in health care in the 1980s, through the work of Tim Porter-O'Grady (Barden, Griffin, Donahue, & Fitzpatrick, 2011). Porter-O'Grady emphasized that **shared governance** "is a professional practice model based clearly in the principles of partnership, equity, accountability and ownership at the unit level where the point of service occurs." In the 1990s, interest in shared governance started to wane. Hospitals where a council structure had been instituted eliminated that structure. Today, however, we are seeing a resurgence of interest in shared governance, due to the nursing shortage and the increased interest in acquiring the Magnet designation. Shared governance may differ in practice in each organization, but essentially it is a structure that allows staff nurses to have more control over their practice. This is an area that traditionally has been in the hands of administration. The goal of shared governance is to increase nurses' satisfaction and retention rates. Nursing shortages are always a concern for hospitals. Currently the United States has an aging nursing workforce. Many experienced nurses will be retiring in the next decade, and there are not enough new nurses coming through the schools to take their place. It should be noted that it is not just the reduction in the overall number of nurses that is a grave concern but the vast wealth of knowledge that the retiring nurses are taking with them.

When hospital nursing departments change to a shared governance approach, they usually choose to follow a councilor model (Anthony, 2004). A **councilor model** involves establishing subcommittees such as a nursing practice council, a recruitment and retention council, and a policy and procedure council, which then meet independently and report up to a central or nursing executive council. Moving to a shared governance model is not always an easy task. It requires a nurse executive who believes in nurse empowerment and is willing to invest the time and energy needed for the conversion, as well as support from the hospital's administration and its management team. If the leadership is transactional and unwilling to relinquish control of decision making, the effort to change will be hampered. The institution must have a definitive, strategic plan that is presented to the staff, along with specific timelines and ongoing education for the staff regarding the shared governance model and professional development (Hendren, 2011). Being dissatisfied with working conditions and management can lead to the staff forming a union. Many in management have the mistaken conception that wages are the most important factor in determining employee satisfaction (Sullivan & Decker, 2004). This is untrue. If you are in a management or administrative role in an organization with a collective bargaining unit, you will be involved in negotiating contracts and dealing with employee grievances.

shared governance
A governance model based on partnership, equity, accountability, and ownership at the point of service.

councilor model
A type of shared governance involving multiple subcommittees and a centralized committee that provides oversight.

Staffing

Staffing a hospital is complex and complicated. It is a 24/7, 365 days per year operation that does not allow for holidays, weekends, or inclement weather. Hospital staff members include not only nurses and physicians but also the individuals who work in all the numerous other departments, and all these individuals must operate in concert with one another. Many of these departments provide direct patient care but there are others that do not. The value of the departments that are not involved in direct patient care must not be minimized for they provide the structure and support without which the facility could not function. The staffs of departments not directly involved with patient care are frequently referred to as ancillary staff.

As previously stated, the largest department in a hospital is nursing. Nursing is also the largest health care profession in the United States. Currently, there are more than 2.4 million registered nurses actively employed, and 56 percent of them work in hospitals (Alichnie, 2012). The nursing department consists of registered nurses (RNs), licensed practical or vocational nurses (LPNs or LVNs), and nurse's aides. These caregivers deliver direct patient care at the bedside. It is crucial to have the right amount of staff and the right skill mix available to take care of patients. Skill mix refers to the different levels of provider available and needed to care for patients. What is the best nurse-to-patient ratio in hospitals? This is a difficult question to answer as the staffing of inpatient units depends on the acuity of the patients in each particular unit and the expertise of the nurses. **Patient acuity** refers to how sick patients are and how much

patient acuity
The intensity of a patient's illness, which indicates the care that he or she requires.

care they require. According to the Medicare CoPs, hospitals are required to "have adequate numbers of licensed registered nurses, licensed practical (vocational) nurses and other personnel to provide nursing care to all patients as needed" (CoP 482.23). This is very vague. In determining the number of nurses needed to staff a particular unit, there are two major areas of concern. First and foremost is patient safety. Without a suitable number of staff with the appropriate skill mix, the safety of the patient is at risk. Second is the health and safety of the staff caring for the patients. An understaffed unit places an increased burden on staff, both physically and mentally. The federal requirement to provide adequate staff to care for patients is vague; therefore it has been left to the states to determine what they consider enough staffing. Some states have enacted legislation to address nurse staffing in hospitals. In 1999, California became the first and so far only state to mandate specific licensed nurse-to-patient ratios (California Department of Public Health, 2014). While state-mandated ratios have their supporters, they are not necessarily the best answers to the staffing dilemma. **Mandatory staffing ratios** are inflexible and do not take into account

mandatory staffing ratios
Nurse-to-patient ratios required by law.

rapidly changing patient needs, the technology available, or the education and experience of the staff. Two other avenues that states have taken are, first, to require hospitals to have a nurse-driven staffing committee whose responsibility it is to create staffing plans based on the needs of the patient population and to match these needs with the skill and expertise of the staff, and second, to require hospitals to disclose their staffing levels to the public and/or a regulatory body (American Nurses Association, 2012).

Many hospitals use the **nursing hours per patient day (NHPPD)** method of staffing. This method takes into consideration patient acuity and nursing skill mix to calculate the amount of time nurses spend with each patient each day. Generally the nursing skill mix includes RNs, LPNs (or LVNs), and aides. Both the RNs and LPNs have scopes of practice that are regulated by the board of nursing in the state in which they are licensed to work, and each nurse must work within that scope of practice. The RN has the greatest scope, while the LPN must work under the supervision of an RN. It is the responsibility of the hospital to ensure that each licensed individual is working within his or her scope of practice when staffing individual units and making patient assignments. Failure to do so can result in citations for the hospital and sanctions to the individual nurse's license.

nursing hours per patient day (NHPPD)
A method for calculating the amount of time the various types of nurses must spend with each patient each day.

Traditionally nursing units have been staffed in three eight-hour shifts (day shift, evening shift, and night shift), with staff working every other weekend and every other holiday. Cyclical nursing shortages have demanded more creative staffing plans to attract nurses to the profession and to retain nurses who were already employed. Many hospitals have begun to offer ten- and twelve-hour shifts, weekend programs, job sharing, and "mother's hours." Twelve-hour shifts have become increasingly popular as they provide more days off and, in some cases, allow a nurse to actually work another full-time job. These longer shifts have come under greater scrutiny of late. In a study completed at the University of Pennsylvania School of Nursing on the relationship between nurse shift length and patients' assessment of care received, it was determined that when nurses worked shifts of ten hours or more, they were up to 2.7 times more likely to report burnout, up to 2.4 times more likely to report job dissatisfaction, and up to 2.8 times more likely to report an intention to leave their job within a year (Brown, 2012). On December 14, 2011, The Joint Commission (TJC) issued a Sentinel Event Alert titled "Health Care Worker Fatigue and Patient Safety." This alert calls on hospitals to do a self-evaluation to determine their risk for fatigue-related incidents that threaten patient safety and to put into place suggested evidence-based actions to mitigate these risks from the fatigue that can result from long work hours (TJC, 2011). Many states have overtime laws that mandate the circumstances under which direct patient caregivers can work overtime and the number of hours.

At the core of the nurse staffing issue is how nursing care is paid. The nursing department is not revenue producing; it is a cost center. In the early hospitals, unpaid nursing students provided most nursing care. Most hospitals used to have schools of nursing, which provided them with an endless pool of free labor. The graduates of these programs usually did not go to work in a hospital but were privately employed to take care of patients in the home. As technology advanced, regulations changed, and nursing programs transitioned from the hospital diploma model to university-based baccalaureate programs, the free labor market dried up. Hospitals then had to staff their facilities with paid nursing staff. This cost for providing nursing care was then lumped in with "room and board." Interestingly, it is said that room and board charges were originally made to be similar to hotel room charges, so that people would have some frame of reference, even though the services provided were not at all similar (Welton, 2007)! Today, room and board charges vary in a hospital depending on the type of patient unit. Intensive care or specialty units charge more per day for room and board than a general medical surgical unit does, but the charge within any particular unit does not vary with the intensity of care required by the patient. For example, a patient who is newly transferred out of an intensive care unit to a general medical or surgical floor will generally need more care than a patient who is being discharged to home the next day. The newly transferred patient may need an RN assigned to take care of him or her, as opposed to an LPN (this is where understanding the skill mix needed comes into play when staffing a unit). Using an RN rather than an LPN costs the hospital more, but there is no way for the hospital to recoup this cost in the standard room and board charge (Welton, 2007).

The average hospital patient today is also much sicker than in years past. With the advent of managed care in the 1990s, many procedures that had previously required a hospital stay were moved to the outpatient arena. Thus the patients who are admitted to the hospital are those who require more intense care. These inpatients are also staying in the hospital for shorter periods of time than formerly. It is reported that average hospital lengths of stay have decreased from seven to eight days in the 1980s to four to five days currently (Welton, 2007). With sicker patients and the need for more complex and intense care comes the need for more highly educated and skilled nurses. As the cost of staffing the nursing department has increased, and with no way to recoup any of those costs through charges, most hospitals have cut costs in other ways. This has usually been accomplished by decreasing the number of unlicensed staff, such as nurse's aides or people in nondirect patient care departments such as housekeeping. These reductions may save dollars on the balance sheet, but they increase the workload on the nurse at the bedside.

So what is the best ratio of nurses to patients? Research suggests the least expensive is 1:8 (one RN per eight patients), but this 1:8 ratio has also been associated with the highest patient mortality rate. Each decrease in the ratio increases the nurse labor cost per patient and decreases overall mortality. It has been estimated that the cost associated with saving one life by changing from a 1:8 to a 1:7 ratio is $46,000. If the ratio is changed to four patients per nurse, the cost is $142,000 per life saved (Rothberg, Abraham, Lindenauer, & Rose, 2005). This is something that must be looked at very carefully by the organizational leadership. The immediate financial benefits must be weighed against the long-term benefits in patient outcomes.

Horizontal and Vertical Integration

According to the Pan American Health Organization (2008), **horizontal integration** is "the coordination of activities across operating units that are at the same stage in the process of delivering services." **Vertical integration** is "the coordination of services among operating units that are at different stages of the process of delivering patient services." How does this apply to health care, and why would a hospital want to become integrated? Health care organizations have been consolidating or integrating since the 1990s. Examples of horizontal integration include care organization mergers, strategic alliances between neighboring hospitals in order to form local networks, and formation of multihospital systems. Examples of vertical integration include hospitals' acquisition of physician practices, strategic alliances with physicians in physician-hospital organizations, and alliances with management service organizations.

horizontal integration
Coordination of activities across operating units at the same stage of the service delivery process.

vertical integration
Coordination of services among operating units at different stages of the service delivery process.

Horizontal integration and vertical integration result in a consolidation of services. Integrated delivery systems in health care produce horizontal and vertical combinations of providers (Kim, 2004). There is some disagreement among researchers as to whether or not integration of health care has a positive effect on their financial performance. According to Kim (2004), among hospitals with vertical integration, the revenue per discharge is significantly higher than it is for hospitals without any integration strategy. However, hospitals with only horizontal integration showed no significant difference in revenue when compared to hospitals without any integration strategy.

Vertical integration, as stated previously, is the merging of units that are at different stages or points in delivering services. Some of the reasons a hospital would consider vertical integration are to increase its efficiency, to form large patient and provider pools to diversify risk, to reduce the cost of payer contracting, to reach quality goals, to offer a seamless continuum of care, and to assume responsibility for the health status of local populations

(America's Essential Hospitals, Essential Hospitals Institute, 2013). For example, in order to achieve a degree of vertical integration, a hospital might seek to purchase physician practices. As a result, the physicians in these practices become salaried employees of the hospital. Many physicians view this as advantageous as they no longer have the burden of running an office as well as tending to patients, and they also can decrease their on-call time. The downside of this to some physicians is a loss of autonomy in the way they choose to practice. When physicians are employed by a hospital, it is easier for the hospital to require the physicians to follow certain best practices or protocols that have been adopted in order to achieve quality goals.

Vertical integration through the employment of physicians is also seen as a way to provide a continuum of care to patients. The **continuum of care** has been defined by Evashwick (2005) as "a client-oriented system composed of both services and integrating mechanisms that guides and tracks clients over time through a comprehensive array of health, mental health, and social services spanning all levels of intensity of care" (p. 4). In other words, it provides the patient with the right services, at the right time, and at the right level of care. Vertical integration should provide seamless access to services along the continuum.

Hospitals may have more private agendas in seeking to vertically integrate. As health care has become more competitive and more hospitals have vertically integrated, there is a fear of losing referral bases. Some hospitals have thought that they will be able to control referrals if they purchase primary care physician practices. Many also have held the view that a common operating infrastructure will result in economies of scale and scope. According to Burns and Pauly (2002), this has not been the case.

Despite some opinions and research suggesting vertical integrations have not been successful, the period between 1995 and 2007 saw the percentage of hospitals employing physicians grow from 17 percent to 35 percent (Mutti & Stensland, 2009). This increase in integration has not gone unnoticed by the federal government. The **Medicare Payment Advisory Commission (MedPAC)** is an independent agency established by Congress as part of the Balanced Budget Act of 1997. The commission has a statutory mandate to advise Congress on payments to private health plans participating in Medicare and to providers in Medicare's traditional fee-for-service program. MedPAC is also tasked with analyzing access to care, quality of care, and other issues affecting Medicare (MedPAC, 2012). MedPAC has viewed vertical and horizontal integration as leading to increased prices and increased costs for health care services. These increases may then increase pressure to raise Medicare rates because of the disparity between private and Medicare payments (Mutti & Stensland, 2009).

continuum of care
The comprehensive array of health, mental health, and social services available to patients over time and varied levels of care.

Medicare Payment Advisory Commission (MedPAC)
An independent federal agency that advises Congress on Medicare and Medicaid payments to providers, and also on care access and quality.

Horizontal integration, as previously stated, is the coordination of activities across operating units that are at the same stage in the process of delivering services. Increased efficiency, access, and utilization of economies of scale are the major goals in horizontal integration (Burns & Pauley, 2002). Horizontal integration results in multihospital systems or in mergers and strategic alliances between neighboring hospitals to form local networks (America's Essential Hospitals, Essential Hospitals Institute, 2013). According to MedPAC (2012) horizontal integration increases prices by at least 5 percent, which is thought to be the result of these integrated organizations' better negotiating leverage.

Research on the effects of integration on quality is mixed. Horizontal integration appears to decrease the quality of care, while vertically integrated hospitals are more likely to use care management processes and information technology (IT) to improve quality of care (Mutti & Stensland, 2009). Both types of integration seem to increase prices to insurance companies or patients.

Quality and Safety in Hospitals

It has been estimated that as many as 98,000 people die in U.S. hospitals each year as a result of medical errors that were preventable. According to the Institute of Medicine (IOM) (1999), a medical error is "the failure of a planned action to be completed as intended or the use of a wrong plan to achieve an aim." Errors that commonly occur in the course of providing health care are adverse drug events, improper transfusions, surgical injuries and wrong-site surgery, suicides, restraint-related injuries or deaths, falls, burns, pressure ulcers, and mistaken patient identities. High error rates with serious consequences are most likely to occur in intensive care units, operating rooms, and emergency departments (IOM, 1999). In addition to the cost in human lives, it is estimated that preventable medical errors cost between $17 billion and $29 billion per year nationwide (IOM, 1999). How do we change this?

In September 1999, the Quality of Health Care in America Committee of the Institute of Medicine published its first report, titled *To Err Is Human: Building a Safer Health System*. It set as a goal a reduction in errors of 50 percent over the next five years. One of the main conclusions of this report is that the majority of medical errors do not result from recklessness on the part of any one individual or group. Mistakes are more often a systems failure; the result of flawed processes and conditions that have set up a person or group to fail. The report points out that health systems must be designed to be safer and to make it harder for people to make an error. While health care workers still need to be vigilant and to be held responsible for their actions, the IOM report encourages health care organizations to create a *culture of safety* rather than one of finger-pointing and blame.

The 1999 IOM report recommends a four-tiered approach to achieve a better safety record:

1. Establish a national focus on creating leadership, research, tools, and protocols to enhance the knowledge base about safety. It is estimated that the health care industry is about a decade behind other high-risk industries in its attention to basic safety.

2. Identify and learn from errors by developing a nationwide, public, mandatory reporting system and by encouraging health care organizations and practitioners to develop and participate in voluntary reporting systems.

3. Raise performance standards and expectations for improvements in safety through the actions of oversight organizations, professional groups, and group purchasers of health care.

4. Implement safety systems in health care organizations to ensure safe practices at the delivery level. Organizations must develop a "culture of safety." This should be an explicit organizational goal.

culture of safety
An environment in which mistakes and near misses can be reported by employees without fear of retaliation.

Hospitals go to great lengths to create a **culture of safety** where employees are encouraged to report mistakes and near misses without fear of retaliation. When employees fear that they will face disciplinary action for a mistake made, they will rarely report it. This leads to an underreporting of errors and a false sense of security. When employees report errors, it is then the responsibility of the organization to investigate the mistake or near miss to determine what in the process likely caused the mistake. Was a multidose vial used when a single dose vial should have been available? Was the correct equipment available and in good working order? Depending on the seriousness of the event, a root cause analysis may be in order. The Joint Commission defines a **root cause analysis (RCA)** as a process for identifying basic or causal factor(s) underlying variation in performance, including the occurrence or possible occurrence of a sentinel event. The analysis results must then be carefully looked at and the processes fixed to ensure that the likelihood of the error occurring again is reduced.

root cause analysis (RCA)
A process for identifying basic or causal factor(s) underlying variation in performance.

When we are in the hospital, most of us believe we are in a safe place to be treated, recover from an illness or surgery, and then go home. However, a person is at greater risk of developing an infection while in the hospital than in the community. Hospitals and other health care facilities have become harbors for some of the worst pathogens in recent history, such as methicillin-resistant *Staphylococcus aureus* (MRSA), vancomycin-resistant enterococci (VRE), carbapenem-resistant Enterobacteriaceae (CRE), and *Clostridium difficile* (C. diff), to name a few. These infections may manifest themselves as, for example, bloodstream infections (BSIs), catheter-related urinary tract infections (CAUTIs), or ventilator-associated pneumonia (VAP). As of 2012, all three of these outcomes were placed on the Centers for Medicare & Medicaid Services list of *never events*. A **never event** (that is, one that should never occur) is an adverse event that is serious, preventable, and of concern to both the public and health care providers for the purpose of public accountability. Never events were first identified in the IOM's 1999 report *To Err Is Human*.

never event
A medical event that is both serious and preventable and thus should never occur.

While the day-to-day management of a hospital falls to the facility's leadership, regulatory agencies play a major role in how hospitals are managed and their quest for quality. The agency with the most authority is the CMS. Recent quality initiatives developed and implemented by both the CMS and The Joint Commission have had a great impact on hospitals and health care organizations. For example, for years hospitals were paid on a fee-for-service basis. Outcomes, be they good or bad, held no reward or consequence in terms of payment. That has changed. First with the introduction of the payment system involving DRGs, and then on October 8, 2008, when CMS announced that it would no longer pay for treatment required because of never events that happened to patients while hospitalized. These costs have now become each hospital's responsibility.

The Joint Commission (TJC), an independent, not-for-profit organization founded in 1951, is the predominant standards setting and accrediting body in health care. TJC accredits and certifies more than 20,500 health care organizations and programs in the United States (TJC, 2014). In order to attain and maintain TJC's Gold Seal of Approval, an organization must undergo an onsite survey by a Joint Commission survey team every three years. Depending on the size of the facility, the survey can last anywhere from three to five days, with a number of surveyors onsite. The survey process is intense, focusing on processes and patient outcomes as well as compliance with CMS regulations. In 2004, TJC began a transition to unannounced accreditation surveys. Before that time a health care facility would receive prior notice of the exact survey dates and the names of the surveyors who would be onsite. Facilities still have a "window" when TJC can be expected, based on the expiration date of the organization's accreditation certificate, but the exact dates remain unknown. The reason for changing to unannounced surveys was to avoid the "ramping up" that most facilities went through in the weeks just prior to the survey. TJC feels that health care organizations should be survey-ready every day, regardless of when the TJC team or any other survey team is expected.

The Joint Commission (TJC)
An independent, not-for-profit organization that is the predominant standards setting and accrediting body in health care.

Magnet Recognition Program

Magnet recognition is awarded to hospitals by the American Nurses Credentialing Center (ANCC) through its Magnet Recognition Program®. The ANCC is an independent, nonprofit organization that is a subsidiary of the American Nurses Association (ANA). The **Magnet Recognition Program**® recognizes health care organizations for quality patient care, nursing excellence, and innovations in professional nursing practice. It is the leading source of successful nursing practices and strategies worldwide. A hospital seeking to receive Magnet recognition is described as being on a Journey to Magnet as it develops the fourteen Forces of Magnetism.

The 1980s saw a significant nursing shortage. Many hospitals also had very high turnover rates, meaning that nurses hired did not stay in one hospital very long. While a certain amount of turnover is always expected, a high turnover rate can take a toll on staff morale and on the expertise of the staff, as well as add a financial burden. Each time a nurse resigns and has to be replaced, it costs a hospital between $22,000 and $64,000 (Jones & Gates, 2007). In 1983, the American Academy of Nursing Task Force on Nursing Practice in Hospitals conducted a study that looked at forty-one hospitals identified as having high nurse retention rates to determine what characteristics these hospitals had in common. These hospitals were not only able to retain the nurses they hired, but they were also able to fill any vacancies quickly. Filling vacancies quickly is also important because the longer a position is vacant, the longer overtime or agency staffing may have to be used to staff a unit. These forty-one hospitals were found to have fourteen characteristics in common that drew nurses to them. These fourteen characteristics later became known as the **Forces of Magnetism** (for the description of each characteristic, see ANCC, 2014):

1. Quality of Nursing Leadership
2. Organizational Structure
3. Management Style
4. Personnel Policies and Programs
5. Professional Models of Care
6. Quality of Care
7. Quality Improvement
8. Consultation and Resources
9. Autonomy
10. Community and the Health Care Organization

Magnet Recognition Program®
A program that recognizes health care organizations for quality patient care, nursing excellence, and innovations in progessional nursing practice.

Forces of Magnetism
The fourteen characteristics displayed by hospitals that retain nurses.

11. Nurses as Teachers

12. Image of Nursing

13. Interdisciplinary Relationships

14. Professional Development

In 1994, the American Nurses Credentialing Center gave the first Magnet recognition award to the University of Washington Medical Center in Seattle, Washington. As of 2011, 6.61 percent of the registered hospitals in the United States were Magnet accredited (ANCC, 2014). A number of benefits result from achieving Magnet status. Magnet status is awarded to a hospital's nursing department in recognition of nursing excellence. The original goal of Magnet was to improve the work environment of nurses, thereby improving nurses' satisfaction and increasing retention rates. The research is mixed on whether or not Magnet has been successful in achieving this goal, but even those whose research has not found success in this area agree it is the model that should be followed. According to the ANCC, the benefits of the Magnet designation are an increased ability to attract and retain top talent; improved patient care, safety, and satisfaction; the fostering of a collaborative culture; advanced nursing standards and practice; and the ability to grow business and achieve financial success. *US News and World Report* uses the Magnet Recognition Program as a competence indicator in assessing the hospitals that it ranks in order to report the best medical centers in the nation. The Leapfrog Hospital Survey automatically gives a hospital full credit for meeting Leapfrog's Safe Practice #9 (which addresses the nursing workforce), if that hospital has Magnet designation (ANCC, 2014).

In 2007, the ANCC developed a new model for the Magnet Recognition Program that organized the fourteen Forces of Magnetism into five model components. This new model focuses on measurement of outcomes and has streamlined the documentation process. The five components and the Forces of Magnetism they consist of are (ANCC, n.d.)

1. Transformational Leadership
   - Quality of Nursing Leadership
   - Management Style
2. Structural Empowerment
   - Organizational Structure
   - Personnel Policies and Procedures
   - Community and the Health Care Organization
   - Image of Nursing
   - Professional Development

3. Exemplary Professional Practice
   - Professional Models of Care
   - Consultation and Resources
   - Autonomy
   - Nurses as Teachers
   - Interdisciplinary Relationships

4. New Knowledge, Innovation and Improvements
   - Quality Improvement

5. Empirical Quality Results
   - Quality of Care

Journey to Magnet
The process of achieving Magnet recognition.

The process of achieving Magnet recognition is referred to as the **Journey to Magnet**. And a journey it truly is. The process is lengthy, the criteria specific, and there must be strong support from throughout the hospital for embarking on this journey. First and foremost, the decision to go on the Journey to Magnet must be fully supported by the nursing staff. It cannot be an idea that comes from the top down without buy-in or support from staff. If the staff members do not believe in the journey, it will fail.

There are strict criteria the hospital must first meet in order to even apply for Magnet designation. There must be a chief nursing officer (CNO) who oversees and is responsible for nursing in the organization. The Magnet model is very focused on the educational preparation of nurses and nursing leaders within Magnet organizations. The CNO must possess a master's degree and must serve on the organization's highest governing, decision-making, and strategic planning body. In addition, effective January 1, 2013, 100 percent of the nursing managers must have either a bachelor's or master's degree in nursing, as must any other nurse leaders who fall organizationally between the nurse manager and the CNO. The organization must also be in compliance with the requirements of all regulatory organizations, such as the Occupational Safety and Health Administration (OSHA), the Department of Health and Human Services (HHS), and the Department of Labor and the National Labor Relations Board (NLRB) as they relate to registered nurses in the workplace. The organization must collect *nurse-sensitive quality indicators* at the unit level, that is, indicators whose outcomes are directly affected by nursing care. These data must then be benchmarked at the highest and broadest level possible in order to support research and quality improvement initiatives. There is also a lengthy document to be written and submitted that shows how the organization integrates each of the Forces of Magnetism. All documentation and data submitted must come from the two-year period prior to submission. Once the documentation is submitted and accepted, a team of Magnet surveyors completes an onsite visit to validate the documentation. If all goes well, Magnet recognition is awarded for a four-year period. During this four-year period the organization must continuosly collect and submit data in order to stay in compliance and be prepared for redesignation (ANCC, 2014).

Preparing for and maintaining the Magnet designation is a tremendous undertaking, and it demands that the organization be dedicated to providing the manpower and finances to achieve this status. The average health care organization spends approximately 4.25 years on its initial Magnet journey. Initially, it conducts a gap analysis to identify areas that need attention. Keeping staff engaged over this period of time can be a challenge. If the nursing department does not already have a shared governance structure, this must be initiated. Financially, it has been reported that the annual cost of the journey to Magnet designation can be anywhere from $100,000 to $600,000, depending on the size of the organization. So why, with health care organizations being so financially strapped, would they want to undertake this project? Because the benefits both financially and in terms of quality are so great. Remember that the initial study that led to the Magnet Recognition Program looked at increased nurse retention rates, decreased turnover, and increased nurse satisfaction. According to the Studer Group (a consulting organization), every 1 percent decrease in turnover translates to a direct cost savings of $250,000 and indirect cost savings of $500,000. Magnet hospitals generally have better patient outcomes, which leads to a decreased average length of stay and fewer adverse or never events, outcomes that also affect the organization's balance sheet (Russell, 2010).

Challenges and the Future

Hospitals have evolved from cots in monasteries and almshouses with patients being tended by members of religious orders to vast bastions of technology. They have gone from places where the only comfort to be offered was food and relief of pain and discomfort to places of hope and the reality of being cured of disease. The journey has not been an easy one, and hospitals will continue to face many challenges in the future. Decreased reimbursement and the Affordable Care Act, an aging population and aging workforce, consumer-driven health care plans, and competition for physicians are just a few of these challenges. The health care industry faces pressure to increase efficiency, improve quality and overall performance, and remain compliant with government mandates. Many hospitals are looking toward increased automation and electronic systems to aid in this endeavor; others are streamlining services as ways to work smarter. Where will it all lead? What will hospitals look like ten or twenty years from now?

They will probably be very different from the hospitals we know today. Regardless, the goals will always be the same: to continue to improve patient outcomes and provide the best care possible.

SUMMARY

From the convents and monasteries of early religious communities in Europe to the ultramodern, state-of-the-art bastions of technology we know today, hospitals have undergone enormous change. Once a place where only the poor and infirm were treated, hospitals are now the place where all seek care and treatment. Early hospitals were not-for-profit organizations and were financed primarily through charitable contributions. The advent of modern medicine and technology and an increased demand for services have made health care one of the largest industries in the United States and also one of the most highly regulated. The introduction of the federal Medicare program in the 1960s has been a major factor in the increase in government oversight. In addition to government oversight many private organizations, such as The Joint Commission and the Leapfrog Group, have arisen to ensure public safety and monitor quality outcomes.

Finances and reimbursement are currently, and will be for the foreseeable future, the major concern for health care organizations. Reductions in Medicare reimbursement and changes included in the Affordable Care Act will influence how health care is delivered and paid for in years to come. In this rapidly changing industry one thing never changes—the need for competent and accessible quality care.

KEY TERMS

Centers for Medicare & Medicaid
    Services (CMS)

committee of the whole

conditions for coverage (CfCs)

conditions of participation (CoPs)

continuum of care

councilor model

culture of safety

diagnosis related group (DRG)

Forces of Magnetism

governing board

Hill-Burton Act

horizontal integration

The Joint Commission (TJC)

Journey to Magnet

Magnet Recognition Program®

mandatory staffing ratios

Medicaid

medical executive committee (MEC)

medical staff bylaws

Medicare

Medicare Payment Advisory
Commission (MedPAC)

never event

not-for-profit organizations

nursing hours per patient day
(NHPPD)

patient acuity

patient care department managers

root cause analysis (RCA)

shared governance

vertical integration

DISCUSSION QUESTIONS

1. How would you describe the governance structure of a typical hospital?

2. What are the advantages of vertical integration and of horizontal integration, including the expected effect on financial performance?

3. What effects has the introduction of the Centers for Medicare & Medicaid Services had on health care?

4. What is the Journey to Magnet, and why is it beneficial for an organization?

5. What are mandatory staffing ratios, and are they beneficial? Why or why not?

REFERENCES

Alichnie, C. (2012). The cost of nursing. *Pennsylvania Nurse, 67*(4), 3, 23–24.

American Association of Colleges of Nursing. (2011). *Nursing fact sheet*. Retrieved from http://www.aacn.nche.edu/media-relations/fact-sheets/nursing-fact -sheet

American Medical Association. (2009). *Physician's guide to medical staff organiza- tion bylaws* (4th ed.). Chicago, IL: Author.

American Nurses Association. (2012). Nurse staffing plans and ratios. Retrieved from http://www.nursingworld.org/MainMenuCategories/Policy-Advocacy /State/Legislative-Agenda-Reports/State-staffingPlansRatios

American Nurses Credentialing Center. (2014). Forces of Magnetism. http://www .nursecredentialing.org/Magnet/ProgramOverview/HistoryoftheMagnet Program/ForcesofMagnetism

American Nurses Credentialing Center. (n.d.). Magnet Recognition Program model. Retrieved from http://nursecredentialing.org/Magnet/ProgramOverview /New-Magnet-Model

America's Essential Hospitals. (n.d.). History of public hospitals in the United States. Retrieved from http://essentialhospitals.org/about-americas-essential -hospitals/history-of-public-hospitals-in-the-united-states

America's Essential Hospitals, Essential Hospitals Institute. (2013). Types of integration. Retrieved from http://66.101.198.47/Share/Research/Integrated -Health-Care/Types-of-Integration.aspx

Anthony, M. K. (2004). Shared governance models: The theory, practice, and evidence. *Online Journal of Issues in Nursing, 9*(1), manuscript 4. Retrieved from http://www.nursingworld.org/MainMenuCategories/ANAMarketplace /ANAPeriodicals/OJIN/TableofContents/Volume92004/No1Jan04/Shared GovernanceModels.html

Barden, A. M., Griffin, M. T. Q., Donahue, M., & Fitzpatrick, J. J. (2011). Shared governance and empowerment in registered nurses working in a hospital setting. *Nursing Administration Quarterly, 35*(3), 212–218.

Brown, T. (2012, November 8). Nurses and patients both suffer from longer nursing shifts. *Medscape Medical News.* Retrieved from http://www.medscape.com /viewarticle/774191

Burns, L. R., & Pauly, M. V. (2002). Integrated delivery network: A detour on the road to integrated health care? *Health Affairs, 21*(4), 128–143. Retrieved from http://content.healthaffairs.org/content/21/4/128.full.html

California Department of Public Health. (2014). Nurse-to-patient staffing ratio regulations. Retrieved from http://www.cdph.ca.gov/services/DPOPP/regs /Documents/R-37-01_Regulation_Text.pdf

Centers for Medicare & Medicaid Services. (2013). Conditions for coverage (CfCs) and conditions of participation (CoPs). Retrieved from http://www .cms.gov/Regulations-and-Guidance/legislation/CFCsAndCops/index.html

City of New York. (2013). Bellevue: About Bellevue: Facts. Retrieved from http://www.nyc.gov/html/hhc/bellevue/html/about/facts.shtml

Cutter, J. B. (1922). Early hospital history in the United States. *California State Journal of Medicine, 20*(8), 272–274.

Domrose, C. (2012, November 12). History lesson: Nursing has evolved over the decades. *Nurse.com.* Retrieved from http://news.nurse.com/article/20121112 /HL02/311120010

Electronic Code of Federal Regulations, Title 42 [Public Health], Chapter IV, http://www.ecfr.gov/cgi-bin/text-idx?SID=b725a13be55b4e2ccb5421932e257 163&tpl=/ecfrbrowse/Title42/42tab_02.tpl

Evashwick, C. J. (2005). *The continuum of long-term care* (3rd ed.). Retrieved from https://www.nelsonbrain.com/content/evashwick96375_1401896375_02.01 _chapter01.pdf

Feigenbaum, E. (2012). Organizational structure of hospitals. *Houston Chronicle.* Retrieved from http://smallbusiness.chron.com/organizational-structure -hospitals-3811.html

Goldin, G., National Library of Medicine, & National Institutes of Health. (1984). *Historic hospitals of Europe, 1200-1981: An exhibit of photographs by Grace Goldin.* Retrieved from https://archive.org/details/101237629.nlm.nih.gov

Health Resources and Services Administration. (2012). Hill-Burton free and reduced coast health care. Retrieved from http://www.hrsa.gov/gethealthcare /affordable/hillburton

Hendren, R. (2011, May 31). *Boost nurse responsibility with shared governance.* HealthLeaders Media. Retrieved from http://www.healthleadersmedia.com /page-1/NRS-266757/Boost-Nurse-Responsibility-with-Shared-Governance

Institute of Medicine. (1999). *To err is human: Building a safer health system.* Retrieved from http://www.iom.edu/~/media/Files/Report%20Files/1999/To-Err-is-Human/To%20Err%20is%20Human%201999%20%20report%20brief.pdf

The Joint Commission. (2011, December 24). Health care worker fatigue and patient safety. Sentinel Event Alert Issue 48. Retrieved from http://www.joint commission.org/sea_issue_48

The Joint Commission. (2014). About The Joint Commission. Retrieved from http://www.jointcommission.org/about_us/about_the_joint_commission _main.aspx

Jones, C. B., & Gates, M. (2007). The costs and benefits of nurse turnover: A business case for nurse retention. *Online Journal of Issues in Nursing, 12*(3). Retrieved from http://www.nursingworld.org/mainmenucategories/anamarketplace /anaperiodicals/ojin/tableofcontents/volume122007/no3sept07/nurse retention.aspx

Kim, Y. K. (2004). *The influence of vertical integration and horizontal integration on hospital financial performance.* Paper presented at the 9th Asia-Pacific Decision Sciences Institute Conference. Retrieved from http://iceb.nccu.edu.tw /proceedings/APDSI/2004/pdf/078.pdf

Medicare Payment Advisory Commission. (2012). About MedPAC. Retrieved from http://www.medpac.gov/about.cfm

Moore, J. D., & Smith, D. G. (2005–2006). Legislating Medicaid: Considering Medicaid and its origins. *Health Care Finance Review, 27*(2), 45–52. Retrieved from https://www.cms.gov/Research-Statistics-Data-and-Systems/Research /HealthCareFinancingReview/downloads/05-06Winpg45.pdf

Mutti, A., & Stensland, J. (2009, October 9). *Provider consolidation and prices* [Slide presentation]. Retrieved from http://www.medpac.gov/transcripts/Provider _consolidation_and_prices1.pdf

National Bipartisan Commission on the Future of Medicare. (2012). *Medicare from the start to today.* Retrieved from http://rs9.loc.gov/medicare/history.htm

Pan American Health Organization. (2008). *Integrated delivery networks: Concepts, policy options and road map for implementation in the Americas. Renewing primary health care in the Americas* series. Retrieved from http://www.paho.org /sur/index.php?option=com_docman&task=doc_view&gid=88&Itemid=

Rothberg, M. B., Abraham, I., Lindenauer, P. K., & Rose, D. N. (2005). Improving nurse-to-patient staffing ratios as a cost-effective safety intervention. *Medical Care 43*(8), 785–791. Retrieved from http://vwvw.massnurses.org/files/file /Legislation-and-Politics/Cost_Effectiveness_Study.pdf

Russell, J. (2010). Journey to Magnet: Cost vs. benefits. *Nursing Economic$, 28*(5), 340–342. Retrieved from http://www.medscape.com/viewarticle/735385

Sullivan, E. J., & Decker, P. J. (2004). Handling collective bargaining issues. In *Effective leadership and management in nursing* (6th ed.). Upper Saddle River, NJ: Pearson Prentice Hall.

Wall, B. M. (2012). History of hospitals. In University of Pennsylvania School of Nursing, *Nursing history & health care*. Retrieved from http://www.nursing .upenn.edu/nhhc/Pages/History%20of%20Hospitals.aspx

Welton, J. M., (2007). Mandatory hospital nurse to patient staffing ratios: Time to take a different approach. *Online Journal of Issues in Nursing, 12*(3). Retrieved from http://gm6.nursingworld.org/MainMenuCategories/ANAMarketplace /ANAPeriodicals/OJIN/TableofContents/Volume122007/No3Sept07 /MandatoryNursetoPatientRatios.aspx

CHAPTER 5

AMBULATORY CARE SERVICES

Tina Marie Evans

This chapter explores the current information on the vast array of health care diagnostic and treatment services provided in U.S. communities to outpatients. In particular, it discusses **ambulatory care**, which allows a patient to receive personal health care consultation and treatment, surgery, or other interventional services using advanced medical technology on a strictly *outpatient* basis (meaning that the duration of care from the time of registration to discharge from the facility is contained within a single calendar day, without overnight accommodations). Ambulatory care is quickly emerging as the fastest growing segment of the U.S. health care market, and this trend toward providing health care services in the less expensive outpatient settings, as opposed to providing hospital-based services to inpatients, is predicted to continue steadily in the coming years. The number of existing ambulatory care centers in the United States increases each year, and the types of services provided in these outpatient centers grow more numerous and diverse as well. New and innovative technologies have made ambulatory care not only a popular and growing choice but also a setting where outpatients can receive needed care in a more convenient and less expensive way.

The National Ambulatory Medical Care Survey (NAMCS) defines an ambulatory care patient as "an individual presenting for personal health services who is neither bedridden nor currently admitted to any health care institution" (Fiebach, Kern, Thomas, & Ziegelstein, 2007, p. 3). The focus in ambulatory care settings is mostly on short-term medical consultation, diagnostics, and treatment. These facilities are designed to serve the needs of acute

LEARNING OBJECTIVES

After reading this chapter you should be able to

- Understand the reasons for the rapid expansion of ambulatory care settings.

- Name some of the most common diagnosis groups that lead patients to visit ambulatory care providers.

- Explain the advantages and disadvantages of receiving care in outpatient settings rather than inpatient settings.

- Explain the advantages and disadvantages of receiving a surgical procedure in an ambulatory surgery center rather than an inpatient hospital.

- Describe the services that home health agencies provide.

- Explain the philosophy behind hospice care, the indications for that care, and the common services available to hospice patients.

- Discuss the various types of accreditation services available for ambulatory care centers.

ambulatory care
Personal health care consultation, treatment, surgery, or other health care services provided on an outpatient basis.

care patients as well as the needs of those with chronic yet medically stable conditions that can be managed with long-term outpatient care. An extremely broad and diverse range of services can now be provided in the ambulatory care settings—services that range from routine medical examinations, dental care, and diagnostic testing to simple surgeries, acute injury consultations, and chemotherapy. As technology continues to advance and pressure on reimbursement grows, it is becoming more and more possible as well as financially advantageous to perform diagnostic and interventional procedures (including an impressive array of minor surgical procedures) in the outpatient setting. Ambulatory care settings are numerous and diverse. Here are some examples:

Ambulatory Care Settings

- Solo physician practices
- Group physician practices
- Hospital emergency departments
- Centers for same-day surgery
- Diagnostic imaging centers
- Endoscopy centers
- Hospital-based outpatient clinics
- Community health clinics
- Physical and occupational therapy clinics
- Home health care services (nursing, therapy, hospice, spiritual counseling)
- School health services
- College and university health centers
- Prison health services
- Family planning clinics
- Women's health care centers
- Childbirth centers
- Renal dialysis centers
- Oncology centers
- Lithotripsy centers
- Cosmetic surgery centers
- Migrant health centers
- Veterans' health system and military health services

- Industrial clinics
- Vision services
- Hearing services
- Dental services
- Medical laboratories
- Mental health services
- Poison control centers
- Community-sponsored hotlines
- Telephone and email communications with health care providers

History of Ambulatory Care Services

Let's review how the ambulatory care settings came into existence, and grew into what they are today. Long before the advent of hospitals and hospital-based care, most health care services were provided in what we now define as ambulatory care settings. In the early 1900s, much of the medical care in the United States was provided either by solo medical practitioners who worked in privately owned offices or by physicians who traveled to provide care in their patients' homes. At that time some physicians chose to locate their offices in their own homes or in small office buildings, as opposed to today's large medical office buildings and medical clinics. The limited amount of technology used in the past allowed physicians to easily pack their supplies and travel from patient to patient.

Home care was not only common but also very popular at that time—especially among wealthier patients, who could afford to request house calls to obtain their needed care. Physicians often visited homes via horse and buggy, and the time spent in travel between patients seriously limited the number of patients that one provider could visit in a single day. For the poor and indigent patients of that time, the scenario was much different. They did not have the benefit of affording home care or private physician care; rather, they sought care at community health care clinics that were established specifically to serve their needs. Their health care—when care was available—was usually limited to such public and philanthropic clinics (Williams & Torrens, 2008).

Sultz and Young (2009) describe the steady development since the nineteenth century of outpatient clinics owned by acute care hospitals, especially in urban settings where indigent populations did not have access to private medical services. Once the growth of not-for-profit hospitals began in the early twentieth century, outpatient clinics became a means for the hospitals to fulfill part of their charitable mission to serve the indigent populations who needed better access to private medical care. The number of hospitals grew quickly at that time as sanitation increased, hospital infections decreased, and antiseptic surgery began to be practiced (Raffel & Barsukiewicz, 2002).

By 1916, 495 hospitals had opened ambulatory outpatient clinics (Roemer, 1981). These hospital outpatient clinics also became popular settings for teaching and training young physicians, who commonly agreed to staff the ambulatory clinics in return for hospital admitting privileges. The image of the time was that the outpatient clinics were the "stepchild" of the acute care hospitals and that the patients there were given low priority. The staff at these clinics were almost exclusively young professionals in training, reinforcing this inferiority. J. H. Knowles, the director of Massachusetts General Hospital during this time, wrote: "Turning to the outpatient department of the urban hospital, we find the stepchild of the institution. Traditionally, this has been the least popular area in which to work, and as a result, few advances in medical care and teaching have been harvested here for the benefit of the community" (Knowles, 1965, p. 68). In the early 1900s, hospital outpatient clinics were busy helping with a wide variety of complex medical and social problems among their mostly indigent patients. It was common to see poor levels of compliance with recommended treatment regimens and serious discontinuities in care—with serious improvement in the chain of care needed.

As cars became popular and other types of transportation also improved after World War II, travel became much easier for physicians, and some patients were able to travel to physicians' offices as well (Raffel & Barsukiewicz, 2002). Advances in medical knowledge and the expansion of medical technology allowed some dramatic changes to begin to take hold. Hospitals expanded and diversified their services in the 1970s and 1980s to accommodate the demand linked to the increase in Medicare, Medicaid, and privately insured patients, which led hospital bills to rise. It did not take the third-party payers long to figure out that it would be less costly to test, diagnose, and treat patients as outpatients instead of admitted inpatients—which shifted the emphasis from inpatient-based care to outpatient-based care. Many medical centers responded to this shift by increasing their ambulatory care service offerings and expanding their outpatient care departments. Groups of medical providers also began organizing and going into business at satellite locations (i.e., locations outside hospital property), setting up new outpatient facilities in local shopping centers and in freestanding medical clinics. This move allowed them to offer services at a lower cost than the hospitals charged and in settings that were more convenient for patients to access (Gottfried, 2008).

During the 1980s, the status of hospital outpatient clinics also changed in a dramatic way. The "stepchild" image had all but disappeared, and the outpatient clinics began to earn recognition as vital portions of the U.S. health care system—portions that were a source of inpatient admissions and of a solid revenue stream from the use of hospital ancillary services. The earnings of outpatient clinics were only approximately 13 percent of total hospital revenues in the year 1980, but that number increased dramatically throughout the decade and into the 1990s to 35.2 percent of total hospital revenues. Once a setting that was used only for young physicians and medical students who needed to refine their skills, outpatient clinics now became well organized and staffed by private physician groups who transformed the ambulatory settings into well-equipped, aesthetically pleasing locations for competent medical care that emphasized excellence in customer service (Sultz & Young, 2009).

The 1990s continued to be a period of growth in both the number of ambulatory care centers and also in the types of care services that were offered. Some ambulatory settings have continued to be general practice clinics, and some (such as cancer care centers and endocrinology clinics) have evolved to meet the needs of patients who have specialized medical requirements. Many facilities have now expanded to offer outpatient chemotherapy, diagnostic imaging, dialysis, pain management services, physical therapy, cardiac rehabilitation programs, outpatient same-day surgery, occupational therapy, women's health care, and wound care services (Sultz & Young, 2009). These specialty outpatient clinics have been attractive to private physicians and to researchers because they draw a narrow clientele with common needs. These clinics then have the opportunity to truly advance the knowledge and care in their specialty areas, and their patients benefit from having access to the highly trained professionals who have researched and developed innovative ways to diagnose and care for the patients' conditions.

Centers for Disease Control and Prevention (CDC) data published in 2011 show that from the years 1997 to 2007 (Figure 5.1), the number of ambulatory care visits continued to grow by 25 percent (Schappert & Rechtsteiner, 2011). Sultz and Young (2009) also recently noted that ambulatory care is now the predominant mode of health care delivery in the United States. Hospital outpatient clinics, especially those located in urban areas, continue to function as the community's safety net for poor and marginalized populations. Regardless of the type of patient to be served, the historical growth and professional development of physicians, the technological advances in medical equipment, and the advent of specialty clinics allow patients of all means and conditions the potential for excellent medical care in outpatient settings.

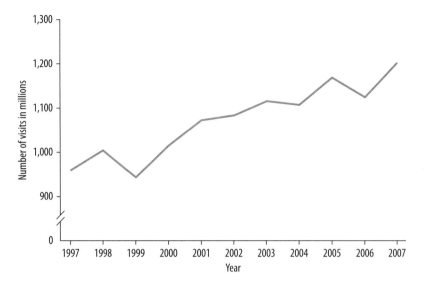

Figure 5.1   Annual Number of Ambulatory Care Visits: United States, 1997–2007

Source: Schappert & Rechtsteiner, 2011. Data from CDC, National Center for Health Statistics; National Ambulatory Medical Care Survey; and National Hospital Ambulatory Medical Care Survey.

Reasons for the Expansion of Ambulatory Care

One of the primary reasons for the shift from the traditional inpatient setting to the outpatient ambulatory setting has been the rising cost of medical care in the United States and the consequent attempts to control and also lower these costs. A role for government mandates in lowering costs became clear in the 1980s when prospective hospital reimbursement replaced retrospective payment on a national level with the introduction of Medicare's **diagnosis related group (DRG)** payment system. This new system offered financial incentives to those institutions that decreased the duration of inpatient care stays and also raised the efficiency level of the services being provided. In response to this, many hospitals (and also many groups of medical care providers) began to migrate their services to the outpatient setting, where types of care similar to inpatient care could be provided in a less expensive yet safe manner (Sultz & Young, 2009). In many cases it was found that the costs of receiving care in outpatient ambulatory settings were indeed lower than the costs incurred by patients who had the same procedure or treatment in an inpatient hospital setting. This outpatient cost savings (which is in part related to the lower overhead expenses of an outpatient center compared to a traditional hospital) holds benefits for both patients and the insurance companies or other payers. The elimination of some overnight hospital stays not only lowers the financial

diagnosis related group (DRG)
A classification system, based on ICD diagnoses and procedures, for paying specific amounts for treatment of specific diagnoses.

burden on the payers, but it also allows patients to return to their home environments and their usual life commitments and activities sooner.

New technologies that support diagnostic and interventional medicine also play a central role in the growing popularity of outpatient care. Even ten years ago, many surgical procedures required hospital care on one or more days, but now many of the same procedures can readily be handled in the ambulatory setting. Innovative advances in equipment, pharmacology, and anesthesiology have made it possible for minor surgery patients to receive their procedures on a same-day outpatient basis, with a low risk of complications. Instead of the traditional overnight (if not two- or three-day) stay in the hospital, ambulatory care is now viewed as an ideal and often preferred setting for patients who require minor surgical procedures that do not involve prolonged anesthesia or extended observation. Examples of such procedures are laser eye surgery, colonoscopies, certain plastic surgery cases, some gynecological procedures, and minor orthopedic surgeries. In addition to the technological advances that have greatly expanded the list of diagnostic and interventional procedures available outside the hospital setting, advances in care have also made these outpatient options both safe and effective—with a respectable level of quality.

Another important reason for the expansion of ambulatory care lies in the fact that compared with the traditional hospital care settings, ambulatory care locations are generally more convenient to access and use. Sultz and Young (2009) describe the 1980s and 1990s as a period of increasing consumer demand for "conveniently located, easily accessible facilities and services—two factors frequently lacking on hospital campuses and the large building complexes associated with them" (p. 122). This is of particular concern in large urban settings, where inner-city congestion, traffic, and parking play a role in reducing accessibility. At most ambulatory facilities the appointment is scheduled in advance (with some walk-in care allowed), and the patient simply enters the front door of the center directly from the center's parking lot—which eliminates the need for the ill or injured patient to walk through a maze of hallways to reach the correct hospital department. More important, routine scheduled outpatient testing does not get rescheduled, or "bumped" due to higher priority emergency diagnostic evaluations, as is sometimes necessary in the traditional hospital setting. And from the hospital's point of view, the availability of outpatient ambulatory care serves to free up hospital resources for the more critical cases that require the immediate attention of highly trained medical personnel and quick access to diagnostic or interventional medical equipment.

Time is also a central factor in the demand for ambulatory services, as ambulatory care clinics usually have operating hours that extend well beyond the typical nine to five schedule—frequently offering evening, weekend, and even holiday hours to accommodate patients' needs. Additional conveniences include shorter waiting times and greater privacy during the visit. Hospital emergency departments triage and prioritize patients by the level of care needed in each case, and that priority ranking system determines how soon a physician will see each patient. Obviously, those with the most critical needs are seen first, which may cause patients who have less critical needs to wait a bit longer (or sometimes a lot longer). Ambulatory urgent care centers are a valid alternative source of medical care for patients with noncritical or non-life-threatening injuries or illnesses, as their waiting times are likely to be shorter in these settings.

Hospital-Based Ambulatory Care

Hospital outpatient departments are settings where patients can access ambulatory care for both emergency and nonemergency medical issues. Many hospitals operate one or more ambulatory clinics to offer walk-in **hospital-based care** that is separate from the traditional emergency department and that can handle nonemergency cases. Of course the hospital emergency department will also handle nonemergent cases, especially during the hours when the ambulatory clinics are not open. The emergency department of a hospital is considered an outpatient service setting of the hospital, since its patients are most often provided with care and then allowed to return home on the same day. This continues to be the most familiar and also the most appropriate setting for most of the acute and all of the life-threatening medical circumstances that may arise. However, there is great concern over the high numbers of patients who continue to inappropriately present at hospital emergency departments for care of noncritical issues or for follow-up care of routine illnesses. This practice slows the chain of care by increasing the number of cases that the emergency department must triage, and it is also a particularly expensive way to handle noncritical injuries and illnesses, which makes it a practice that payers are actively working to curb.

hospital-based care
Health care services provided in the hospital setting.

From 1999 to 2009, the number of visits to hospital emergency departments increased by 32 percent, from 102.8 million visits in 1999 to 136.1 visits in 2009 (McCaig & Burt, 2001; National Center for Health Statistics, 2009a). Those over age seventy-five are the most frequent visitors (by age category), and African American patients had higher visiting rates (about 61 per 100 persons) than did Caucasian patients (about 38 per 100 persons). The emergency department of a hospital continues to serve a wide variety of important functions, including care to the critically ill and injured, and it is also a setting that doubles as a well-equipped physician's office and that provides a vital source of patient admissions for the hospital (Jonas, 2003). Hospital emergency departments are well equipped to treat discrete incidences of illness and injury, but they are not a good setting in which to receive routine and nonemergent care. This care setting is much more expensive than nonhospital ambulatory settings because it consumes the time and skills of specialty medical personnel—regardless of the level of care actually needed by the patient. Moreover, as previously mentioned, waiting times to receive care for nonemergent issues are often long, as patients with life-threatening conditions are appropriately cared for first—often leaving the many patients with not-so-critical conditions to wait several hours before being attended to (Sultz & Young, 2009).

In some cases hospital emergency department personnel will refer patients with nonemergent or routine care conditions to a hospital out-patient clinic, thereby encouraging the patients to use a more appropriate setting for care and preserving the hospital's emergency resources for those who truly need such care. National Hospital Ambulatory Medical Care Survey data are very useful for tracking outpatient department utilization over the years. Table 5.1, for example, displays the twenty leading primary diagnosis groups for outpatient department visits in 2009.

Like other ambulatory clinics, those operated by hospitals may offer either general care or specialized care; for example, in children's services, oncology, or pain management. As discussed earlier, hospital clinic services were traditionally established to meet the needs of the community and also to provide teaching and research opportunities for physicians—which is why many hospital-based clinics tend to be organized around body systems (for example, dermatology, cardiology, or pulmonology) or specialties (for example, orthopedics or neurology). For patients these clinics provide excellent access to physician researchers who are skilled in particular areas of need—and who are especially interested in their conditions. For physicians these clinics offer access to a large number of patients with the conditions they find of particular interest (Sultz & Young, 2009).

Outpatient settings continue to expand, owing to the increased competition between hospitals and the decreasing reimbursement for inpatient hospital services. The push to have nonemergent and routine care cases handled in the more appropriate outpatient setting has led to an increase in the number of hospital-sponsored ambulatory care clinics. These clinics are also an excellent place for hospitals to attract middle-income patients, who are a good source of additional income for the hospital through their clinic visits and hospital admissions when necessary (Raffel & Barsukiewicz, 2002).

Table 5.1   Leading Primary Diagnosis Groups for Outpatient Department Visits: United States, 2009

Principal Reason for Visit and RVC Code[1]		Number of Visits in Thousands (standard error in thousands)		Percentage Distribution (standard error of percentage)	
All visits	—	96,132	(9,381)	100.0	—
Progress visit, not otherwise specified	T800	9,052	(1,420)	9.4	(1.2)
General medical examination	X100	5,762	(892)	6.0	(0.7)
Cough	S440	2,638	(423)	2.7	(0.3)
Counseling, not otherwise specified	T605	2,550	(400)	2.7	(0.3)
Prenatal examination, routine	X205	2,410	(546)	2.5	(0.5)
Medication, other and unspecified kinds	T115	2,282	(351)	2.4	(0.3)
Symptoms referable to throat	S455	1,773	(286)	1.8	(0.3)
Back symptoms	S905	1,,630	(327)	1.7	(0.3)
Postoperative visit	T205	1,593	(258)	1.7	(0.2)
Diabetes mellitus	D205	1,568	(440)	1.6	(0.4)
Fever	S010	1,341	(244)	1.4	(0.2)
Knee symptoms	S925	1,331	(303)	1.4	(0.3)
Earache or ear infection	S355	1,326	(217)	1.4	(0.2)
Stomach pain, cramps and spasms	S545	1,231	(185)	1.3	(0.1)
Well-baby examination	X105	1,198	(203)	1.2	(0.2)
Headache, pain in head	S210	1,091	(159)	1.1	(0.1)
Low back symptoms	S910	*1,078	(453)	*1.1	(0.5)
Hypertension	D510	1,078	(242)	1.1	(0.2)
Skin rash	S860	1,053	(181)	1.1	(0.2)
Gynecological examination	X225	1,032	(155)	1.1	(0.1)
All other reasons	—	53,115	(5,265)	55.3	(1.5)

Note: Numbers may not add to totals because of rounding; — = Category not applicable.
* Figure does not meet standards of reliability or precision.
[1] Based on *A Reason for Visit Classification* (RVC), defined in the 2009 National Hospital Ambulatory Medical Care Survey Public Use Data File Documentation. Reason for visit is defined by the patient.
Source: National Center for Health Statistics, 2009b.

Non-Hospital-Based Ambulatory Care

non-hospital-based care
Health care services provided in a variety of settings not directly affiliated with a hospital or a local or regional health care system.

The rapidly growing ambulatory care segment of health care also includes **non-hospital-based care**, which occurs in a variety of settings that are not directly affiliated with a hospital or a local or regional health care system of care; for example, schools, prisons, community clinics, vision clinics, dental clinics, and mental health clinics. Patients who choose to receive care in these ambulatory settings will enjoy the convenience of both scheduled and walk-in care, while the care is provided at a lower cost than hospital-based care.

It is also important to recognize community health centers' dedication to needs of underserved populations. These federally funded primary care centers are critical in providing targeted primary care services to "minorities, women of childbearing age, infants, persons with HIV/AIDS, substance abusers, and individuals and families who experience health service access barriers for any reason" (Sultz & Young, 2009, p. 146). Community health centers also provide important information about and links to other supportive programs for these populations—programs such as public assistance; Medicaid; the Women, Infants, and Children supplemental nutrition program; and the respective state-sponsored Children's Health Insurance Programs. It is now common for community centers to offer in-house laboratory testing, health education, and radiology and pharmacy services, as well as some transportation and translation services. Workers in the community health center outpatient setting are often trained not only to provide health care services, but also to serve as social service outreach workers who can competently perform needs assessments, advocate well for early interventions, and protect the continuity of medical care (Sultz & Young, 2009). Not all insurance policies cover vision, dental, and mental health services, and these aspects of care, even though they are a vital segment of any patient's health care, are sometimes overlooked. Some community health centers are beginning to fill the gap in these essential service areas.

Many educational institutions, from primary schools to universities, now provide some type of organized ambulatory health care to their students during school hours. Although at the primary and secondary school level most of this care is confined to addressing the basic needs of acutely ill and injured students, some schools provide routine vision and hearing screenings as well. Most college and university health clinics now go beyond this basic level of care to offer a higher level of general diagnostic service and treatment, including screening and referrals for mental health issues and substance abuse. Some primary and secondary school health care centers are run by the local board of education or in cooperation with the local health department (Jonas, 2003). Students who are seen by a school-based care provider are usually then referred to their personal primary care physician (or if the student has no personal physician, to a provider who is connected with the institution) for follow-up, additional monitoring, or interventional care.

Freestanding Emergency Centers and Urgent Care Centers

Another fast-growing segment of the ambulatory care market consists of freestanding emergency centers and urgent care centers or clinics. An

urgent care center

A walk-in clinic that provides outpatient medical care services.

urgent care center is a walk-in clinic that provides outpatient medical care when patients are unable to reach their primary care physicians or when they do not wish to visit the emergency department. According to the Urgent Care Association of America (UCAOA, 2011), there are currently over 8,700 urgent care centers in the Unites States, and this number increases by approximately 300 new centers per year (332 between 2008 and 2009, and 304 between 2009 and 2010). Freestanding urgent care centers see patients on a walk-in (no appointment necessary) basis, with extended hours access for the care of acute illnesses and injuries that are either beyond the scope or the availability of the typical primary care practice or storefront clinic. For urgent (but non-life-threatening) conditions, ambulatory urgent care has come to be known as a faster and possibly more convenient option than a visit to a traditional hospital emergency department. In many areas of the United States, urgent care centers are usually open twenty-four hours per day to provide consistent access for their communities.

It is critical to make the distinction that even though urgent care centers will provide a more extensive scope of services than retail clinics do, they are still not equal to the comprehensive level of care that is given at hospital emergency departments. True life-threatening medical conditions are still more appropriately treated at the hospital emergency department, where all hospital resources and necessary equipment are available, including quick access to interventional care by other medical specialists. Urgent care centers generally do not treat life-threatening conditions—so if a patient's condition is such that an ambulance is required, the hospital emergency department is probably the more appropriate place.

Typically, freestanding urgent care centers employ at least one physician and additional staff consisting of physician assistants, nurses, and other supportive medical professionals. The specific types of medical services provided vary by location and also by the level of training of the staff. From the managerial perspective, careful marketing will assist potential patients in understanding the types of care provided at certain locations. Such marketing may be especially important in an area where freestanding urgent care is a new option for the community. These centers are often built in high-visibility areas; they may be located in standalone buildings or in other storefronts or local shopping malls.

Regardless of their location, most urgent care centers provide routine medical examinations as well as basic diagnostic procedures and vaccinations, and can easily care for common medical needs such as minor lacerations, burns, flu, strep throat, and sinus infections. Diagnostic testing is also a common reason for patients to seek outpatient care at one of these centers. Technological advances have now made many forms of diagnostic testing available outside the hospital setting—magnetic resonance imaging, computed tomography scans, X-rays, electrocardio-grams, sonography, blood testing, mammograms, and biopsies are among these available methods. In contrast to walk-in emergency departments, some urgent care centers allow patients to make appointments for diagnostic services, and these centers are often outfitted with the most current, state-of-the-art equipment for diagnostic procedures. In addition to routine and diagnostic care, many centers also offer pharmacy services onsite, allowing the patient to have a one-stop shopping experience and thereby streamline the necessary care.

There is another key difference between traditional hospital emergency departments and the urgent care centers. Unlike hospital emergency departments, urgent care centers often require full payment at the time that services are provided (usually by cash, credit card, or check). Some urgent care centers will bill insurance for the patient, but in many cases patients are given copies of the documents that they must submit to their insurance carrier for reimbursement. Patient information should be available at the center about the treatments that insurance payers are likely or not likely to cover.

In our current competitive health care market, urgent care centers allow physicians and for-profit organizations a unique opportunity to compete with hospitals and office-based physicians for patients (Raffel & Barsukiewicz, 2002). They also provide a significant level of assistance in filling the gap between local retail clinics and hospital emergency departments—which is truly important for various reasons, including reserving the resources of emergency departments for the more critical and life-threatening injuries and illnesses.

The long waiting times in most emergency departments continue to be a concern for both health care managers and clinicians alike. Recent research by Hing and Bhuiya (2009) found that between 2003 and 2009, the mean waiting time in emergency departments in the United States had increased by 25 percent—from 46.5 minutes to 58.1 minutes. This study also provided important numbers regarding geographic variations in average hospital emergency department waiting times, which were found to be 62.4 minutes in urban areas, and 40.0 minutes in nonurban areas. These numbers can be compared to the finding of a recent study by the UCAOA (2011) that 57 percent of patients seeking care at ambulatory urgent care centers wait 15 minutes or less to be seen. This clearly illustrates the shorter waiting time urgent care center patients enjoy versus the likely longer wait time for those who either must or who choose to utilize traditional hospital emergency departments for urgent care.

More patients choosing an urgent care setting for non-life-threatening conditions may serve to free up the traditional hospital emergency departments and also to reduce the overall wait time for care in those departments, thereby allowing patients with emergency medical needs to be seen without delay. The consistent positive growth in the number of urgent care centers is a clear sign that patients see these centers as valid alternatives to visiting hospital emergency departments. In addition, for patients who do not have a personal primary care physician, urgent care centers provide an important safety net in times of need (Sultz & Young, 2009).

Retail Clinics

retail clinic
A basic care walk-in clinic located in a drugstore or other retail store.

The **retail clinic** came onto the ambulatory care scene in 2000 as an additional setting for outpatient health care. These clinics, typically located inside large retail stores such as Walgreens, Target, CVS, Rite Aid, and Walmart stores, offer a basic level of health care on a walk-in basis. Most often the care is provided by either physician assistants or nurse practitioners, who staff the clinic and routinely see both adult and pediatric patients who suffer from nonemergent illnesses. Colds, flus, and minor infections are common reasons for patients to seek care at a retail clinic. Others stop by to receive routine immunizations, especially patients who do not have a consistent relationship with a primary care physician.

Retail clinics have been successful in offering short waiting times without appointments being necessary, which has helped them to grow in popularity. The additional convenience of being able to shop for personal, grocery, and home care items in the same store where the retail clinic is located is also a plus for this care setting. In past years most retail clinic care was paid by the patient out of pocket; however, many large insurers, including Medicare and Medicaid, have now begun to offer covered benefits for retail clinic care. The convenience factor in combination with the relatively low cost and rising level of insurance coverage make this a setting that is highly likely to continue its growth trend in the upcoming years (Mehrotra, Wang, Lave, Adams, & McGlynn, 2008).

Ambulatory Surgery Centers

In every area of the United States, hospitals are experiencing an increase in the number of surgical patients who enter the hospital, receive surgical care, and go home on the same day. This shift toward outpatient surgical care began in the 1970s, and such care continues to be an option that is growing in popularity. In 1981, the American College of Surgeons began a process to approve freestanding ambulatory surgical centers. This further reinforced the shift toward ambulatory surgical care and the establishment of many more outpatient surgical centers in the United States. An additional reason for the quick growth of outpatient surgical centers in recent years is the demand by insurance companies as well as the government to provide patients with needed surgical care at a lower cost. Outpatient surgical centers have a financial advantage over the traditional hospital setting because they have lower overhead expenses than hospitals usually have (Raffel & Barsukiewicz, 2002). It is estimated that 70 percent of surgical procedures are now performed as ambulatory, or outpatient, surgeries (Sultz & Young, 2009), including many endoscopies, laser surgeries, biopsies, and arthroscopies.

For most patients, having a surgical procedure at an outpatient ambulatory surgical center is a choice, but in some cases it is a necessity. Some third-party payers now require that certain surgical procedures be completed on an outpatient basis. This requirement has in some cases significantly affected hospitals' utilization of beds and also the overall organizational design of hospitals. In addition, independent ambulatory surgical centers can now effectively compete with hospitals because Medicare is one of the third-party payers that will cover certain surgical procedures only when they are performed as outpatient procedures. It is also not uncommon to see ambulatory surgical centers affiliating directly with various HMOs and PPOs, which further increases the level of competition that the surgical centers have with hospitals for the same patient base. In response to this competition, some hospitals have chosen to open their own freestanding ambulatory surgical centers, have formally partnered with existing surgical centers, and/or have increased the effort and budgetary resources spent on marketing their own hospital-based surgical services (Raffel & Barsukiewicz, 2002).

Ambulatory surgical facilities may be owned by a hospital and operated as extensions of that hospital, or a surgeon or a group of surgeons may own them independently, sharing the expenses and profits. Depending on the geographic location and specialty of the surgical practitioners involved, much variation is currently seen in types of facility ownership. When surgeons open and operate a surgical center that is independent of a hospital, they incur start-up costs as well as the ongoing costs for staff wages; rental or lease of real estate (if they have not purchased real estate, a start-up cost); medical equipment; medical supplies; and insurance premiums for malpractice and liability. However, with reimbursement for outpatient surgical procedures growing at a respectable pace, many centers are profitable despite the high start-up costs and continuing expenses. Health care managers are enjoying this new employment prospect as well, because well-managed facilities become profitable quickly.

Regardless of the type of facility ownership, ambulatory surgery offers a few advantages over in-hospital surgical care. In addition to lower costs, patients have noted attractive surroundings, easy accessibility, and the opportunity to better customize the scheduling of care in the absence of hospital bureaucracy. Patients typically see these facilities as "far more user friendly and responsive to their needs than their hospital-based counterparts" (Sultz & Young, 2009, p. 144).

Most ambulatory surgical centers comply with their respective state's licensure, certification, and accreditation requirements. If a center serves Medicare beneficiaries (which most do), it must be Medicare certified on aspects of care involving patient safety and quality of surgical care. Although accreditation is currently voluntary, many centers also choose to undergo accreditation reviews by The Joint Commission (formerly known as the Joint Commission on Accreditation of Healthcare Organizations), the American Association for the Accreditation of Ambulatory Surgery Facilities, or the Accreditation Association for Ambulatory Health Care (Sultz & Young, 2009). It is currently expected that the trend toward moving as many surgical procedures to outpatient care as is safely possible will continue as technologies advance further and reimbursement pressures continue. There is also significant and realistic concern on the part of community hospitals, which are not connected or formally affiliated with freestanding ambulatory surgical centers, regarding the large portion of revenue that can and likely will be lost by the shift toward ambulatory surgery and away from inpatient surgical care.

Primary Care Management

Comprehensive primary care is the cornerstone for ensuring that patients receive optimal integration of all available medical services. Coordination of outpatient care by primary care physicians is critical for emphasizing preventive services, as prevention is a fundamental part of primary care. The advice of a primary care physician has been shown to have a positive influence on patients' behaviors, thereby not only helping individual patients enjoy a better state of health but also lessening the burden of disease that affects society and the health care system as a whole (Fiebach et al., 2007). Correctly applied primary care management also prevents "fragmentation of care and the hit-or-miss nature of patient self-referral to specialists and promotes comprehensive care, for the patient as a whole person, not merely a set of parts" (Jonas, 2003, p. 70). It is also believed that the level and quality of primary care provided (or lack thereof) is a clear indicator of the quality of the nation's health care delivery system altogether (Starfield, 1996).

The importance of proper primary care was recognized back in the 1960s, and emphasis was placed on revitalizing the role of the primary care physician in an attempt to raise the level of continuity of care and better address all needs of patients. The building of a trusting professional relationship between patient and physician was also emphasized as an essential part of primary care. This relationship that a patient optimally develops with his or her primary care physician allows the physician to develop a clearer understanding of the patient as well as his or her family. It also facilitates the physician's job of developing a plan for the patient's long-term health and wellness—a plan that recognizes the patient's physical, social, psychological, and spiritual dimensions.

Most visits that patients make to a physician's office or to a dental group are considered ambulatory care, including those for routine well adult and well child visits, sick visits, and consultations regarding specific signs and symptoms. Common preventive measures promoted by primary care physicians include personal lifestyle or behavioral changes, immunizations, prenatal screenings and services, and periodic physical examinations for the prevention or early diagnosis of various diseases. In the fast-paced, ambulatory primary care setting, other health care professionals commonly assist physicians, including nurse practitioners, advanced practice nurses, and physician assistants. Mundinger (2002) notes that these highly trained ancillary professionals can help to provide primary care services that are equal to those provided by physicians. Ambulatory care nursing has recently begun to evolve into an additional specialty area of the nursing profession to further support the needs of this popular outpatient setting. And nursing education programs are beginning to build didactic and clinical experiences into their curricula to ensure that future nursing graduates are proficient and well equipped to be successful in meeting the high-paced demands of the various ambulatory care settings.

Primary care physicians, whether in solo or group practice, still provide much of a patient's routine care today, but they also serve as a source of proper referrals to specialists in particular types of injuries and illnesses. Office-based physicians receive an estimated 787.4 million visits per year, or approximately three visits per person per year (Raffel & Barsukiewicz, 2002). These care providers are recognized as the ones who provide the majority of the important preventive care services, such as healthy lifestyle counseling, immunizations, and regular screening for illness detection (Raffel & Barsukiewicz, 2002). These services are all critical in allowing treatment interventions to take place before illnesses become more serious and also at a point when they are less costly to treat.

Home Health Care Services

Home health care services are provided to patients and families who need assistance with promoting, maintaining, or restoring a patient's health and level of independence and minimizing the consequences and effects of

home health care services
Services provided in the patient's home by traveling health care professionals.

hospitals without walls
Home health care agencies that bring care and medical technology to a patient's home.

injury, disability, and illness. Home health care agencies are often referred to as **hospitals without walls**, since technological advances allow them to pack the items needed for care and bring them into a patient's place of residence. Home care services can be used as either a form of long-term care and service provision for chronically ill persons (thereby avoiding institutionalization) or as a form of short-term care for those who have been discharged from hospitals following acute illness or surgery.

These formal, regulated programs of care offer a wide range of medical, therapeutic, and also nonmedical services that are provided by a variety of health care professionals and also social workers and nonmedical volunteers in a patient's home (Jones, Harris-Kojetin, & Valverde, 2012) and are usually coordinated by a nurse case manager. This effectively allows many patients who in the recent past would have been hospitalized for continuing care to return home and have needed services brought directly to them as they convalesce (Jonas, 2003). Nursing services are the most frequently used home health service, and this care is often critical in easing the transition from hospital to home. The duration and frequency of home visits is dependent on the level of a patient's needs and the orders of the patient's physician (Barnett & Mayer, 1992). In addition to basic medical and personal care assistance services, home health care personnel may be trained to perform specimen collection, radiographs, electrocardiograms, physical therapy, speech therapy, occupational therapy, mental health counseling, and social work services. In recent years home health agencies have begun employing nurse practitioners, enterostomal therapists, and clinical pharmacy consultants to provide more extended and sophisticated care. Advanced services such as intravenous therapies and ventilator support, which in the past were available only in an inpatient setting, may now take place in the comfort and familiar surroundings of the patient's home (Fiebach et al., 2007).

This sector of the health care industry enjoyed a great period of growth at the end of the twentieth century, as cost-effectiveness initiatives imposed by managed care organizations led many to explore home care services as a less costly alternative to inpatient nursing or hospital care. In many cases home care services can minimize the need for admission to acute care or long-term skilled nursing facilities. As of 2007, more than 1 million U.S. men and women aged sixty-five years and over were receiving home health care services each day. Currently over 20,000 home health care agencies exist in the United States, with over 80 percent of them operating on a for-profit basis and total expenditures on their services amounting to more than $34.5 billion per year (Jones et al., 2012).

Demographically, among individuals aged sixty-four to eighty-five, women had significantly higher rates of home care service utilization than

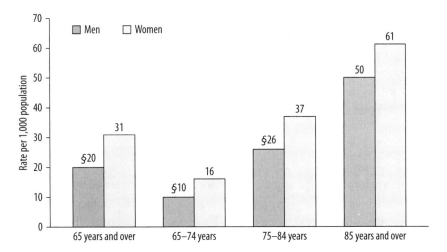

Figure 5.2 Rate of Receipt of Home Health Care per 1,000 Civilian Noninstitutionalized Population Aged Sixty-Five and over by Sex: United States, 2007

Note: § Statistically significant difference *p* < 0.05 by sex.

Source: Jones et al., 2012. Data from CDC, National Center for Health Statistics, National Home and Hospice Care Survey, 2007.

men (Figure 5.2). However, men over age sixty-five were more likely to receive skilled home health care services for wound care and physical therapy immediately after an inpatient stay, whereas women in that age group received homemaker services more frequently than men and were also found to require home health services for longer periods of time. Male patients over age sixty-five were found to be almost three times as likely as female patients of that age to have their spouse as their primary caregiver, whereas female patients in the same age group had a child or other nonspousal relative as their primary source of caregiving twice as often as the male patients did. Common services required by home health care patients aged sixty-five years and over include "skilled nursing services (84%), physical therapy (40%), assistance with activities of daily living (37%), homemaker services (17%), occupational therapy (14%), wound care (14%), and dietary counseling (14%)" (Jones et al., 2012).

Any patient or patient's family can purchase the services of a home health care agency, but most of the cost is typically covered by Medicare, Medicaid, or another third-party or managed care organization. Medicare remains the dominant payer for home care services, paying approximately 38 percent of the overall home health care expenditures annually (Sultz & Young, 2009). Ongoing cost-containment initiatives have led to stricter control of the amounts and types of services that are authorized for payment, and reimbursement for all services requires the approval of the patient's physician. Moreover, for this setting of care to be effective, consistent and thorough communication between the physician and the home health care workers is necessary (Fiebach et al., 2007). This care setting continues to be an integral part of the U.S. health care delivery system, providing an "effective, safe and humane alternative to institutional care for the medical treatment and personal care of individuals of all ages" (Sultz & Young, 2009, p. 303).

Hospice Services

hospice
A specialized approach to coordinating the care of terminally ill patients.

palliative care model
Health care that emphasizes controlling pain, lessening anxiety, and relieving symptoms rather than curative care.

Hospice is a specialized approach to coordinating the care of terminally ill patients. It works to improve patients' quality of life while supporting their various needs through the end of life. This specialized approach to delivering care is organized around an interdisciplinary team of professionals and other helpful volunteers. The hospice team commonly employs physicians, nurses, social workers, chaplains, therapists, and counselors. Instead of the traditional medical model of curative care used in the rest of the U.S. health care system, hospice employs the palliative care model. The **palliative care model** emphasizes controlling pain, lessening anxiety, and relieving symptoms rather than supplying curative care, in light of a patient's likely terminal condition. The goal of prolonging life is set aside, which allows care to focus on interventions that support and improve quality of life as defined and decided on by the patient and his or her family (Fiebach et al., 2007). Medical interventions during the final stages of a patient's life are often traumatic and invasive and typically also involve moving the patient from home to hospital or from nursing facility to hospital over and over and over. In many cases the result of this is unnecessary pain, discomfort, and stress on the dying patient, with no significant overall benefit to the patient's condition. The patient's overall well-being is at risk of being lost in the medical shuffle at a time when control of pain, reduction of stress, and ensuring peaceful surroundings should be the focus of care efforts (Matthews, 2010).

Outside the United States, hospice care began as a nonprofit, volunteer effort. Although several models of care for the dying exist, St. Christopher's Hospice in England is commonly recognized as the primary model that influenced hospice development in the United States. Another strong influence on the growth and development of hospice in this country was Elisabeth Kubler-Ross's book *On Death and Dying* (1969). This book, especially during the late 1960s and early 1970s, was particularly powerful in bringing attention to the experience of dying and the stages of dying, as it detailed those experiences for both terminally ill patients and their caregivers.

Since the introduction of the palliative model of care and the founding of the first hospice in the United States in 1974, hospice teams have provided care to many patients in their homes, in skilled nursing facilities, in hospitals, or in other residential hospice facilities. Despite the many care settings offered, the majority of hospice services continue to be supplied in the patient's home. This allows the continuation of familiar home surroundings of peace and comfort, while the necessary services are brought to the patient and are provided with dignity and respect. Family members and friends are usually encouraged to participate in supportive care if they are willing to do so (Wolper, 1999).

The different perspective used by hospice workers has challenged the traditional curative medical model by insisting that the personhood of a dying patient be recognized and not be lost in a maze of science and technology. Under this new model, palliative care and psychosocial support have grown in popularity, as many terminally ill patients and families are choosing supportive comfort care and opting to forego advanced medical interventions at the end of life. The palliative care model has challenged the traditional paternalistic role of the physician as well. Physicians on hospice teams must accept rather limited roles because they are serving as only one member of an interdisciplinary team bringing specialized care to the dying patient—care that at times delivers more spiritual and emotional guidance and support than actual medical care (Raffel & Barsukiewicz, 2002). The decision to "give up" on curative care can be very difficult for these physicians, and some have great difficulty in agreeing to stop treatments even when the odds of survival become extremely poor.

Hospice care providers are experiencing a steady rate of growth, of approximately 19 percent annually for agencies that are Medicare certified, with freestanding hospices being the fastest growing segment among the hospice care providers (Wolper, 1999). Data from the CDC's 2007 National Home and Hospice Care Survey reveal that the most common diagnoses of hospice care patients in that year were "malignant neoplasm (46.4%) . . . heart disease (32.2%), including congestive heart failure (15.4%); essential hypertension (23.5%); dementia (21.3%); . . . chronic obstructive pulmonary disease and allied conditions (14.8%); diabetes mellitus (12.2%); and cerebrovascular disease (10.9%)" (Caffrey, Sengupta, Moss, Harris-Kojetin, & Valverde, 2011, p. 7).

With the rapid growth of demand for hospice services, most third-party payers, including Medicare Part A, now provide hospice benefits. To qualify for hospice benefits under Medicare, a patient must meet the following criteria: "the patient must be terminally ill with a life expectancy of six months or less, must be unable to benefit from or have refused further aggressive (curative) therapy for his or her terminal illness, must be able to receive most care at home, and must have a caregiver who will assume the responsibility for custodial care of the patient and be the decision maker in the event the patient becomes incompetent to make decisions" (Fiebach et al., 2007, p. 196). Bereavement services in the form of grief counseling, educational support, and pastoral care support for the families of deceased hospice patients are provided for up to thirteen months following the death. Additional counseling services can also be obtained using a caregiver's own insurance plan if he or she has difficulty coping with the death of a loved one. Because of the high level of hospice coverage by Medicare and many other insurance providers, hospice care should be considered by anyone who is nearing the end of life.

Quality Assurance in Ambulatory Care

As the settings for ambulatory health care continue to grow in number and in diversity, quality assurance is and will continue to be a vital part of ensuring excellent patient experiences and outcomes. Accreditation for some ambulatory care settings is still voluntary at this time but is nonetheless highly recommended. Many ambulatory centers now choose to submit voluntarily to accreditation reviews by The Joint Commission, the Accreditation Association for Ambulatory Health Care, or the American Association for the Accreditation of Ambulatory Surgery Facilities (Sultz & Young, 2009). It is also becoming more common for payers to make reimbursement for services dependent on facility accreditation by an agency approved by the Centers for Medicare & Medicaid Services. In addition, most ambulatory surgical centers comply with state licensure and certification requirements, but Medicare must also certify those that provide services to Medicare patients on standards related to patient safety and quality of care. One option for satisfying Medicare's requirements is to obtain accreditation by The Joint Commission.

The Joint Commission began its Ambulatory Care Accreditation Program in 1975 and has since given accreditation approval to over 1,900 freestanding ambulatory care organizations. The settings that seek this accreditation generally fall into the broad categories of surgical services, medical or dental services, or diagnostic or therapeutic services. The standards put in place by The Joint Commission relate to the performance of ambulatory care facilities in specific and defined areas, including detailed requirements to ensure patient safety. In order for accreditation to be earned and subsequently maintained, an ambulatory care organization must undergo an onsite survey every three years by one of The Joint Commission survey teams. The objective of this onsite survey is to "not only to evaluate the organization, but to provide education and guidance that will help staff continue to improve the organization's performance" (The Joint Commission, 2011, pp. 1–2).

Another organization that provides accrediting services for ambulatory care is the Accreditation Association for Ambulatory Health Care (AAAHC), which was founded in 1979 to "encourage and assist ambulatory health care organizations to provide the highest achievable level of care for recipients in the most efficient and economically sound manner." This organization has since accredited over 5,000 ambulatory care organizations (the process must be repeated every three years) and continues to promote a commitment to developing national standards to "advance and promote patient safety, quality, value and measurement of performance for ambulatory health care through peer based accreditation processes, education and research." Peer-based assessment of standards, consultation, education, and a helpful handbook are offered to assist care providers in staying on the leading edge of ambulatory care knowledge and practices (AAAHC, 2012).

One of the greatest continuing concerns as ambulatory care has grown and evolved is patient safety. Most diagnostic and treatment procedures now performed in the outpatient settings are ones with a low risk of complications. However, proper managerial oversight, proper training of medical personnel, and correct and up-to-date equipment are still needed to ensure good quality of care. The Joint Commission has taken the initiative to increase people's awareness of the quality of ambulatory care in their communities by providing online information about the safety and quality of its accredited ambulatory care organizations. This information is available on the QualityCheck website, www.qualitycheck.org. Using this wonderful resource, consumers can quickly access a comprehensive listing for each Joint Commission–accredited ambulatory care facility, including the facility name, address, telephone number, accreditation decision, current accreditation status, effective accreditation date, and also a copy of the facility's most recent quality report (The Joint Commission, 2011, p. 3).

SUMMARY

In recent years, increases in both the number and diversity of ambulatory facilities have allowed a significant number of patients to receive care outside the more costly hospital setting. This trend away from the hospital setting is being driven largely by innovations and advances in diagnostic and treatment technologies; cost-reduction demands and initiatives by government payers, private insurance payers, and managed care organizations; and also patients' demands for more accessible, accommodating, and convenient locations for medical care. Care that once was provided only in the inpatient hospital setting has now been successfully shifted to the outpatient setting, with the health care literature now documenting ambulatory care as the predominant mode of health care delivery in the United States.

Ambulatory care is predicted to expand even further in the next few decades, and it will certainly continue to play a vital role in the U.S. health care system. Understandably, this causes concern among traditional hospitals in terms of their bottom line; however, much potential exists for successful partnership and collaboration among inpatient and outpatient facilities.

KEY TERMS

ambulatory care

diagnosis related group (DRG)

home health care services

hospice

hospitals without walls

hospital-based care

non-hospital-based care

palliative care model

retail clinic

urgent care center

DISCUSSION QUESTIONS

1. What are some specific reasons for the growth of ambulatory care settings?

2. What are some of the specific types of home health care services that are available for patients?

3. What specific types of care are available in ambulatory surgical centers?

4. What is the primary care physician's role in a patient's continuum of care, and how important is this role?

5. What are the differences between the hospice model of care (palliative care model) and the traditional medical model of care?

REFERENCES

Accreditation Association for Ambulatory Health Care. (2012). A history of AAAHC. Retrieved from http://www.aaahc.org/en/about/history

Barnett, A. E., & Mayer, G. G. (Eds.). (1992). *Ambulatory care management and practice*. Gaithersburg, MD: Aspen.

Caffrey, C., Sengupta, M., Moss, A., Harris-Kojetin, L., & Valverde, R. H. (2011, April 27). *Home health care and discharged hospice care patients: United States, 2000 and 2007* (National Health Statistics Reports, no. 38). Retrieved from http://www.cdc.gov/nchs/data/nhsr/nhsr038.pdf

Fiebach, N. H., Kern, D. E., Thomas, P. A., & Ziegelstein, R. C. (Eds.). (2007). *Principles of ambulatory medicine* (7th ed.). Philadelphia, PA: Lippincott, Williams and Wilkins.

Gottfried, D. (2008). *Too much medicine: A doctor's prescription for better and more affordable health care*. St. Paul, MN: Paragon House.

Hing, E., & Bhuiya, F. (2009). *Wait time for treatment in hospital emergency departments: 2009* (NCHS data brief, no. 102). Hyattsville, MD: National Center for Health Statistics.

The Joint Commission. (2011). Facts about ambulatory care accreditation. Retrieved from http://www.jointcommission.org/assets/1/18/Ambulatorycare_1_112.pdf

Jonas, S. (2003). *Introduction to the U.S. health care system* (5th ed.). New York, NY: Springer.

Jones, A. L., Harris-Kojetin, L., & Valverde, R. (2012, April 13). *Characteristics and use of home health care by men and women aged 65 and over* (National Health Statistics Reports, no. 52). Retrieved from http://www.cdc.gov/nchs/data/nhsr/nhsr052.pdf

Knowles, J. H. (1965). The role of the hospital: The ambulatory clinic. *Bulletin of the New York Academy of Medicine, 41*, 68–70.

Kubler-Ross, E. (1969). *On death and dying*. New York, NY: Macmillan.

Matthews, J. L. (2010). *Long-term care: How to plan and pay for it* (8th ed.). Berkeley, CA: Nolo.

McCaig, L. F., & Burt, C. W. (2001, June 25). National Hospital Ambulatory Medical Care Survey: 1999 emergency department summary. *Advance Data, (320)*, 1–34.

Mehrotra, A., Wang, M. C., Lave, J. R., Adams, J. L., & McGlynn, E. A. (2008). Retail clinics, primary care physicians and emergency departments: A comparison of patient visits. *Health Affairs, 27*(5), 1271–1282.

Mundinger, M. O. (2002). Through a different looking glass. *Health Affairs, 21*(1), 163–164.

National Center for Health Statistics. (2009a). National Hospital Ambulatory Medical Care Survey: 2009 Emergency department summary tables. Retrieved from http://www.cdc.gov/nchs/data/ahcd/nhamcs_emergency/2009_ed_web_tables.pdf

National Center for Health Statistics. (2009b). National Hospital Ambulatory Medical Care Survey: 2009 Outpatient department summary tables. Retrieved from http://www.cdc.gov/nchs/data/ahcd/nhamcs_outpatient/2009_opd_web_tables.pdf

Raffel, M. W., & Barsukiewicz, C. K. (2002). *The U.S. health system: Origins and functions* (5th ed.). Albany, NY: Delmar.

Roemer, M. I. (1981). *Ambulatory health services in America*. Gaithersburg, MD: Aspen.

Schappert, S. M., & Rechtsteiner, E. A. (2011). Ambulatory medical care utilization estimates for 2007. National Center for Health Statistics. *Vital and Health Statistics, 13*(169). Retrieved from http://www.cdc.gov/nchs/data/series/sr_13/sr13_169.pdf

Starfield, B. (1996). Public health and primary care: A framework for proposed linkages. *American Journal of Public Health, 86*(10), 1365.

Sultz, H. A., & Young, K. M. (2009). *Health care USA: Understanding its organization and delivery* (6th ed.). Sudbury, MA: Jones & Bartlett.

Urgent Care Association of America. (2011). About urgent care. Retrieved from http://www.ucaoa.org/home_abouturgentcare.php

Williams, S. J., & Torrens, P. R. (2008). *Introduction to health services* (7th ed.). Clifton Park, NY: Delmar/Cengage Learning.

Wolper, L. W. (1999). *Health care administration: Planning, implementing, and managing organized delivery systems*. Gaithersburg, MD: Aspen.

CHAPTER 6

HEALTH INSURANCE AND PAYMENT FOR HEALTH CARE SERVICES

Jeffrey R. Helton
Bernard J. Healey

Health care is a big business in the United States, consuming 17.9 percent of the nation's gross domestic product (GDP) in 2009 and 2010. Our nation spends a great deal of money on health care services, and these costs continue to increase despite numerous efforts by government and employers to control them. The amount that a U.S. consumer of health care services must pay for those services can be a significant portion of his or her personal income and may be more than the consumer can afford to pay out of pocket. Because of this, many people in the United States rely on health insurance plans to pay for health care services (Folland, Goodman, & Stano, 2005), and many of these plans are employer sponsored. According to Schimpff (2012), the cost of health care insurance has increased 140 percent in the last decade, with the employer and employee together paying premiums of over $13,000 for family coverage and $7,500 for individual coverage on an annual basis. These costs continue to rise every year, for a variety of reasons, and are not sustainable for the government, the employer, or the employee in the long term. As these costs increase so do an employer's expenses. These increases can be passed on to the consumer of the business's products through higher prices, but these higher prices then hurt the business's ability to compete in domestic and international markets.

In order to justify the need for comprehensive health reforms in our country, it is helpful to look at the escalation of health care costs over the last several years. The inflation rate for health care costs has exceeded that for the broader U.S. economy as measured by the consumer price index.

LEARNING OBJECTIVES

After reading this chapter you should be able to

- Understand the relative proportion of the U.S. economy devoted to health care services, the rate of growth of health care spending, and some of the causes of that increase.

- Describe the concept of health insurance and discuss how health insurance has functioned to date in the U.S. health care system.

- Describe the factors contributing to increased health care spending in the United States.

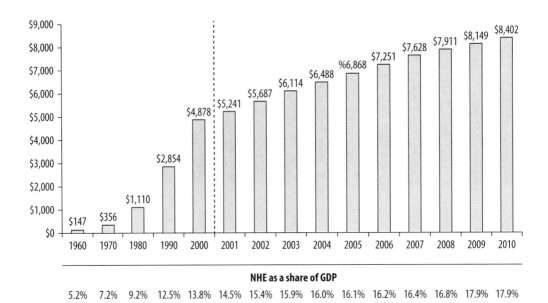

Figure 6.1   National Health Care Expenditures per Capita, 1960–2010

Note: Population is the U.S. Bureau of the Census resident-based population, less armed forces overseas.

Source: Henry J. Kaiser Family Foundation, n.d. Data from Centers for Medicare & Medicaid Services (CMS), Office of the Actuary, National Health Statistics Group, at http://www.cms.hhs.gov/NationalHealthExpendData (see Historical; NHE summary including share of GDP, CY 1960-2010).

Figure 6.1 shows the rapid growth of health care expenditures on a per capita basis over time. Health care expenditures continue to grow faster than the other sectors of our economy, rising from a per capita expense in 1960 of only $147 to $8,402 in 2010. Per capita health care costs for a country are determined by spreading the total amount spent on health in a year over the entire population. In 2010, a total of $2.6 trillion was spent on health care in the United States. These cost increases are passed on to those who pay for health insurance premiums and are predicted to increase from 17.9 percent of our current gross domestic product (GDP) in 2009 and 2010 to 19.6 percent by the year 2021. This means that in a very short time, one out of every five dollars produced by our economy each year will be paid to the health care sector. Health care costs will continue to rise into the distant future, due to the large number of elderly people, increases in the costs of technology and drugs, and the epidemic of expensive chronic diseases and their complications.

Figure 6.2 shows the average annual growth rate for the U.S. national health expenditure (NHE) and GDP, per capita, for selected time periods. As inflation of health care costs exceeds inflation in the overall economy, the share of GDP that health care takes will increase. This will result in health care taking resources from other parts of the nation's economy, as there are finite resources available. If health care's share increases, then

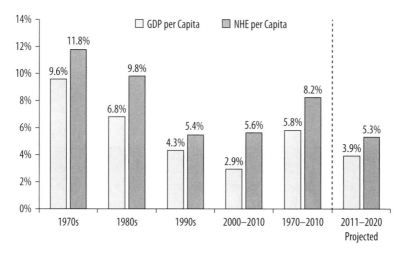

Figure 6.2 Average Annual Growth Rate for NHE and GDP, per Capita for Selected Time Periods

Source: Henry J. Kaiser Family Foundation, n.d. Data from CMS, Office of the Actuary, National Health Statistics Group, January 2012, at http://www.cms.hhs.gov/NationalHealthExpendData (see Historical; NHE summary including share of GDP, CY 1960-2010). Projections from CMS, Office of the Actuary, National Health Statistics Group, July 2011, tbl. 1, http://www.cms.hhs.gov /NationalHealthExpendData/downloads/proj2010.pdf

the share of other goods or services (such as education or defense) must decrease. This cannibalization of resources by health care will soon be a significant problem as U.S. lawmakers begin to make difficult decisions on the services that will be cut to pay for health care.

For most of people, illness, hospitalization, and large health care bills are things they usually do not experience until later in life. However, other people do not have this good fortune and become ill at a young age or are born with medical problems that can become expensive. Many Americans also practice high-risk health behaviors—such as smoking or excessive alcohol consumption—that can result in poor health and a need for medical care. For the most part, individuals cannot predict when they will need health care or how much care they will require to restore health. Also, health care is unlike other goods in that people rarely if ever know what the price is for their health care services. Physicians or hospitals do not usually publish a "menu" with prices. So for the most part, Americans do not know when health care will be needed, or if needed, how much it will cost. So, how do individuals pay for these costs if they occur? The mechanism of payment for these unpredictable and unknown costs involves the well-known concept of insurance, in this case health insurance.

According to Starr (2011), the United States is unique among industrialized countries in the world because it does not have a national health insurance program, leaving a large segment of its population without health insurance coverage. Other countries made a decision long ago that health care services are a *public good* that is distributed by the government and paid for with higher taxes. The United States has instead decided that only certain groups are to be covered by government-financed health insurance and that the rest of the country must deal with a market system for its health insurance, which is usually financed by people's employers. Unfortunately, neither government-financed health insurance nor the market system of health insurance is available for a large segment of the U.S. population.

The United States currently has over 50 million individuals without health insurance, despite the fact that we spend much more on health care than the countries that have provided health care insurance for all their citizens. Again, Starr (2011) points out that this deep and very political health insurance divide is not found in any other country. Other countries have made the decision that health care is a right of citizenship. In the United States only the elderly and the poor receive government-sponsored health insurance, through Medicare and Medicaid, respectively.

The recently passed **Patient Protection and Affordable Care Act of 2010 (ACA)** is intended to increase the availability of health insurance coverage in the United States; however, the ACA specifically excludes certain persons, such as undocumented immigrants and persons with demonstrated hardships in obtaining health insurance, from its requirements. In addition, the ACA calls for persons who do not have health insurance to pay financial penalties. However, the penalty amounts are generally less than the cost of health insurance for the consumer. So the number of persons who will get health insurance under the ACA is currently difficult to predict.

Patient Protection and Affordable Care Act of 2010 (ACA)
Signed into law on March 23, 2010, the ACA seeks to increase the quality and availability of health care coverage for most Americans.

Basics of U.S. Health Insurance

The most important component of insurance is the transfer of risk. **Insurance** is a form of risk management in which the risk is transferred to the insurance company in exchange for payments. An economic market has developed around the demand for health insurance and the suppliers of health insurance, who agree to assume the risk for a monetary payment called a **premium**. When individuals or companies purchase insurance policies, all the money from the premiums is combined into an insurance pool. Insurance companies make a huge profit when money in the pool is unused, which enables them to pay out large claims for the subset of insured people who become ill. Insurance is thus a form of risk management that is designed to protect us from the possibility of an uncertain loss. This risk transfer occurs through the payment of a dollar premium by the entity wanting to avoid the risk of an uncertain event to the entity willing to accept that risk in return for the premium. Insurance agreements are legal contracts that clearly spell out the way insurance payments are made

insurance
A form of risk management in which risk is transferred to an insurance company in exchange for payments.

premium
The price paid by an individual or business for insurance.

and received. This insurance mechanism has become a normal process for protecting people from loss involving their lives, homes, automobiles, and other personal belongings. It seems very natural to address the costs of health care services through this same process.

Barton (2010) describes how those who provide insurance to others conduct a **risk assessment process,** also known as *underwriting*, in order to estimate the probability of loss from varied uncertain events and the likely dollar value of those losses. This estimated cost of loss determines the premium that a consumer will be asked to pay to transfer the risk of loss to the insurer. If this transaction is determined to be potentially profitable, a contract is developed that includes the terms of the agreement along with the costs for insurance protection.

risk assessment process
The determination of all risks present in a given set of events in order to estimate the probability and likely dollar value of losses.

Health insurance can be very beneficial to individual consumers, since the costs of health care services can be extremely high and often unpredictable. Individuals usually do not know when they will be sick, need surgery, or have a heart attack. However, an insurer that looks at a large number of consumers needing health care services can accurately predict the number and cost of health care services in that group of consumers and set premiums based on that prediction. The consumer thus pays for his or her share of the expected cost of medical services to the group served by a given insurer. The price the consumer pays to a health insurer also covers some additional costs for profit and administrative overhead, known collectively as the **loading cost**. When it comes to potential losses from health care costs, consumers thus face a trade-off between their risk of paying an unpredictable but possibly large amount out of pocket for health care services or smaller, predictable amounts for health insurance that transfers that risk to an insurer.

loading cost
The dollar amount that covers the insurer's overhead and profit.

History of Health Insurance

Before the 1930s, very little care was available from any health care system other than making ill people comfortable until they died. In 1900, the life expectancy in the United States was only forty-nine years, with many individuals dying at an early age from influenza, tuberculosis, and even diarrhea because no highly effective treatments were available. There was little medical technology available; antibiotics for acute illness were not discovered until the mid-1930s. Most medical care was supplied in the home and not the hospital. Moreover, medical care was inexpensive, and therefore there was little need for health insurance. If you became ill you would simply pay out of pocket for what medical care was available. Health care services were affordable because when you became ill you were cared for in the home by family members or by charitable organizations. Buying health insurance or providing health insurance simply did not make any sense when the risk of a catastrophic financial loss (a key determinant of demand for insurance) was low. A market for health insurance comes into being when potential profits from supplying insurance can be seen because large numbers of people are demanding insurance. Such was not the case during that period of time.

Health insurance for the majority of the American population began its long-term growth phase shortly after World War II. As health care costs began to increase, a market for private health insurance (also known as commercial health insurance) developed. This insurance was initially a very inexpensive product and large numbers of people demanded it. Some organizations offering commercial health insurance were nonprofit and some were for-profit, and they usually offered both group and individual insurance plans.

The wage and price controls of the 1940s limited the ability of employers to raise wages to attract and retain employees. So employers started to use health insurance and other nonsalary benefits to lure workers. Labor unions also were in a strong position to demand and receive health insurance as part of a comprehensive, employer-funded benefit package. Starr (2011) points out that federal authorities allowed companies to add health insurance as a benefit for employees despite the wage and price controls that were in place. The cost of this new benefit of health insurance was allowed to be tax deductible for employers and eventually was treated as nontaxable income for the employees receiving the insurance. Under these conditions, health insurance coverage expanded rapidly across the United States. Newly insured employees were now able to afford more expensive health services, which became the incentive required to create new ways to treat illnesses; demand then increased for hospital construction and expansion to deliver the new medical technologies.

Medicine became big business with the expansion of new, higher-cost treatments and the increased numbers of physicians and hospitals in the United States. As more health care providers entered the market, competition increased among them, which, interestingly, increased the amount of services provided. This reflects a unique feature in the health care industry—**provider-induced demand**. The average consumer of health care does not know how to diagnose his or her medical condition and does not have a license to order services or prescribe medications. So consumers rely on the knowledge of a health care provider to determine what services are needed, even though that provider stands to make more money by ordering more services. As competition increased, providers could maintain their incomes by recommending more services to the persons they served.

provider-induced demand
Demand not made by the consumer but induced by a third party.

Insurance benefits may not be very valuable to the person covered by insurance in the short run unless they are used. Insurance made patients insensitive to the cost of medical procedures and hospitalization because they would now have to pay only a small part, if any, of the cost of medical services. This leads to the condition known as **moral hazard** (discussed in Chapter One), in which an individual is more likely to take risks when the costs associated with the risk are borne by another. In this case, the very existence of health insurance coverage creates an incentive for the insured individual (also known as the **beneficiary**) to use the benefit.

Thinking to reduce moral hazard, many insurers attempted to share some costs of care with the insured person. Cost sharing happens in three different ways. First, the insurance policy may specify a **deductible**, where the insured person pays a specified amount before the insurer pays. Second, the patient may be asked to pay **coinsurance**, which is a percentage of the payment for services. Third, the patient may have a **copayment**, where the patient pays a flat amount each time he or she obtains services. Insurance plans may have one or more of these cost-sharing mechanisms. For example, an insurance plan may have a $500 deductible with a $25 copayment for physician's office visits.

As providers continued to increase the volume of services provided and the prices paid for those services, the escalation of health care costs mentioned earlier in this chapter began to manifest itself. Health care providers began to operate more like businesses, with profit and market share expectations, which further fueled this upward trend in health care costs in the United States. As insurers and consumers began to push back against inflation in health care costs, reductions in payment rates and mechanisms to limit the volume of services provided, an approach known as managed care (described later in this chapter and in more detail in Chapter Seven) came into vogue.

As costs have increased, so has interest in the financing of health care services. Providers of health care services in the United States have worked hard at fighting efforts to reduce payments and in fact have made concerted efforts to see that their payments continue to increase. Because the government has become one of the largest payers and the only regulator of the health care industry, it has become a major goal of health providers to gain the attention of the various legislators through lobbyists. Stiglitz (2012) points out that there are more than 3,100 lobbyists working at the federal level on behalf of various health care interests, or six for every one of our federal legislators. These lobbyists work to influence the health care legislation that in turn influences provider payment for services. Therefore health care finance is a result of political forces as much as economics.

moral hazard
A condition that exists when an individual is more likely to take risks because the costs associated with the risk are borne by another.

beneficiary
An individual who receives proceeds or benefits from, for example, an insurance policy.

deductible
An amount paid by the insured before the insurer pays.

coinsurance
A percentage of the service costs paid by the insured.

copayment
The amount paid by the insured each time the service is utilized.

The success story of improving health care technology has led to an increased life expectancy in the United States. However, this success has also had the secondary effect of increasing the prices of health care services beyond the reach of the average American. The need for reform of our health care delivery system has never been greater but this reform will involve much more than finance. Developing reforms that will affect the cost of health insurance requires gaining a better understanding of how the health insurance market works.

How Health Insurance Markets Work

There is a market composed of supply and demand for health insurance that is similar to many other markets in the U.S. economy. However, the health insurance market also has some important differences from other markets found in a capitalist system. On one hand the individuals demanding health insurance are those who believe they may be at risk for large medical bills over a given period of time. It is obvious that individuals who are already ill and those who are older will have a much greater demand for health insurance coverage. On the other hand the young and those who are in good health will usually not have a great demand for the protection afforded by health insurance and will usually shy away from purchasing this product if it is expensive. Having a mix of younger, healthier persons and older, sicker persons who are all paying insurance premiums would help to keep health insurance affordable. Because younger persons have a lower likelihood of needing coverage, they would tend to pay more into the pool than they use, and this would subsidize the costs incurred by the older and sicker persons. In actuality, however, their lower risk tends to steer younger persons out of the nation's insurance pool. Because not everyone is buying into the insurance pool, insurance becomes much more expensive for those who really need it. This problem is termed **adverse selection** (Gapenski & Pink, 2011). This problem can lead to the pool of individuals covered by the insurer consisting of those most likely to utilize their insurance because of poor health, eventually bankrupting the insurance company.

There are two ways that an insurer can spread the risks of losses among persons in an insurance pool. The first method used in the early days of commercial health insurance was **community rating**. In this method the risk of poor health is spread over a large number of individuals, with each required to pay the same premium no matter what their health status. However, as health insurance became more competitive, insurers realized that some employer groups tended to have younger, healthier members and that those people were paying premiums that were much higher than their risk of loss. This led to the use of **group rating**, a method more

adverse selection
What results when individuals' demand for insurance is directly related to their personal risk of loss.

community rating
Spreading the risk over a large number of people, who each pay the same premium whatever their health status.

group rating
Spreading the risk over an employer group, which will lower premiums if the group as a whole is healthy.

in vogue among commercial insurers that sell to employers. Under this approach, premiums are based on the risk of loss within an employer group. So employers who hire younger persons tend to pay lower insurance premiums than employers with an older workforce. In either method the affordability of health insurance depends on having a large number of individuals participating in the insured pool. Otherwise health insurance programs will fail due to premiums being unaffordable. As mentioned earlier, increasing the number of persons participating in the nation's insurance pool is a key goal of the ACA, with the hope of reducing the average insurance premium paid in the United States.

Health insurance then is a legal contract that protects the insured individual from the financial costs likely to result if that individual becomes ill. Unfortunately, it has become a contract that is almost impossible to understand by anyone except those who profit from this challenging component of health care services financing. According to Perednia (2011), "No single aspect of the health care system is more inefficient, destructive, and harmful to the average American than the way in which medical services are currently priced, billed, and paid for" (p. 135). The current method used to reimburse health care providers creates an incentive to provide additional, potentially unnecessary medical procedures, which may harm the patient, or restricts necessary services, which may also hurt the patient.

The business element of health care has driven health care providers to change the way they provide services, in order to increase or maintain their incomes from different forms of payment for services. According to Christensen, Grossman, and Hwang (2009), "because people will predictably do more of what is profitable and less of what isn't, the system of reimbursement in the United States constitutes one of the most powerful and pervasive schemes of macro- and microlevel regulation that humanity has ever devised" (p. xxxii). So a challenge as the United States moves forward with the ACA is to evaluate what type of payment mechanism will give an incentive to providers to render the services necessary while earning a fair income and minimizing use of unnecessary or excessive services.

Health Insurance Providers

According to Perednia (2011), the most important providers of health insurance in our country are private health insurance providers like Blue Cross and government providers of health insurance like Medicare and Medicaid. Private health insurance plans financed by employers still cover the largest proportion of persons with health insurance in the United States, followed by Medicare and Medicaid. Even with the widespread availability of health insurance, 50 million Americans remain without health insurance.

The ACA is intended to reduce this number by about 60 percent, following its full implementation in 2014. The amount of insurance provided by government programs is increasing because of unemployment, the aging of Americans, and the expansion of state Medicaid programs under the ACA.

Health insurance is paid for by the person, company, or other organization that pays the premium for the insured person, be it with government or private funds. This payer-of-premium concept classifies premium payment by the following categories: do you work (benefit of employment), did you use to work (Medicare), or is your income low (Medicaid). The employer or employee, or both, pay for private health insurance, and the government funds, through tax revenues, insurance for the poor and the elderly and for veterans, current members of the military, and other government workers. Conover (2012) points out that over the last eighty years, "the out-of-pocket share of health spending has declined while the portion paid by third parties has increased" (p. 39).

Private insurers can either be for-profit or nonprofit but both operate under the same business model. Perednia (2011) points out that this model requires a belief that all the insured will not become ill at the same time and that their combined premium payments will more than cover the costs for those who do become ill. In fact most health insurance providers not only pay the costs for persons who become ill but also retain some funds for profits (or surpluses if they are nonprofits) on an annual basis. Insurer profits (or surpluses) are necessary to retain funds for future investment or to hedge against future, unpredicted expenses.

Government-financed health care programs tend to pay providers less than the private insurers do, as a result of legislative efforts to balance government budgets and the fact that government entities can to some degree dictate the rates they pay. Providers who see a large proportion of patients covered by government insurance programs may see their incomes fall, thus causing them to increase the fees billed to private insurers. This is a practice known as *cost shifting*, where the provider's costs are shifted from the lower-paying source to the individual who is covered by a private insurance plan. Although this practice seems unfair, it has become the normal way to do business when the government-financed health programs continue to reduce their payments to health care providers. There are several major types of health insurers in the United States. Following is a description of the key characteristics of these insurers.

Blue Cross/Blue Shield

Blue Cross and Blue Shield developed separately, with Blue Cross plans providing coverage for hospital services and Blue Shield plans covering physicians' services. According to Christensen et al. (2009), Blue Cross was born during the Depression when an entrepreneur by the name of Justin Ford Kimball devised a way for 1,300 schoolteachers in Dallas to pay a small monthly fee to Baylor Hospital that would fund twenty-one days of hospitalization if required. The resulting nonprofit company sold prepaid health insurance plans that covered hospital services at a reasonable price. These hospital insurance plans benefited both the individual paying the premium and the hospital. The insurance payment was made whether hospital care was utilized or not. Blue Shield was also started during this time, selling insurance plans that covered physician services. The Blue Shield insurance concept was a response to the dangerous occupations found in the mining and lumber industries when, in order to attract workers, the mining and lumber companies began offering their employees health insurance for physician visits. In 1982, these two insurance entities combined to form the Blue Cross and Blue Shield Association, which has grown over the years to be one of the largest prepaid group insurance plans, directly or indirectly insuring over 99 million Americans.

Medicare

Health insurance became quite common after World War II and, as mentioned earlier, was provided to working adults by their employers as part of their benefit package. This was fine for persons who were young enough and well enough to work, but once they became older and unable to work they no longer had health insurance, probably when it was needed most. There was clearly a need for the provision of health insurance for this segment of the nation's population.

The 1960s ushered in the beginning of large-scale government programs to pay for health care services for distinct groups of individuals. In 1965, Congress passed and President Johnson signed legislation authorizing Medicare and Medicaid health coverage for the elderly and the poor, respectively. The Medicare program, established under Title XVIII of the Social Security Act Amendments of 1965, is focused primarily on payment for health care for persons aged sixty-five years and above but also covers individuals under age sixty-five who receive Social Security Disability Insurance (SSDI) or who have end-stage renal disease (ESRD) or Lou Gehrig's disease. Medicare is a federally administered benefit and comprises four programs, labeled Parts A, B, C, and D.

Medicare Part A covers hospitalization expenses including home health care. There is no charge to the recipient for this part of the program. **Medicare Part B** covers outpatient services, including physician visits, outpatient procedures, and durable medical equipment. Medicare contributes half of the cost of this part of the program with the rest being

Medicare Part A
Part A covers hospital inpatient care and helps to cover the cost of hospice and home health care.

Medicare Part B
Part B helps to cover physician services and outpatient care but requires a monthly premium payment from the insured.

covered by a monthly premium from the recipient of care. Gapenski and Pink (2011) point out that Medicare Parts A and B will not cover all out-of-pocket costs for those insured owing to deductibles, coinsurance, copayments, and coverage limits. This problem created a need for private insurers to offer policies that paid these amounts not covered by Medicare, policies known as Medicare supplement or Medigap plans.

Medicare Part C

Part C, also known as Medicare Advantage, offers recipients an expanded set of options for the delivery of their health care.

Medicare Part C consists of the Medicare Advantage plans; beneficiaries enroll in these private health insurance programs with Medicare paying the premiums. This part of the Medicare program allows private insurers to accept a capitated reimbursement for the total care of the recipient. This option was made available in order to improve the quality of care offered at lower costs through plan efficiency. Unfortunately, although Medicare Advantage plans offer beneficiaries more benefits, the cost reductions promised by these plans have not occurred.

Medicare Part D

Part D provides outpatient coverage for prescriptions.

Medicare Part D consists of Medicare's prescription drug benefit. This part of Medicare was passed by Congress in 2003 and is administered by private insurers, with the cost being shared by the insured and the government. As the Henry J. Kaiser Family Foundation (2008) points out, individuals can obtain this drug benefit coverage through a private plan that offers drug benefit only or a Medicare Advantage plan that covers drug benefits. The legislation does not allow the federal government to negotiate drug prices directly with the drug manufacturers. This legislation also produced a coverage gap, known as the "doughnut hole," a period during which beneficiaries whose drug expenditures have reached a certain level must then pay 100 percent of their drug costs until they reach the yearly out-of-pocket spending limit, after which most of their drug costs are covered again. Reforms under the ACA are aimed at reducing the doughnut hole for Medicare beneficiaries.

Figure 6.3 shows the characteristics of the 45 million enrollees in the Medicare program in 2006. Almost 50 percent are poor and almost 40 percent have three or more chronic diseases. Although many of these individuals still have a fairly long life expectancy, many are ill and will be consuming large amounts of health care resources over their remaining years of life. Moreover, because of their chronic diseases, which may result in complications, their quality of life may not be very good despite their being insured.

Also notable in Figure 6.3 is that 16 percent of Medicare recipients are permanently disabled and 5 percent are housed in a long-term care setting. The Centers for Medicare & Medicaid Services pointed out in 2006 that Medicare is expected to consume 14 percent of the federal budget between 2010 and 2030, with estimates of the number of individuals receiving Medicare benefits rising from 46 million to 78 million.

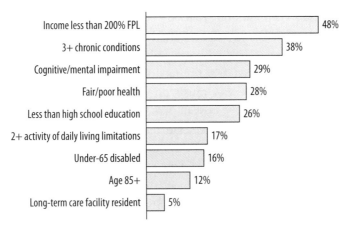

Figure 6.3 Characteristics of Medicare's 45 Million Beneficiaries

Note: FPL = federal poverty limit.
Source: Henry J. Kaiser Family Foundation, 2008. Data from Current Population Survey and CMS Medicare Beneficiary Survey, 2006.

Schimpff (2012) points out that many individuals seem to think that Medicare is a free good to which they have a right. It is not free; in fact it is a very expensive program paid for by current workers and their employers, with each paying 1.45 percent of earned income until retirement. Medicare Part B is partially paid for by a monthly deduction from the retired individual's Social Security payment. The problem that occurs when we think something is free is that we may begin to waste the product or service. This is clearly what has occurred in the context of many third-party payment systems.

Medicaid and the SCHIP Program

The Medicaid program became law in 1965 under Title XIX of the Social Security Act Amendments of that year. This program is also run by CMS and is jointly administered by the federal and state governments. According to Barton (2010) the Medicaid program was initially designed to fund a required set of health services to low-income children and their adult caregivers. The Kaiser Commission on Medicaid and the Uninsured (2013) points out that "Medicaid now covers over 62 million Americans,. . . more than 1 in 3 children and over 40 percent of births. . . . More than 60 percent of people living in nursing homes are covered by Medicaid" (p. 1). Similarly, Harrison and Harrison (2012) note that the federal government sets the minimum standards for the Medicaid program across all states, contributes 43 percent of the cost of the program, and allows individual states to administer the program and determine additional benefits in a manner determined by each state.

Klemm (2000) points out that the cost of the Medicaid program in its first year was only $1 billion but that cost had risen to over $200 billion in fiscal year 2000. This cost will increase substantially when the ACA is fully implemented over the next few years. Future trends that the Medicaid program nationwide must cope with include the increasing cost of long-term care, the rising cost of prescription drugs, the increased use of managed care plans, and Medicaid *maximization*. This maximization is occurring as states adopt innovative strategies designed to achieve the largest amount of federal funding for their Medicaid programs. In 2010, the Medicaid program provided health care to 53.9 million individuals spending $404.1 billion, representing $6,775 on a per capita basis. The federal government has been paying a larger part of this bill than the states have in recent years.

According to the Centers for Medicare & Medicaid Services (2011), the ACA will increase the number of those enrolled in Medicaid by 26 million by 2020. The Medicaid program does offer a low-cost method of increasing the number of people with health insurance because its payment rates and administrative costs are much lower than those in other types of health insurance programs. It must be mentioned that having health insurance does not in itself guarantee the availability of health care. It is also important to point out that the availability of health insurance through Medicaid does not guarantee good health for the individual Medicaid beneficiary. Due to historically low payments by state Medicaid programs, many health care providers have chosen not to accept patients with Medicaid insurance, making it difficult for many with this insurance benefit to get health care services despite their having insurance coverage. Future challenges include getting providers to accept Medicaid patients, and fostering prevention of disease.

State Children's Health Insurance Program (SCHIP or CHIP)

A joint federal and state government program that provides health insurance to uninsured, low-income children not eligible for Medicaid.

The **State Children's Health Insurance Program (SCHIP or CHIP)** was enacted by Congress as part of the Balanced Budget Act of 1997 and was designed to provide coverage to uninsured, low-income children who are not eligible for the Medicaid program. SCHIP funds are available for each state and can be used to expand the state's Medicaid program, to create a new program, or to create a combination approach.

State Health Insurance Exchanges

state health insurance exchanges

Online marketplaces for the comparison and purchase of health insurance plans.

In an effort to increase participation in the nation's health insurance pool, the ACA called for the creation of **state health insurance exchanges**. These exchanges are open marketplaces where insurers offer plans to uninsured persons in each state. These health insurance exchanges are expected to expand access to private health insurance coverage for low- and moderate-income individuals and employees of small businesses. This approach to health insurance is designed to make enrollment easier while allowing easy comparison of insurance costs and benefits among the competing plans involved in the insurance exchange. Also, by pooling large numbers of uninsured persons in these state exchanges, it is expected that insurance premiums will be more affordable to consumers. The ACA also provides for subsidies to low-income consumers who do not qualify for Medicaid to buy insurance in the state exchanges.

Affordability has been a problem for insurers selling to individuals or small employers owing to high administrative costs and the inability to spread the risk over large numbers of individuals. State health insurance exchanges hope to address these problems and make insurance more affordable to individuals and small employers. According to Altman and Shactman (2011), the insurance market for large groups (aimed at employers of more than fifty persons who provide health insurance as a benefit) is not in need of an exchange.

According to the Henry J. Kaiser Family Foundation (2009), the functions envisioned for these new exchanges consist of

- Offering consumers a choice of health plans and focusing competition on price
- Providing information to consumers
- Creating an administrative mechanism for enrollment
- Moving toward portability of coverage
- Reforming the insurance market

Reimbursement for Health Care Providers

It may be hard to believe, but at one time the payment of physicians was not a complicated process. The payment mechanism most utilized by private and public insurers called for fees that were **usual, customary, and reasonable (UCR)**. Under this system, insurers paid a set fee that was determined to be the usual and reasonable price customarily charged by providers in a given area. This system was easy to understand and simple to implement because it was a fee-for-service mechanism. However, this system was an incentive for the provider-induced demand mentioned earlier in this chapter. As health care costs increased, the problem became one of establishing goals for the health care payment system other than simply paying providers for services rendered. When Medicare and Medicaid were passed in 1965 and implemented in 1966, the costs for these programs were insignificant in terms of the federal and state budgets and as a percentage of GDP. As the number and size of health care providers increased, along with an increase

usual, customary, and reasonable (UCR)
A fee for health care services that matches general prevailing costs for the service.

in medical technology, costs increased dramatically. This led to an increase in the number of different payment systems (often different systems for different insurers), regulations, and paperwork that health care providers had to deal with to obtain payments for services provided.

There are now numerous ways to pay health care providers for their services, and it is important that the payer of these bills understands the role that incentives play in patient care. According to Perednia (2011), there are over 800,000 physicians practicing medicine in the United States, both generalists and specialists, who make the decisions that involve approximately 80 percent of total U.S. health care costs. It is obvious that the way we reimburse the physician is a critical component in dealing with the cost and quality of our health care services. Four mechanisms for payment are discussed in the remainder of this section.

Fee-for-Service

fee-for-service
The way most providers are paid when they are paid for each activity performed.

A **fee-for-service** payment system, also called *indemnity coverage*, is a reimbursement system that uses a fee schedule for medical procedures (Harrison & Harrison, 2012). The fee schedule must be negotiated and agreed to by both the payer and the provider. As mentioned earlier, this type of payment system encourages physicians to do more for every patient in order to increase their personal income. The fee-for-service reimbursement system allows the physician to determine how many services are offered to his or her patients, resulting in large numbers of medical services, some of which may be medically unnecessary and possibly even dangerous for the patient. This type of payment system is relatively easy to understand and implement, but it offers the wrong incentives to physicians, encouraging them to do more medical procedures and tests despite the costs in order to increase their personal income.

This type of reimbursement mechanism was originally introduced by Blue Cross and Blue Shield for the purpose of the insured individual purchasing coverage for specific benefits and paying the provider for delivery of these specific services (Buchbinder & Shanks, 2012). This payment system was adopted by the Medicare and Medicaid programs, resulting in a rapid increase in the cost of health care services in our country.

Capitation

capitation
The way providers are paid when they receive a set annual fee for each individual's health care.

In order to repair the abuses found in fee-for-service plans, a new system of provider payment called capitation was begun. The **capitation** reimbursement system offers the provider of health services a fixed fee to provide medical care for an individual for a set period of time, usually a year. Some argue that capitation reimbursement removes the incentive to provide more care than necessary and instead incentivizes the provider to offer fewer health care services (Christensen et al., 2009). The belief is that the provider will also attempt to offer his or her patients wellness and preventive care. Unfortunately, this type of payment system, which is used by most managed care organizations, incentivizes doing less care including preventive services. It also makes it less likely that providers will want to care for ill individuals and will instead "cherry-pick" healthy patients who will not be requesting care except for emergency situations. There really is no incentive to keep patients healthy because next year they may change insurance plans and eventually, when they start to become ill, they will usually be old enough to move on to Medicare coverage.

Resource-Based Relative Value Scale

The **resource-based relative value scale (RBRVS)** represents an attempt to pay physicians based on the costs of the resources required to produce a given medical service. It is a new reimbursement system, adopted by Medicare in 1992 for the payment of physician services. The three components of a physician's cost of service consist of the physician's work, practice expenses, and professional liability insurance. This system is a variant of the UCR system described earlier, where physicians' fees are set based on an estimate of the costs of providing care, but under RBRVS, fees are set less arbitrarily than under a UCR system. In addition, RBRVS payments are made on a fee-for-service basis, and so, while they retain the benefit of ease of implementation, they also retain the incentives to perhaps provide more services than necessary.

resource-based relative value scale (RBRVS)
A means of calculating physician pay based on the costs of the resources required to produce a given medical service.

Pay-for-Performance

Pay-for-performance (P4P) programs are designed to offer financial incentives to health care providers, including physicians, to meet quality health goals, efficiency goals, and other targets. Perednia (2011) argues that the P4P movement is the evolution of the concept of *evidence-based medicine*, which entails utilization of current best evidence in making medical decisions. This type of provider reimbursement system is also called *value-based purchasing*, and several studies are showing some improvement in outcomes and efficiency with the use of this provider payment system. Unfortunately, this payment system has become complicated by the establishment of additional guidelines for its use.

pay-for-performance (P4P)
A system that offers providers of care financial incentives for better patient outcomes.

Rosenthal and Dudley (2007) note that most providers of health care services agree that the current provider reimbursement system does not improve patient quality of care and needs to be reformed. These authors caution that the available research involving pay-for-performance systems suggests there are both opportunities and challenges in implementing this type of reimbursement system. There is no question that carefully designing a payment system for providers that eliminates wasteful services that are expensive and may even be dangerous for the patient is an absolute requirement for ongoing health care reform efforts. The natural extension of a pay-for-performance system with its emphasis on quality would be a *pay-for-outcomes* approach that would highlight patient health outcomes.

Why Health Insurance Is Such a Huge Problem in the United States

As pointed out earlier, every industrialized country in the world other than the United States made the decision long ago that health care is a fundamental right of citizenship. In these countries the medical providers work with the government in the provision of most health care services to the population. This has not been the case in the United States, where the citizens have discouraged government involvement in health care. The question then becomes, Why has health insurance become such a controversial subject for the United States?

The health care industry has become the largest sector of the U.S. economy, consuming about 17.9 percent of the gross domestic product in 2009 and 2010 and resulting in an annual health care bill approaching $3 trillion. This is a very large amount of money, and health care reform means reducing the annual increase. However, many businesses and individuals have become very wealthy and powerful producing health services and products over the years, and they will do everything in their power to preserve their profits and their influence. These special interest groups are concerned about the possibility of change in the way they do business, even if the proposed change will improve the availability of health services for the population.

Lobosky (2012) notes that the largest health insurers in the United States increased their profits by over 50 percent and provided their executives with millions of dollars in bonuses during the period from 2003 to 2006. This was accomplished by raising premiums, denying claims, contracting with health care providers that accepted the lowest fees, and discovering ways to cancel policies when individuals became ill. This has caused many in the United States to question the priorities of health insurers that appear to value profit over the well-being of consumers. Reforms in the ACA include requirements to stop these sorts of practices by commercial insurers.

Creative Destruction of Health Insurance

There is a general agreement that our health care system costs too much and that many of our health quality indices (such as average longevity or birth rate of healthy babies) are too low when compared with indices for other countries that spend much less on health care than we do. High costs and poor outcomes stem from a lack of goals and a lack of appropriate financial incentives to providers of health care. We can use financial incentives to improve outcomes while making better use of scarce resources in health services delivery.

According to Jennings (2012), when money is used in an effort to address current problems, other solutions that could potentially solve the problems are hidden, and therefore the underlying causes of the problems are never evaluated and opportunities for permanent solutions are never discovered. Perednia (2011) points out that approximately 25 percent of U.S. health care dollars spent simply disappear, with little value gained for the expense incurred. It seems that we have developed an unplanned and fragmented system of financing health care that produces enormous waste.

Expansion of the fee-for-service system resulted from the growth of commercial health insurance along with implementation of the Medicare and Medicaid programs. During the legislative process that led to the Medicare and Medicaid programs, the American Medical Association reluctantly supported that legislation in return for the use of fee-for-service payment for the providers of care in those programs. Yet, according to Christensen and colleagues (2009), up to half of all medical expenditures resulting from fee-for-service are medically unnecessary. In view of this finding, future use of the fee-for-service mechanism must be critically reevaluated.

Christensen et al. (2009) argue that fee-for-service payment systems create at least three major distortions in any effort to achieve least-cost goals:

1. They protect costly procedures, along with blocking disruptive innovation.
2. They block incentives to invest in new products and services.
3. They increase, rather than decrease, hospital costs.

The other major approach, capitation, has produced a great deal of backlash among providers of care and even among the original supporters of a capitated integrated HMO like Kaiser Permanente. It was thought that a capitated system would encourage preventive health programs for all enrollees. This did not happen because administrators of the capitated plans realized that individuals change health insurance plans frequently and so one plan's efforts to keep its members healthy would end up benefiting other plans or Medicare.

Topol (2011) argues that the delivery of health care services in our country is about to be creatively destroyed in order to build a better health care system that will work for our entire population. The noted Austrian American economist Joseph Schumpeter popularized the term *creative destruction*. This concept rose out of work completed by Karl Marx, which Schumpeter used to explain economic innovation and business cycles. In its simplest form **creative destruction** involves destroying old products and services in order to create new and better products and services. Major transformation is expected to result from radical innovation. In a capitalist system entrepreneurs produce a disruptive force that creates increased economic growth even as previous vehicles of economic growth are destroyed. This is exactly what is required in the way that we pay providers for health care service delivery.

Along with applying the concept of creative destruction, we also have to encourage the concept of disruptive innovation that has been mentioned in previous chapters. It stands to reason that if we completely destroy our current financing system for health care services, then we must come up with an alternative way to reimburse providers of those services for their work. Disruptive innovation has the capability of changing expensive and complicated products and services into less expensive and less complicated products and services. This is exactly the type of change that is so necessary to incentivize reform in the way health care services are financed.

The current health care system has been developed and protected by those who reap the profits from current reimbursement structures. When change is being considered, it is likely that these same people will be consulted. It is quite natural that these providers will attempt to protect the current system because it is working just fine for them. The regulations in health care should foster innovation, not reward maintaining the current system. The poor results and high costs we currently experience call for significant change in our health care delivery system in order to make it sustainable.

Altman and Shactman (2011) point out that health care already consumes 20 percent of the entire federal budget, which takes resources away from other important priorities, what economists call a *crowding out effect*. The amount we take away from education or other priorities to fund continued growth in health care expenditures must be reconsidered. One of the greatest concerns with the ACA is that it does very little to reduce the cost escalation found in the health care sector of our economy. However, one of the important regulatory components of the ACA is creation of the **Independent Payment Advisory Board (IPAB)**, a fifteen-member federal

creative destruction
Destroying old products and services in order to create new and better products and services.

Independent Payment Advisory Board (IPAB)
A fifteen-member federal agency responsible for achieving savings while maintaining quality in Medicare.

agency responsible for achieving savings in Medicare without reducing quality. The IPAB will establish a target rate of growth for Medicare spending in 2018 as the average previous five-year increase in GDP plus one percentage point. For example, if GDP grows at an average of 3 percent, the target will be 4 percent. If Medicare spending growth exceeds this target (which it has over much of the last ten years), the board is required to issue recommendations to reduce the growth rate to the target rate or at least to reduce it by 1.5 percent. This part of the ACA may very well be one of the answers to controlling health care costs.

Many of the important parts of a good health insurance plan are already found in our current Medicare program, absent the fee-for-service mechanism for paying providers. Individuals receiving Medicare do not experience problems with getting access to care or high expenses as a percentage of income when compared to adults who receive insurance coverage from their employer (Davis, Stremikis, Doty, & Zezza, 2012). Medicare beneficiaries tend to be very satisfied with their insurance coverage. Klein (2009) argues that the Medicare program has achieved this satisfaction from beneficiaries despite having the lowest overhead of any insurance provider, currently reported as 3 percent. Commercial for-profit insurers put from 15 percent to 30 percent of costs toward overhead and profit.

The delivery of health care services is undergoing very rapid change in the United States due to a litany of environmental forces, focused primarily around the magnitude of spending for these services. The way that we pay for these services is also in need of further change. These changes are requiring that those who finance health care services adapt to their ever-changing business environment. McKeown (2012) argues that changes to the way things used to be will provoke resistance rather than adaptation to the changing circumstances. This can happen even when adapting to those changes can produce tremendous opportunities. McKeown also points out that ignorance and self-interest are quite often the reason that organizations fail to adapt to change and respond with a different strategy. Organizations that are failing to achieve their goals are usually failing to adapt to a changing environment. This could be said of the reimbursement system for health care services in our country. Health care finance, whether public or private, has become a rigid bureaucracy that does not encourage or reward creativity and innovation.

The inability to adapt is most likely the reason for our private and public health insurers' inability to correct the way that they have been paying for health care services. There are so many problems found in the way that we currently insure and pay for the delivery of health care services that we are in dire need of changing most parts of the system in order to reduce the burden of our health care system on the nation's overall economy.

SUMMARY

Our current system of health insurance began its development and growth around the end of World War II. Private health insurance allowed Americans to spread the risk of illness over large numbers of individuals in order to make the cost of health insurance affordable for most individuals.

Now, however, the cost of health care services continues to rise every year, and despite various strategies attempted by employers and government, no one has found a way to keep these costs from increasing. With the costs of health care escalating, the price of insurance coverage for individuals also continues to rise. These cost increases are clearly not sustainable in the long term or they will bankrupt our nation.

The concept of creative destruction has been discussed in this chapter in relation to the radical changes needed in the current health insurance system if we are to accomplish our most important health care goals. This creative destruction should result in the much-needed disruptive innovation so necessary to reducing the costs of health services delivery while at the same time improving the health outcomes produced by health care providers.

KEY TERMS

adverse selection

beneficiary

capitation

coinsurance

community rating

copayment

creative destruction

deductible

fee-for-service

group rating

Independent Payment Advisory
    Board (IPAB)

insurance

loading cost

Medicare Part A

Medicare Part B

Medicare Part C

Medicare Part D

moral hazard

Patient Protection and Affordable
    Care Act of 2010 (ACA)

pay-for-performance (P4P)

premium

provider-induced demand

resource-based relative value scale
    (RBRVS)

risk assessment process

state health insurance exchanges

State Children's Health Insurance
    Program (SCHIP or CHIP)

usual, customary, and reasonable
    (UCR)

DISCUSSION QUESTIONS

1. How has health insurance evolved in the United States?

2. What are the parts of the Medicare program, what does each one cover, and how is each one financed?

3. Medicare and Medicaid are two different government insurance programs. What are at least three ways in which they differ from each other?

4. What is provider-induced demand? How can it affect health care costs?

5. What incentives do providers have under a fee-for-service payment system? What incentives do they have under a capitated payment system?

6. What is the concept of creative destruction? How might creative destruction improve the way health insurance pays for health care services in the United States?

7. In what ways are insurance exchanges likely to affect the health insurance market?

REFERENCES

Altman, S., & Shactman, D. (2011). *Power, politics, and universal health care.* Amherst, NY: Prometheus Books.

Barton, P. L. (2010). *Understanding the U.S. health services system* (4th ed.). Chicago, IL: Health Administration Press.

Buchbinder, S. B., & Shanks, N. H. (2012). *Introduction to health care management* (2nd ed.). Burlington, MA: Jones & Bartlett Learning.

Centers for Medicare & Medicaid Services. (2006). *Medicare Current Beneficiary Survey.* Baltimore, MD: Author.

Centers for Medicare & Medicaid Services, Office of the Actuary. (2011). *National health expenditures 1960 –2010.* Retrieved from http://www.cms.gov /Research-Statistics-Data-and-Systems/Statistics-Trends-and-Reports /NationalHealthExpendData/NationalHealthAccountsHistorical.html

Christensen, C. M., Grossman, J. H., & Hwang, J. (2009). *Innovator's prescription: A disruptive solution for health care.* New York, NY: McGraw-Hill.

Conover, C. J. (2012). *American health economy illustrated.* Washington, DC: American Enterprise Institute.

Davis, K., Stremikis, K., Doty, M. M., & Zezza, M. A. (2012). Medicare beneficiaries less likely to experience cost- and access-related problems than adults with private coverage. *Health Affairs, 31*(8), 1–10.

Folland, S., Goodman, A., & Stano, M. (2005). *The economics of health and health care* (5th ed.). Upper Saddle River, NJ: Prentice-Hall.

Gapenski. L. C., & Pink, G. H. (2011). *Understanding healthcare financial management* (6th ed.). Chicago, IL: Health Administration Press.

Harrison, C., & Harrison, W. (2012). *Introduction to health care finance and accounting.* Clifton Park, NY: Delmar.

Henry J. Kaiser Family Foundation. (2008). *Medicare now and in the future.* Retrieved from http://kff.org/health-reform/issue-brief/medicare-now-and-in -the-future

Henry J. Kaiser Family Foundation. (2009, May). *Explaining health care reform: What are health insurance exchanges?* Retrieved from http://www.ct.gov /hix/lib/hix/kaiser_-_what_are_exchanges.pdf

Henry J. Kaiser Family Foundation. (n.d.). *National health expenditures per capita, 1960–2010* [Slides]. PowerPoint file retrieved from http://kaiserfamily foundation.files.wordpress.com/2013/04/health-spending-trends-and-impacts -health-costs-0510121.pptx

Jennings, J. (2012). *The reinventors: How extraordinary companies pursue radical continuous change.* New York, NY: Penguin Group.

Kaiser Commission on Medicaid and the Uninsured. (2013). *Medicaid: A primer: Key information on the nation's health coverage program for low income people.* Retrieved from http://kaiserfamilyfoundation.files.wordpress.com/2010/06 /7334-05.pdf

Klein, E. (2009, June 24). Dr. Klein's health insurance relationship advice. *Washington Post.* Retrieved from http://voices.washingtonpost.com/ezra-klein/2009 /06/dr_kleins_health_insurance_rel.html

Klemm, J. D. (2000). Medicaid spending: A brief history. *Health Care Financing Review, 22*(1), 105–112.

Lobosky, J. M. (2012). *It's enough to make you sick: The failure of American health care and a prescription for the cure.* New York, NY: Rowman & Littlefield.

McKeown, M. (2012). *Adaptability: The art of winning in an age of uncertainty.* Philadelphia, PA: Kogan Page.

Perednia, D. A. (2011). *Overhauling America's healthcare machine: Stop the bleeding and save trillions.* Upper Saddle River, NJ: FT Press.

Rosenthal, M. B., & Dudley, R. A. (2007). Pay-for-performance: Will the latest payment trend improve care? *Journal of the American Medical Association, 297*(7), 740–744.

Schimpff, S. C. (2012). *The future of health-care delivery: Why it must change and how it will affect you.* Washington, DC: Potomac Books.

Starr, P. (2011). *Remedy and reaction: The peculiar American struggle over health care reform.* New Haven, CT: Yale University Press.

Stiglitz, J. E. (2012). *The price of inequality: How today's divided society endangers our future.* New York, NY: W. W. Norton.

Topol, E. (2011). *The creative destruction of medicine: How the digital revolution will create better health care.* New York, NY: Basic Books.

CHAPTER 7

MANAGED CARE

Bernard J. Healey

There is no question that most individuals find the U.S. health care financing system difficult to understand and have become totally confused by the various methods used to pay for health care. Health care has become the largest and most expensive sector of the U.S. economy. This sector has been receiving a very large portion of the U.S. economic pie, and its share of the pie has continued to grow despite government and business attempts to restrain costs. It stands to reason that if health care is receiving a larger share of a fixed amount of money, then other sectors of the economy are receiving less. This also means that some of these increased costs of health care services are borne by those who receive the services, in terms of higher premiums, higher deductibles, and higher copayments.

Perednia (2011) argues that our current financial strategy for health care is not only unsustainable but actually poses a great threat to our freedom and our future wealth. If this system is allowed to continue, we are going to wind up sicker and poorer as individuals and as a nation and be subject to more and more government regulation. Our current financing mechanism represents an inefficient system of payment for health care services, services that are also wasteful in their utilization of scarce resources.

Many reasons for the cost escalations in health care delivery have been discussed in earlier chapters. One of the major reasons is the emphasis on increased use of technology designed to improve patient health. According to Halvorson (2009) in any other industry an increase in the use of technology increases efficiency, usually resulting in lower prices and improved quality. This has not happened in health care; in fact increased technology use in health care delivery has only increased prices, with very little improvement in quality or improved health outcomes.

LEARNING OBJECTIVES

After reading this chapter you should be able to

- Describe the development of managed health care plans in the United States.

- Understand how the various managed health care plans function.

- Identify the ways in which managed care plans attempt to reduce the utilization of health care services.

- Understand how comparative effectiveness research works.

As discussed in Chapter Six and illustrated in Figure 6.1, national health expenditures per capita over the past fifty years have continued to rise, despite efforts at managing health care costs. These costs continued to rise at a rate greater than inflation in every year. This cost escalation gained the attention of business and government in the early 1970s, prodding discussion among health policymakers about finding a method to better control the cost of U.S. health care.

Figure 7.1 shows the total health care expenditure per capita for the United States and selected other countries for 2008, making it clear that the cost for health care services is much higher in the United States than in any other country. Large increases in health care costs in this country over the years have also led to large increases in insurance premiums, and that has produced a market reaction in the form of managed health care. This concept of managed care has reached into every segment of U.S. health care delivery in an attempt to control its costs. In fact managed health care plans have become a subsystem of our health care delivery system.

Shi and Singh (2013) point out that the American health care system is divided into several subsystems of health care delivery: managed care; care for the military; care for vulnerable populations; integrated care delivery, which entails linking care providers' efforts so they all focus on patient outcomes; long-term care delivery; and public health. **Managed care** attempts to maximize efficiency in the delivery of health care services while reducing costs and has become the dominant mode of providing

managed care
A set of techniques designed to reduce the costs of health care services while improving the quality of care.

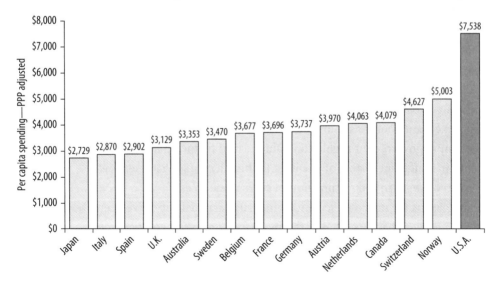

Figure 7.1   Total Health Expenditure per Capita, United States and Selected Countries, 2008

Note: PPP adjustments take into account the purchasing power of different currencies and are calculated by looking at the cost of an identical basket of goods in each currency. Data from Australia and Japan are for 2007. Figures for Belgium, Canada, the Netherlands, Norway, and Switzerland are OECD estimates.

Source: Henry J. Kaiser Family Foundation, 2011, exh. 1.

health care in this country. As discussed in more detail later, there are several types of managed care plans, including the **health maintenance organization (HMO)**, an early form of managed care developed in the U.S. northwest and also known as the prepaid group practice. A **managed care organization (MCO)** has contracts with health care providers and medical facilities to provide care for MCO members at reduced costs. These providers and facilities make up the plan's *network*. Turnock (2012) points out that managed care uses administrative controls designed to reduce costs through managing the utilization of services. The key to success in managed health care plans was seen as becoming efficient through the elimination of waste. The problem posed by this strategy was how to determine what is wasteful and who should make this determination.

Managed care plans were successful in their early attempts to reduce health care costs, although whether they have improved quality is still a matter for debate. They accomplished their objectives by reducing unnecessary hospitalizations along with pressuring providers of health care services to discount their fees. Over the years these tactics have produced a tremendous backlash from providers, government, and those covered by managed health care plans. Despite some setbacks, the concept of managed health care has been able to prove its value by producing some cost savings for a number of health plans.

health maintenance organization (HMO)
An organization that provides managed health care through certain providers for a prepaid insurance premium.

managed care organization (MCO)
An organization that has contracts with health care providers, including hospitals, to provide care for MCO members at reduced costs.

Concepts of Managed Health Care

At its introduction the concept of managed health care revolved around cost-saving applications designed to keep the costs of health insurance reasonable for the majority of Americans. This goal of affordable care has been met in most other countries through government involvement in providing or at least contracting for health services delivery for its population. People in the United States generally do not want a government-run health service sector and prefer that the market control health care delivery, including its costs.

Turnock (2012) points out that MCOs have two reasons for existing: to insure people and to manage the care those people receive. This management of health care involves controlling utilization of health care services and requires saying no to medical testing and other procedures when they will provide little or no value to the patient. This management of care also entails reducing the length of a hospital stay by again saying no to unnecessary days in the expensive inpatient setting.

The major concept behind managed health care plans is to increase efficiency and effectiveness. A more efficient health care plan will cause an increase in productivity, as measured by a reduction in the cost of health care delivery. An increase in effectiveness will enable providers to reach predetermined goals of intervention, which should entail improved health outcomes. Managed care is an attempt to run health insurance and the delivery of health care services like any other business. But this is health care, and many Americans have believed from the beginning of managed care that the provision of health care is much too important to be allowed to act completely like a business enterprise in an open market.

Phelps (2010) describes managed health care as, in part, an attempt to negate the problem of overutilization created by traditional health insurance. This is accomplished by offering the consumer a lower price for health insurance in return for allowing the insurer to constrain the consumer's choices. There are a number of strategies that managed care organizations employ with both the consumer and the provider in order to reduce the utilization of health care services and thus reduce the costs of care. Phelps (2010) argues that traditional insurance plans usually encourage overconsumption of medical care, while managed care plans usually reduce utilization of medical care, causing some inconvenience to patients or providers or both.

History of Managed Health Care

The concept of managed health care originated a century ago as a series of alternative ways to deliver health care services to certain groups of individuals. According to Kongstvedt (2012), the first HMO, in concept if not in name, was established by the Western Clinic in Tacoma, Washington, in 1910, when the clinic began to offer many medical services through its own providers at a predetermined fee of $0.50 per member per month. According to Shi and Singh (2013), it became common in the early 1900s for large businesses like railroads and mining, and lumber companies to contract for health care services directly with physicians at a flat fee per worker for a given period of time. This arrangement worked nicely for the physicians by providing them with a guaranteed stream of income and the ability to budget accurately for the costs of health care services for a given period of time.

The real innovator in managed care plans was Michael Shadid, a physician who was responsible for a type of managed care plan in Elk City, Oklahoma, in 1929. This health insurance plan offered subscribers the opportunity to pay a predetermined fee and receive health services as required. This attempt at managed care incurred tremendous opposition from other physicians for its innovative approach. In fact Shadid was penalized with the loss of his membership in the county medical society and was also threatened with the loss of his medical license. It took this trailblazing physician over twenty years to win an out-of-court settlement in his favor against the various medical societies trying to oust him.

Physicians Donald Roos and H. Clifford Loos also established a comprehensive prepaid health services delivery program in 1929, this one for the Los Angeles Department of Water and Power. This HMO included a focus on prevention and wellness and established the interest of HMOs in keeping subscribers well rather than allowing them to become ill and then seek medical care. In the long run, it was thought, an emphasis on prevention would reduce health care costs.

In 1937, physician Sidney Garfield established the Kaiser Foundation Health Plan to serve the Kaiser Construction Company, which was building an aqueduct to transport water from the Colorado River to Los Angeles. This physician turned a twelve-bed hospital into a clinic for workers. Garfield had difficulty getting paid for his services because he refused to turn away any injured or sick worker and insurance companies were slow to pay. He was finally able to make an arrangement with some insurance companies to be paid to care for all of these workers on a per capita basis at a nickel per day per worker. He also arranged for voluntary deductions from workers' salaries that covered off-the-job care for workers and their families.

This success story of prepaid health care was followed by a new venture involving care for the over 6,000 workers employed to build the Grand Coulee Dam. Garfield improved his facilities and recruited a team of doctors to work in his prepaid group practice. When the construction of the dam was completed, Garfield expanded his practice into Northern California to care for workers at the Richmond, California, shipyards. When World War II came to an end, Garfield stayed in California and in 1945 opened his clinic, now called the Permanente Health Plan, to the general public. Eventually the plan grew to over 300,000 members. In 1952, the name of the health plan was officially changed to Kaiser Permanente, because of its affiliation with the industrialist Henry Kaiser. The Kaiser Permanente HMO represents a prepaid group practice that has been operating successfully for decades and currently has well over 2 million members. The main successes of this program have been health care cost reduction and the provision of preventive health services.

Expansion of the HMO concept at the federal level is credited to physician Paul Ellwood. In 1970, Ellwood was invited to work with President Richard Nixon's staff to create a new national health policy. His idea was to give consumers a choice among health plans that would compete on price and quality. Although he did not invent the HMO model, which already existed in the form of the Kaiser Permanente health plan in California, he is credited with inventing the term *health maintenance organization*, or

HMO, to describe a plan that pays providers of comprehensive services on a per person (capitation) basis rather than a fee-for-service basis.

As Starr (2011) recounts, the Nixon administration's health strategy attempted to restrain health care costs with the use of a capitation reimbursement system for physicians. Controlling health care costs through the expansion of the HMO concept became a top priority for the Nixon reelection campaign. According to Budrys (2012), Nixon's advisors convinced him that prepaid care would result in savings on health care costs by encouraging individuals to seek health services earlier, before health problems became more complicated and therefore more costly. The country was becoming convinced that such management of health care was going to make the population healthier because of its emphasis on the prevention of disease.

Health Maintenance Organization Act of 1973

A federal law that authorized funds to support the development of HMOs for a trial period.

The **Health Maintenance Organization Act of 1973** was signed into law on December 29, 1973, and committed the federal government to a trial period of support in the development of health maintenance organizations. This act was a direct reaction to the escalation of health care costs. It authorized $375 million over a five-year period to support the development of HMOs. The federal government believed that by supporting the growth of HMOs, it would be helping to expand capitation plans to providers and reduce the use of fee-for-service payments. The intent was to create hundreds of HMOs throughout the nation, thereby stimulating competition for subscribers through cost reductions. According to Kongstvedt (2012) this act required employers with twenty-five or more employees who offered indemnity coverage to those employees to also offer two federally qualified HMOs. This action by the federal government made the HMO concept more acceptable as a form of health insurance.

Turnock (2012) describes how MCOs have moved into the publicly financed Medicare and Medicaid programs, insuring one-half of Medicaid beneficiaries and 10 percent of Medicare recipients. Managed care will become even more important as these government entitlement programs continue to grow as more baby boomers move into the Medicare program and larger numbers of poorer Americans move into the Medicaid program due to the Patient Protection and Affordable Care Act (ACA). The Medicaid program in particular has relied increasingly on managed health care to deliver and finance health care services.

Kongstvedt (2012) points out that for decades the core enrollment in Medicare managed care plans has been of low-income, minority beneficiaries, who accept a plan with fewer physician choices in exchange for paying lower health care costs. In fact the passage of the HMO Act of 1973 was a direct result of government concern about controlling the escalating cost of fee-for-service payments in Medicare. On average, Medicare covers about half of the health care costs of its enrollees. Medicare enrollees must cover the rest of the cost themselves, usually through Medicare Advantage Plans, also called Medicare Part C, which began with the passage of the Balanced Budget Act of 1997. These Medicare Advantage Plans are designed both to provide basic Medicare coverage and to fill the gaps in Medicare coverage. Most Medicare Advantage Plans are run through MCOs.

Types of Managed Care Plans

There are three main types of managed health care plans: health maintenance organizations (HMOs), preferred provider organizations (PPOs), and point of service (POS) plans. All of these managed care plans attempt to reduce utilization and to control the amount of money being paid to providers of care.

Health Maintenance Organizations

As in the days of Sidney Garfield, a health maintenance organization is a managed care plan that provides or arranges for the provision of health care services to a group of defined participants on a prepaid basis for a fixed fee. According to Starr (2011) HMOs require substantial capital investment as well as new management capacity and a new vision for physicians and patients. In order to remain solvent, an HMO needs to reduce subscribers' utilization of health care services such as hospital stays. In fact Goodman (2012) argues that HMOs encourage less health care availability to subscribers because physicians are incentivized through salary increases to reduce utilization.

There are several types of HMOs: closed-panel, staff model, group model, and open-panel. The **closed-panel HMO** is a managed care plan that has an exclusive arrangement with physicians that blocks them from seeing patients from another managed care organization. The **staff model HMO** employs providers of health care and these providers practice in common facilities. The unique feature of this model is that the insurance plan and the doctors are working together for the same employer. Physicians employed in the staff model HMO model are salaried employees who are all required to follow the same practices and procedures. The **group model HMO** contracts with a multispecialty group of physicians who agree to provide, on an exclusive basis, all the covered services for the HMO's subscribers. This type of HMO may contract with a group practice or, in some cases, actually own the group practice. The subscribers to this form of HMO usually represent a significant proportion of the group practice's patients and revenues.

closed-panel HMO
An HMO that pays only for health services provided by physicians and hospitals in its network.

staff model HMO
An HMO that employs health care providers directly, so that both insurance and care are provided by the same organization.

group model HMO
An HMO that contracts for medical services with various multispeciality groups and also with one or more hospitals.

open-panel HMO
An HMO that allows insured members to access providers outside the panel, or network, with some restrictions such as higher costs.

independent practice association (IPA)
An association that negotiates a managed care contract with an MCO for the physicians who are its members.

The **open-panel HMO** requires individual physicians to participate in the program through their membership in an independent practice association. A physician who participates in an open-panel HMO is free to see patients who are not connected with the organization and is not committed to taking on a patient simply because he or she is with the HMO. More specifically, an **independent practice association (IPA)** is a collection of independent physicians who are under contract to provide health services to a MCO at a discounted per capita rate, for a flat retainer fee, or for a negotiated fee-for-service. An IPA can negotiate capitated managed care contracts with health plans. According to Shi and Singh (2013), the IPA is involved in risk sharing with the physicians and assumes responsibility for utilization of care along with quality management. The IPA can help private physicians obtain a steady flow of income and can also help with the need to keep costs at a minimum. The IPA is usually paid a capitated amount by the HMO. Thus the IPA is really an intermediary representing a large group of physicians. According to Shi and Singh (2013), the most successful HMO model in terms of enrollment share has been the open-panel model involving an IPA.

Preferred Provider Organizations

preferred provider organization (PPO)
A health plan that contracts with providers to deliver care to plan members at a discount and also allows members to go out of network for a higher copay.

A **preferred provider organization (PPO)** is a health plan that contracts with providers to deliver care to members of the plan. The PPO has become the dominant type of managed care found in the U.S. health care system today. These plans are usually able to demand and receive greater discounts from their providers than other plans can because of very aggressive negotiations. Kongstvedt (2012) points out that PPOs most likely began in Denver, Colorado, where Samuel Jenkins negotiated hospital discounts for care in the 1970s on behalf of his company. This discount concept was expanded to include physicians, who were afraid that if they did not accept the discounts they would lose patients. Starr (2011) points out that PPO subscribers are not restricted to the network but are offered better insurance coverage if they use network providers. Greater subscriber choice was the catalyst that increased the acceptance and growth of the PPO concept.

The PPO contracts with providers for lower fees in return for inclusion in the PPO's preferred provider network. The arrangement includes a promise by the PPO to deliver a large number of patients through referrals. The subscriber is free to choose any of these network providers and is responsible for an annual deductible (the amount depends on the particular plan) along with a copayment for each visit to a provider. The copayment is higher for out-of-network providers (Shi & Singh, 2013), so the incentive to the subscriber is to choose the network preferred providers in order to reduce his or her share of the health care cost. The PPO does not involve financial risk sharing between the insurer and the provider of care, and the PPOs usually have fewer restrictions than HMOs.

The reason for the popularity of these alternatives to HMOs is twofold: the subscriber can choose his or her provider and these plans do not use gatekeepers, allowing subscribers to make appointments directly with specialists, bypassing the primary care doctor. Kongstvedt (2012) points out that over the last few years the number of PPO companies has decreased even though their overall enrollment has grown.

Point of Service Plans

A **point of service (POS) plan** combines an HMO with an indemnity insurance option that is really an open-panel HMO. Budrys (2012) points out that the POS option was created to address consumer concern about the cost of a PPO. The POS requires the subscriber to choose a primary care physician to coordinate care, but the cost will be lower than the PPO cost. This POS option may be offered by any type of HMO and generally involves allowing the subscriber to obtain covered services from providers within or outside the HMO's network. When health services are chosen outside the network, the subscriber will generally have to pay a greater portion of the cost of the service. Services provided by the plan are tightly controlled in order to control costs. However, the services can also be obtained outside the plan for an increased charge. This model, then, allows for greater consumer choice while still keeping an eye on costs through having specialist referrals handled by the primary care physician.

point of service (POS) plan
A managed care plan that allows members to determine at the point of service whether to receive care from a less expensive network provider or a more expensive out-of-network provider.

Figure 7.2 illustrates the position of PPOs as the most popular form of managed care in the United States in 2013, enrolling 57 percent of workers. Another 20 percent are enrolled in a high deductible health plan with savings option (HDHP/SO), the option being either a health reimbursement arrangement or an HSA (health savings account);14 percent are in HMOs; 9 percent are in POS plans; and fewer than 1 percent have indemnity coverage. The high deductible health plan is no longer a novelty, and entails an insurance plan with lower premiums and a very high deductible when the plan is used. The PPO is the most utilized form of managed care because the subscriber retains some choice in the provider of care.

Managed Care Utilization Control

The main goal of managed health care is to reduce the cost of health care services through some form of utilization control. This can be accomplished by reducing unnecessary health care costs through providing incentives

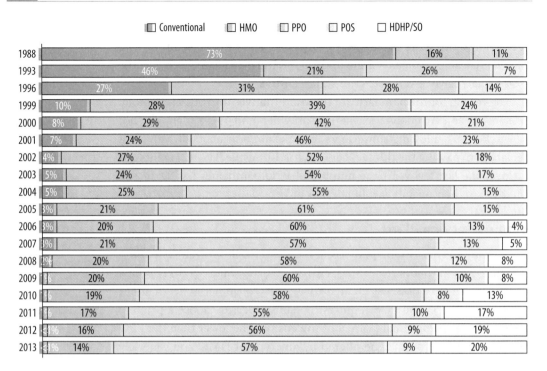

Figure 7.2 Distribution of Health Plan Enrollment for Covered Workers, by Plan Type, 1988–2013

Note: Information was not obtained for POS plans for 1988. A portion of the change in plan type enrollment for 2005 is likely attributable to incorporating more recent Census Bureau estimates of the number of state and local government workers and removing federal workers from the weights.
Source: Henry J. Kaiser Family Foundation, 2013, exh. 5.1. Data from Kaiser/HRET Survey of Employer-Sponsored Health Benefits, 1999–2013; KPMG Survey of Employer-Sponsored Health Benefits, 1993, 1996; and The Health Insurance Association of America, 1988.

for physicians and patients to select less costly forms of care. Although this seems an obvious strategy for health plan administrators to use to reduce health care costs, reducing the utilization of health care services has remained a formidable challenge for U.S. managed health care plans. The main reasons this challenge is proving so difficult are the aging of Americans, increased life expectancy, the chronic disease epidemic, increased availability of new technology, slow acceptance of prevention programs, and fee-for-service payment of providers. An MCO can attempt to reduce utilization by using medical experts who are given the responsibility of determining what services are medically necessary. This strategy can be supplemented with a concerted effort to determine how to reduce the costs associated with the provision of health care services. In order to be successful in these efforts, organizations need a constant review of the course of medical treatment.

One of the major MCO features employed to reduce physician fees is capitation. As described previously, a capitation system pays the provider a fixed amount for each subscriber for a given period of time, whether or not the subscriber uses the health services. The rate paid is dependent on the average expected utilization by the patient. For example, patients who have used greater than average amounts of health care services in the past would most likely be capitated at a higher rate.

These capitation payments are utilized by managed care plans because they place the physician at financial risk if he or she provides too many services to the plan subscribers. At the same time, in order to reduce the possibility that these physicians will provide too little care and reduce quality, MCOs measure the resource utilization of the physicians in the plan and make the results available to the public. Managed health care plans should also encourage preventive services in order to reduce the possibility of patients incurring higher health costs as they age. These capitation plans also provide bonuses or penalties for the physicians under contract, depending on the appropriateness of their resource utilization.

Table 7.1 identifies many of the factors that may decrease or increase health services utilization. The increased use of expensive technology, the aging of Americans, and the epidemic of chronic diseases explain most of the increased utilization found in the American health care system. This table also displays at least three factors that successfully reduce the utilization of care but that also require consumer involvement: a better understanding of the risk factors of disease, prevention programs to prevent disease and to change physicians' in-practice patterns to include a focus on healthy lifestyles, and changes in consumer preferences for different types of medical care.

Shi and Singh (2013) argue that one of the methods commonly used in utilization control is gatekeeping. The gatekeeper is usually a primary care physician who has the responsibility to manage the health care services that are provided to a patient who subscribes to a given health care plan. This gatekeeper has the responsibility to determine specialist referrals along with necessary testing and medical procedures. Having such a gatekeeper offers numerous advantages to both the managed care plan and its subscribers. The reduction in the utilization of expensive testing and medical procedures along with long hospital stays is an obvious advantage to the plan but may also protect the patient from unnecessary medical testing and procedures along with exposure to a possibly unnecessary and sometimes dangerous hospitalization. The other major advantage of utilizing a primary care doctor is found in the fact that having one doctor responsible for coordinating patients' care can mean better overall health care outcomes, especially when patients have multiple chronic diseases. When a patient is under the care of multiple specialists, quite often no one is paying attention to possible drug interactions and the overall health of the patient.

Table 7.1   Forces That Affect Overall Health Care Utilization

Factors That May Decrease Health Services Utilization	Factors That May Increase Health Services Utilization
Decreased supply (e.g., hospital closures, large numbers of physicians retiring)	Increased supply (e.g., ambulatory surgery centers, assisted living residences)
Public health/sanitation advances (e.g., quality standards for food and water distribution)	Growing elderly population
Better understanding of the risk factors of disease and prevention initiatives (e.g., smoking prevention programs, cholesterol-lowering drugs)	• more functional limitations associated with aging
Discovery/implementation of treatments that cure or eliminate diseases	• more illness associated with aging
Shifts to other sites of care may cause declines in utilization in the original sites:	• more deaths among the increased number of elderly (which is correlated with high utilization)
• as technology allows shifts (e.g., ambulatory surgery)	New procedures and technologies (e.g., hip replacement, stent insertion, MRI)
• as alternative sites of care become available (e.g., assisted living)	Consensus documents or guidelines that recommend increases in utilization
	New disease entities (e.g., HIV / AIDS, bioterrorism)
Payer pressures to reduce costs	New drugs, expanded use of existing drugs
Changes in practice patterns (e.g., encouraging self-care and healthy lifestyles; reduced length of hospital stay)	Increased health insurance coverage
	Consumer / employee pressures for more comprehensive insurance coverage
Changes in consumer preferences (e.g., home birthing, more self-care, alternative medicine)	Changes in practice patterns (e.g., more aggressive treatment of the elderly)
	Changes in consumer preferences and demand (e.g., cosmetic surgery, hip and knee replacements, direct marketing of drugs)

Source: Bernstein et al., 2003, tbl. 7.1.

Managed Care Quality Issues

There is not any question that health care costs are too high and need to be reduced. It is also no secret that the way to reduce these costs is through the control of health service utilization. In fact managed care plans attempt to incentivize physician behavior through the provision of bonuses if physicians restrict medical testing and procedures. It is a known fact that a great number of medical testing and procedures are useless and should be restricted. It is also known that a number of these medical testing procedures are dangerous for the patient. The problem has been how to determine a universal value for medical tests and procedures, so that both the consumer and the provider of health care services can tell when the restriction of care would be detrimental to the patient's overall health outcome.

According to Berwick, Nolan, and Whittington (2008), improvement of our system of health care delivery requires the simultaneous accomplishment of three goals (known as the *triple aim*): improving the health care experience, achieving population health, and reducing the per capita costs of health care delivery. The U.S. health care system has been unable to achieve this triple aim, even though our nation is expending over 17 percent of the largest GDP of any other country in the world on a yearly basis. These authors argue that the managed care strategy was developed to be the integrator that could successfully pursue the triple aim but that for many reasons it has not been successful in this attempt. It seems to these authors and others that managed care has become a method of managing money rather than managing care, thus failing in its attempt to improve health outcomes.

Figure 7.3 displays an overview of many of the drivers of quality, both inside and outside the health care organization, that are capable of leading to the improvement of health services delivery. It is important for managed health care plans to understand all the forces that are capable of affecting the quality of the health services they deliver. In managed care plans the consumers (subscribers) are more interested in quality and improved health outcomes than they are in costs. They also want to be equal partners in decisions regarding their health care.

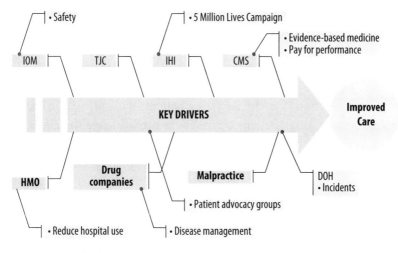

Figure 7.3 Drivers of Quality
Note: IOM = Institute of Medicine; TJC = The Joint Commission; IHI = Institute for Healthcare Improvement; CMS = Centers for Medicare & Medicaid Services; DOH = Department of Health.
Source: Dlugacz, 2009, p. 10.

Managed Care and Prevention of Disease

Turnock (2012) argues that managed care offers great opportunities for the improvement of public health in our country. Population health can be improved by the structured format an MCO imposes on the delivery of health care services, which is better than the fragmented way in which health services are delivered in other contexts. MCOs can also provide databases for public health surveillance and evaluation purposes, in order to better determine the real health care problems facing the nation.

The major premise of managed care plans has been to save money for the plan by keeping its members healthy. According to the Centers for Disease Control and Prevention (1995), MCOs usually focus their efforts on population-based medicine, attempting to achieve desired outcomes that include prevention activities. Clarke (2010) notes that managed care organizations of the 1980s and 1990s were interested in applying insurance coverage to health services that provided disease prevention and health education for their subscribers. Platt and Caldwell (2001) point out that because most of the U.S. population receives health services through managed care, these organizations have a tremendous opportunity to affect the incidence and management of infectious disease. This form of prevention involves the concept of population-based medicine. Disease prevention offers an answer to the cost escalation of health care and the less than adequate health outcomes being produced by our health care system today.

Preventive medicine offers a challenge to the traditional model of health care delivery. Clarke (2010) points out that the traditional focus of the U.S. health care delivery system has been reactive, providing services to patients only when they became symptomatic. In recent years this delivery system has slowly begun to better understand the value of proactive health care delivery and to act on that idea by seeing patients for well visits in order to prevent disease through helping them reduce high-risk health behaviors.

According to Schimpff (2012) unhealthy behaviors are responsible for 40 percent of U.S. deaths each year and 70 to 80 percent of U.S. health care costs. These unhealthy behaviors (like poor diet, sedentary lifestyle, and tobacco and alcohol use) and also stress are considered precursors to the development of chronic disease and, ultimately, complications from these diseases. Despite the enormous expense associated with chronic diseases, less than 3 percent of the total U.S. health care budget is spent on prevention programs designed to avert the development of chronic diseases and their complications. Addressing chronic diseases is of major importance in any attempt at reducing utilization of health services (Chapter Twelve is devoted to a discussion of chronic diseases).

Platt and Caldwell (2001) argue that managed care organizations offer a tremendous opportunity for improvement in the prevention and management of disease. An MCO provides services to a defined population and it has up-to-date information about this population. It can provide health promotion and it is able to make comprehensive changes in care. In many instances the MCO could resemble a public health department by delivering population-based medicine and encouraging its members to use preventive health care services.

The recent passage of the ACA has prioritized the role of prevention in lowering the cost of health care. Clark (2010) notes that several sections of this new law deal specifically with wellness issues, offering proof that the U.S. Congress and the president recognize the value of prevention in the reform of the American health care system.

According to Field (2005) the increased life expectancy of many Americans is becoming one of the greatest challenges to face our nation. Many aging Americans are developing one or more chronic diseases and the associated complications. The only effective answer to this threat is population-based prevention of chronic diseases, rather than individual treatment. Unfortunately, this strategy will take a long time to provide benefits because many aging people are already incubating or have chronic diseases. For those who have one or more chronic diseases, education programs should be offered to help prevent disease complications as these individuals grow older.

Managed care and public health departments are both involved in providing health care services to a population. This makes them interested in the health of the population and interested in interventions that might prove able to improve the health of an entire community. Both are interested in the expansion of health education programs for the young and the old and the targeted reduction of high-risk health behaviors throughout the community. In fact many managed care plans employ the services of epidemiologists to better track the incidence and prevalence of disease in the geographic areas they cover. These health plans also have the resources necessary to develop, implement, and even more important, evaluate the successes and failures of disease prevention activities in a given community.

Comparative Effectiveness Research

In 1967, John Wennberg, currently with the Dartmouth Institute for Health Policy and Clinical Practice, began analyzing Medicare data to determine how well hospitals and physicians were performing. He and his researchers found tremendous variation in every aspect of health care delivery, even in communities serviced by academic medical centers. A basic premise of the time was that medicine was driven by science and by physicians capable of making clinical decisions based on well-established facts and theories, and that therefore medicine should be consistent in its application and practice. This is not what the data revealed.

It turned out instead that geography is a major determinant of health care utilization and therefore costs. This variation in medical practice by geography was considered to be due to a lack of evidence-based medicine. Wennberg (2010) argued that local opinions and levels of medical resources are as important to the use of medical services as the level of illness or the preferences of patients in a given area. He pointed out that if we could reduce this geographic variation, we could increase the quality and reduce the costs of health care services delivery. His research led to a renewed interest in cost-benefit and cost-effectiveness analysis, evidence-based medicine, and most recently, **comparative effectiveness research (CER)**, which is designed to inform health care decisions by providing evidence on the relative effectiveness, benefits, and harms of different treatment options. The evidence is generated from research studies that compare drugs, medical devices, tests, surgeries, or ways to deliver health care (Agency for Healthcare Research and Quality, n.d.).

comparative effectiveness research (CER)
Research into the relative effectiveness, benefits, and harms of different treatment options.

One of the major problems found in the U.S. health care delivery system has been limited information for the consumer of health care and in most cases for the provider of that care too. With limited information a great deal of medical decision making is based on anecdotal evidence, conjecture, and the personal experience of each physician. This lack of information about medical tests and procedures results in overuse of scarce health resources, medical errors, and cost escalation. The answer to this serious problem is found in the expansion of unbiased research into what medical care is best for each type of patient condition. Because this research is expensive and time consuming, it is rarely conducted in the private sector. Therefore the government needs to step in and not only conduct the research but also make certain that the research results are widely disseminated to the medical community.

The United Kingdom, which provides national health insurance for all its citizens, has set a precedent for government-conducted medical research. The National Institute for Health and Care Excellence (NICE), established in 1999, is part of the U.K.'s National Health Service (NHS). This agency has the responsibility for evaluating the clinical and cost effectiveness of medical treatments and procedures in order to determine the best medical interventions for various diseases. NICE has provided evaluations for over 100 specific technologies, 250 medical procedures, and about 60 sets of treatment guidelines. Once a device, drug, or procedure is approved by NICE, then it must be covered by the NHS.

CER represents an attempt to constrain health care costs without producing adverse effects for patients. According to the Congressional Budget Office (CBO) (2007), the evidence that supports the need for comparative effectiveness research is found in the significant differences in health care costs in different areas of the United States, differences that do not translate into higher life expectancy or improved health indices in the higher-spending areas. CER may involve comparisons of similar treatments or of different approaches to medical interventions, such as surgery versus drug treatment. It may focus on benefits and risks or on costs and benefits of each potential option. According to Mushlin and Ghomrawi (2010), research that evaluates what works and does not work well in health services delivery has been practiced for many years. In the past it has been called clinical epidemiology, health services research, and outcomes research. The secret to a successful evaluation is found in the methodology and the rigor employed by the researchers. It is interesting to note that when common medical interventions are thoroughly evaluated, it is often discovered that not only do they add little or no benefit but they may actually be dangerous for the patient. The CBO (2007) points out that currently, while some information about the effectiveness of many medical interventions like new drugs, medical devices, and medical procedures is usually available, in-depth evaluations that compare different treatment options are less common. Of course, when only limited research information is available, then medical decision making is forced to revert to anecdotal evidence, conjecture, and the experience of the physician.

MCOs have attempted to restrain health care costs for decades with only limited success. Schimpff (2012) points out that health care costs represented 5 percent of gross domestic product (GDP) in 1960, 12 percent of GDP in 1990, and 17.9 percent of GDP in 2012, and are predicted to reach 20 percent of GDP in 2020. Health care costs are not only increasing at a rapid rate but are becoming a much larger part of everything we produce as a nation. Health care costs continued to rise even with the addition and expansion of managed health care plans. In some ways it seems that managed health care has actually helped health care costs to increase, despite its emphasis on reducing health care costs. This has happened because screening tests are getting more and more expensive, and for many individuals their costs are far greater than their benefits.

Because the federal government is so heavily involved in paying for health care services for many Americans, it also has an enormous interest in containing these costs. In fact about half of overall health spending in this country is publically financed. According to the CBO (2007) there is currently very little evidence available to indicate which treatments work best for which patients. It is difficult if not impossible to answer the question of whether expensive services provide benefits that are worth their costs, yet our health care system uses these treatments without rigorous evaluation of the value of the interventions and, most important, the safety of the interventions.

The latest attempt at controlling these costs is found in Title VIII of the American Recovery and Reinvestment Act of 2009. This act includes money for comparative effectiveness research. Mushlin and Ghomrawi (2010) point out that this research is meant to help us determine the individual tests and treatments that work best so we can improve our health care system. Unfortunately, very few people understand the concept of CER and what this process can accomplish if done properly. In fact many individuals believe that CER is the starting point for the federal government to stop paying for expensive treatments with only marginal benefits.

In 2009, the Institute of Medicine (IOM) published this definition of CER, which is widely used and which also addresses the purpose of this research: CER is "the generation and synthesis of evidence that compares the benefits and harms of alternative methods to prevent, diagnose, treat and monitor a clinical condition or to improve the delivery of care. The purpose of CER is to assist consumers, clinicians, purchasers, and policy makers to make informed decisions that will improve health care at both the individual and population levels" (p. 1).

Future of Managed Health Care

There's no question that the delivery of health care services in our country must be better managed. This can only be accomplished through collaborative efforts involving health policy experts, businesses, government, and the consumer. According to Alpert (2013) the wealth wasted in health care is beyond belief, averaging thirty cents of every health care dollar spent. This wasted money is going to unneeded procedures, excessive overhead, and many other expenditures that produce no improved health for the individual. This waste represents hundreds of billions of dollars that is being taken away from other government and personal expenditures that could result in real value for our population. Making matters worse is the fact that some of these wasteful expenditures pay for tests and medical procedures that are actually dangerous for the patient. The answer to this problem lies in the reduction of the utilization of health services that have little if any value in the improvement of health outcomes. Managed health care seems to offer a very good start toward solving the health care cost disease, but more intervention is required.

The concept of managed health care is a workable strategy but it requires additional components before it can reduce wasteful utilization of scarce and expensive health care resources while also improving the quality of health services. A vision of how to reduce costs and improve health care outcomes has been put forth by John Torinus in his book *The Company That Solved Health Care*. According to Torinus (2010), reform of the U.S. health care system needs to be supported by these three pillars: consumer responsibility, centers of value, and a primary role for primary care. These pillars need to become part of managed health care plans.

Consumer Responsibility

If managed health care plans are to reduce health care costs while improving health care outcomes, the consumer has to become an active decision maker in his or her own medical care. Without that decision making, there will be no solution to our health care challenges. The best way to involve the consumer in health care decision making is to offer improved incentives along with consumer education.

Many of the monetary incentives are already in place, with the consumer paying a larger part of his or her health care bill every year. Because most consumers no longer consider health care services to be free goods, they are now much more interested in the price and the value of health care services. Although it is unfortunate that health care costs had to rise to such a great extent to get patients' attention, that cost escalation has changed the patient into a price-sensitive consumer of health care services. These consumers are now interested in shopping around for value in their health care purchases, just as they do when they purchase other goods and services. What is now needed is the availability of consumer education about health care services, allowing the consumer to become a real decision maker in the purchasing and consuming process.

Centers of Value

The businesses of our country have to be able to purchase health services from companies that continuously deliver value-based health care. Unfortunately, in the process of focusing on cost, sometimes necessary but expensive medical care that would improve the long-term outcome for some patients gets eliminated. The concept of centers of value includes health care insurance plans that offer cost-effective care that also improves health outcomes. These health care plans will focus their attention and resources on providing value to their subscribers while achieving predetermined health outcomes for every subscriber. Torinus (2010) defines value as the ideal combination of service, quality, and price. The recipients of health care services who get this kind of value will receive improved health outcomes from their care providers. For physicians and patients to achieve these improved outcomes, quality indices must be readily available and understood by the consumer of the care.

Torinus (2010) points out that many approaches have been tried to improve the U.S. system of care while controlling costs. For the most part these ideas have not had very much success, and in many cases health costs continued to rise while the quality of the product being delivered diminished. These flaws can be corrected through increased transparency that allows the patient to become an informed consumer of health care services.

Prime Role for Primary Care

Primary health care delivery and primary care physicians have to be the central components of our health care delivery system. In many cases MCOs have already established the primary care physician as the gatekeeper of health care services for plan subscribers. The primary care physician has the capability to add wellness, prevention, and chronic disease management to the medical care of each patient, thereby reducing the costs of health care delivery and at the same time improving the patient's health outcomes.

Torinus (2010) points out that companies that have given primary care physicians a central role in their health insurance plans have reduced their overall health care costs by one-third. Reliance on specialists rather than primary care doctors increases health costs while fragmenting the care of patients, especially those with one or more chronic diseases. Schimpff (2012) observes that the United States does not have enough primary care providers to provide quality health care while reducing the enormous cost of those services. We have a glut of specialists and a severe shortage of primary care physicians. We need to reverse these numbers in order to improve health care outcomes at a sustainable cost. Berwick et al. (2008) point out that political barriers have replaced the technical barriers that were present for attempts to achieve the triple aim goals. These barriers have to be removed so managed health care in the United States can continue to reduce health care costs and still retain a strong focus on the improvement of the health of our population.

SUMMARY

The U.S. health care system has become the largest and most expensive sector of the U.S. economy, demanding more and more of our GDP every year with no change in sight. This increased cost of health care services is not sustainable in the long run, requiring our nation to make tough decisions about the utilization of health care services. It was determined by health policymakers that managed care plans that linked health services and health financing would reduce utilization of health services while also improving the quality of those services. These MCOs were designed to reduce the quantity of health care services consumed and also to restrict the amount being paid to the providers of care.

The first MCOs were established in the early 1900s, and MCOs began to expand shortly after the establishment of the Medicare and Medicaid programs and the passage of the Health Maintenance Organization Act of 1973. They continued their growth thanks to federal support throughout the 1980s and 1990s. In the beginning they were very successful at reducing the utilization of health care services and restricting payments to providers of health care. However, these successes resulted in a tremendous backlash from subscribers, providers, and government.

There are many ways that utilization of expensive health care services can be reduced. It seems obvious that if we can devise methods to keep people well, the use of services will be reduced. Along with this greater emphasis on prevention, the use of comparative effectiveness research can help patients and providers to make better decisions concerning the use of expensive services that may produce low value for the patient.

Some businesses are now becoming proactive in their attempts to reduce the utilization of health care services by giving consumers responsibility for their health care, creating centers of value for improved outcomes, and making primary care physicians gatekeepers for health care services.

KEY TERMS

closed-panel HMO

comparative effectiveness research (CER)

group model HMO

health maintenance organization (HMO)

Health Maintenance Organization Act of 1973

independent practice association (IPA)

managed care

managed care organization (MCO)

open-panel HMO

point of service (POS) plan

preferred provider organization (PPO)

staff model HMO

DISCUSSION QUESTIONS

1. What are the major reasons for cost escalation in health services delivery over the last fifty years?

2. What are the major types of managed health care plans being used in our country today? How would you describe each of them?

3. How does comparative effectiveness research work?

4. Will the increased use of primary care physicians along with the increased use of prevention programs reduce the cost of health care delivery in the United States?

REFERENCES

Agency for Healthcare Research and Quality. (n.d.). What is comparative effectiveness research. Retrieved from http://effectivehealthcare.ahrq.gov/index.cfm/what-is-comparative-effectiveness-research1

Alpert, D. (2013). *The age of oversupply: Overcoming the greatest challenge to the global economy*. New York, NY: Penguin Group.

Bernstein, A. B., Hing, E., Moss, A. J., Allen, K. F., Siller, A. B., & Tiggle, R. B. (2003). *Healthcare in America: Trends in utilization*. Hyattsville, MD: National Center for Health Statistics.

Berwick, D. M., Nolan, T. W., & Whittington, J. (2008). The triple aim: Care, health and cost. *Health Affairs, 27*(3), 759–769.

Budrys, G. (2012). *Our unsystematic healthcare system* (3rd ed.). New York, NY: Rowman & Littlefield.

Centers for Disease Control and Prevention. (1995). Prevention and managed care: Opportunities for managed care organizations, purchasers of health care, and public health agencies. *Morbidity and Mortality Weekly Report, 44*(RR-14), 1–12.

Clarke, J. (2010). Preventive medicine: A ready solution for a healthcare system in crisis. *Population Health Management, 13*(10), S-3–S-11.

Congressional Budget Office. (2007). *Research on the comparative effectiveness of medical treatments*. Retrieved from http://www.healthpolicyfellows.org/pdfs/CBO12-18-2007ComparativeEffectiveness.pdf

Dlugacz, Y. D. (2009). *Value-based health care*. San Francisco, CA: Jossey Bass.

Field, R. (2005). Introduction. The future of public health: What will it take to keep Americans healthy and safe? *Managed Care, 14*(9 Suppl.).

Goodman, J. C. (2012). *Priceless: Curing the healthcare crisis*. Oakland, CA: The Independent Institute.

Halvorson, G. (2009). *Health care will not reform itself*. New York, NY: CRC Press.

Henry J. Kaiser Family Foundation. (2011, April 12). *Snapshots: Health care spending in the United States & selected OECD countries.* Retrieved from http://kff.org/health-costs/issue-brief/snapshots-health-care-spending-in-the -united-states-selected-oecd-countries

Henry J. Kaiser Family Foundation. (2013, August 20). *2013 Employer Health Benefits Survey.* Retrieved from http://kff.org/report-section/ehbs-2013-section-5

Institute of Medicine. (2009). *Initial national priorities for comparative effectiveness research.* Washington, DC: Author.

Kongstvedt, P. R. (2012). *Essentials of managed care* (6th ed.). Burlington, MA: Jones & Bartlett Learning.

Mushlin, A. I., & Ghomrawi, H. M. K. (2010). Comparative effectiveness research: A cornerstone of healthcare reform? *Transactions of the American Clinical and Climatological Association, 121,* 141–145.

Perednia, D. A. (2011). *Overhauling America's healthcare machine: Stop the bleeding and save trillions.* Upper Saddle River, NJ: FT Press.

Phelps, C. E. (2010). *Health economics* (4th ed.). New York, NY: Addison-Wesley.

Platt, R., & Caldwell, B. (2001). Can managed healthcare help manage health care–associated infections? *Emerging Infectious Diseases, 7*(2), 358–362.

Schimpff, S. C. (2012). *The future of health-care delivery: Why it must change and how it will affect you.* Washington, DC: Potomac Books.

Shi, L., & Singh, D. A. (2013). *Essentials of the U.S. health care system* (3rd ed.). Burlington, MA: Jones & Bartlett Learning.

Starr, P. (2011). *Remedy and reaction: The peculiar American struggle over health care reform.* New Haven, CT: Yale University Press.

Torinus, J. (2010). *The company that solved health care.* Dallas, TX: BenBella Books.

Turnock, B. J. (2012). *Public health: What it is and how it works* (5th ed.). Burlington, MA: Jones & Bartlett Learning.

Wennberg, J. E. (2010). *Tracking medicine: A researcher's quest to understand health care.* New York, NY: Oxford University Press.

CHAPTER 8

LONG-TERM CARE

Tina Marie Evans

As advances in public health, medical technology, and pharmaceuticals continue, the life expectancy of Americans continues to increase to unprecedented numbers. This has led to a rapidly growing elderly population that will likely need assistance with personal and medical care. This proliferation of older persons is not unique to U.S. society; it is a demographic change that is currently taking place around the world but particularly in industrialized nations. The current societies in these nations are the first to experience such large numbers of elderly. Although some elderly people will enjoy continued good health despite their advancing age, many will experience debilitating illnesses that require supportive care.

Long-term care refers to a wide range of medical and social services that are necessary to accommodate persons with functional disabilities. Persons served by long-term care may be of any age, with conditions such as "birth defects, spinal cord injuries, mental impairment, or other chronic debilitating conditions—but most often they are the very elderly whose ability to function independently is deteriorating" (Raffel & Barsukiewicz, 2002, p. 151). This type of extended care may be provided either in the home or in residential facilities, and is generally quite expensive. Individuals' potential need for long-term care services rises greatly after age sixty-five and then continues to increase throughout the lifespan (Figure 8.1). Given the sharp increases that are forecast in the numbers of older Americans, it is important to consider the needs of this rapidly growing population now. The long-term care system in the United States has evolved significantly in the past few decades and now offers a greater diversity of settings as well as

LEARNING OBJECTIVES

After you read this chapter you should be able to

- Articulate the reasons why Americans are now enjoying longer life expectancies.

- Discuss how the aging of the population will affect the future of the health care system.

- Explain the highlights of the history of long-term care in the United States.

- Describe the three categories of long-term care services, including their settings and typical patients or clients.

- Explain the common methods of payment for long-term care services.

- Discuss the most common chronic conditions that affect Americans, including how many people they affect.

- Articulate each of the five challenges facing long-term care in the near future.

long-term care
Medical care and social services that accommodate persons with functional disabilities.

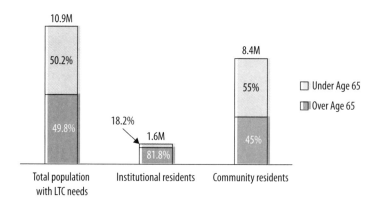

Figure 8.1 People with Long-Term Care (LTC) Needs

Source: Kaiser Commission on Medicaid and the Uninsured [KCMU], 2012, fig. 1. Data from 2007 American Community Survey and the 2005 Survey of Income and Program Participation.

specialized care options, but there are further challenges it must address to be well prepared to serve the elderly and meet their long-term care needs (Olson, 1994).

The Aging of Americans

In a recent study, the population of *older Americans* (persons aged sixty-five years and older) numbered 40.2 million. This represents 13.1 percent of the U.S. population—or just over one out of every eight Americans. The number of older Americans is growing significantly, and has increased by 5.4 million (or 15.3%) since the year 2000—which is a very high and disproportionate rate of growth when compared to the increase in the numbers of the under sixty-five population in the same time period (8.7%). Given these numbers, it is also important to recognize that the number of Americans who are aged forty-five to sixty-four (and who will all reach age sixty-five at various times within the next two decades) has increased by 31 percent during the same period.

Breaking these data down further by gender reveals that there were 23.0 million older women and 17.5 million older men, or a gender ratio of 132 women for every 100 men. This ratio of women to men has been shown to only increase further with age, ranging from 112 to 100 for the sixty-five to sixty-nine age group to a high of 206 to 100 for women eighty-five and over (U.S. Department of Health and Human Services [HHS], Administration on Aging, 2011).

Historically, since the year 1900, the percentage of Americans aged sixty-five years and over has more than tripled (from 4.1% in 1900 to 13.1% in 2010), and the actual number of persons in the country has grown by almost thirteen times (from 3.1 million to 40.4 million). Approximately 2.6 million Americans celebrated their sixty-fifth birthday in the year 2010, while in the same year, almost 1.8 million persons aged sixty-five or older died. The figures for 2010 illustrate a net population increase in older persons of 814,406 in only one year. An additional factor that contributes to the growing number of older Americans is that the death rates of the older population are decreasing—especially for men (HHS, Administration on Aging, 2011). This is due to a massive rise in life expectancy that is clearly one of humanity's crowning achievements as, after 200,000 years of no or very slow increases in life expectancy, a remarkable shift in the numbers has occurred. Many of the extrinsic causes of death (such as accidents, infectious diseases, and contagious conditions) that once commonly took the lives of many people in their early years of life have been dramatically reduced thanks to magnificent advances in public health, medical technology, and pharmaceuticals. The once common outbreaks of highly lethal infectious diseases are now under control, which has greatly enhanced survival rates and contributed to increased life expectancy (Binstock & George, 2011). In addition, new life-sustaining measures as well as an increased emphasis on preventive care and healthy lifestyles have contributed to the increase in the population of older Americans (Sultz & Young, 2009).

Table 8.1 shows current trends in life expectancy. For the total population, life expectancy at birth increased from 70.8 years in 1970 to 78.3 years in 2010. A person who reached the age of 65 in 2009 can expect to live (on average) another 18.8 years. More specifically, males who reached 65 in 2009 can expect to live another 17.3 years and females another 20.0 years. As life expectancy has increased, it has also changed the meaning of chronological age—some now consider 75 to be the new 65! Looking at the 2009 data regarding children, an infant born in 2009 can expect to live (on average) 78.2 years—mostly due to the lower death rates in children and adolescents resulting from technological and public health advances (HHS, Administration on Aging, 2011).

Another factor to consider in painting a current picture of the aging of Americans is that our older population (as a whole) is becoming increasingly older. In the year 2010, the sixty-five to seventy-four age group (20.8 million persons) was ten times larger than it was back in the year 1900. More surprisingly, the seventy-five to eighty-four age group (13.1 million persons) was found to be seventeen times larger and the eighty-five and older age group (with 5.5 million persons) was forty-five times larger than in the year 1900. Furthermore, the United States is also observing a wonderful increase in the number of centenarians (persons who live to or beyond the age of one hundred years). In 2010, there were 53,364 centenarians, which

Table 8.1   Life Expectancies at Birth, 1970–2007, and Projections, 2010–2020

Year	Total			White			Black		
	Total	Male	Female	Total	Male	Female	Total	Male	Female
1970· · · · · · · · · · · · · ·	70.8	67.1	74.7	71.7	68.0	75.6	64.1	60.0	68.3
1980· · · · · · · · · · · · · ·	73.7	70.0	77.4	74.4	70.7	78.1	68.1	63.8	72.5
1981· · · · · · · · · · · · · ·	74.1	70.4	77.8	74.8	71.1	78.4	68.9	64.5	73.2
1982· · · · · · · · · · · · · ·	74.5	70.8	78.1	75.1	71.5	78.7	69.4	65.1	73.6
1983· · · · · · · · · · · · · ·	74.6	71.0	78.1	75.2	71.6	78.7	69.4	65.2	73.5
1984· · · · · · · · · · · · · ·	74.7	71.1	78.2	75.3	71.8	78.7	69.5	65.3	73.6
1985· · · · · · · · · · · · · ·	74.7	71.1	78.2	75.3	71.8	78.7	69.3	65.0	73.4
1986· · · · · · · · · · · · · ·	74.7	71.2	78.2	75.4	71.9	78.8	69.1	64.8	73.4
1987· · · · · · · · · · · · · ·	74.9	71.4	78.3	75.6	72.1	78.9	69.1	64.7	73.4
1988· · · · · · · · · · · · · ·	74.9	71.4	78.3	75.6	72.2	78.9	68.9	64.4	73.2
1989· · · · · · · · · · · · · ·	75.1	71.7	78.5	75.9	72.5	79.2	68.8	64.3	73.3
1990· · · · · · · · · · · · · ·	75.4	71.8	78.8	76.1	72.7	79.4	69.1	64.5	73.6
1991· · · · · · · · · · · · · ·	75.5	72.0	78.9	76.3	72.9	79.6	69.3	64.6	73.8
1992· · · · · · · · · · · · · ·	75.8	72.3	79.1	76.5	73.2	79.8	69.6	65.0	73.9
1993· · · · · · · · · · · · · ·	75.5	72.2	78.8	76.3	73.1	79.5	69.2	64.6	73.7
1994· · · · · · · · · · · · · ·	75.7	72.4	79.0	76.5	73.3	79.6	69.5	64.9	73.9
1995· · · · · · · · · · · · · ·	75.8	72.5	78.9	76.5	73.4	79.6	69.6	65.2	73.9
1996· · · · · · · · · · · · · ·	76.1	73.1	79.1	76.8	73.9	79.7	70.2	66.1	74.2
1997· · · · · · · · · · · · · ·	76.5	73.6	79.4	77.2	74.3	79.9	71.1	67.2	74.7
1998· · · · · · · · · · · · · ·	76.7	73.8	79.5	77.3	74.5	80.0	71.3	67.6	74.8
1999· · · · · · · · · · · · · ·	76.7	73.9	79.4	77.3	74.6	79.9	71.4	67.8	74.7
2000 [1]· · · · · · · · · · · · · ·	76.8	74.1	79.3	77.3	74.7	79.9	71.8	68.2	75.1
2001 [1]· · · · · · · · · · · · · ·	76.9	74.2	79.4	77.4	74.8	79.9	72.0	68.4	75.2
2002 [1]· · · · · · · · · · · · · ·	76.9	74.3	79.5	77.4	74.9	79.9	72.1	68.6	75.4
2003 [1,2]· · · · · · · · · · ·	77.1	74.5	79.6	77.6	75.0	80.0	72.3	68.8	75.6
2004 [1,2]· · · · · · · · · · ·	77.5	74.9	79.9	77.9	75.4	80.4	72.8	69.3	76.0
2005 [1,2]· · · · · · · · · · ·	77.4	74.9	79.9	77.9	75.4	80.4	72.8	69.3	76.1
2006 [1,2]· · · · · · · · · · ·	77.7	75.1	80.2	78.2	75.7	80.6	73.2	69.7	76.5
2007 [1,2]· · · · · · · · · · ·	77.9	75.4	80.4	78.4	75.9	80.8	73.6	70.0	76.8
Projections: [3]									
2010· · · · · · · · · · · · · ·	78.3	75.7	80.8	78.9	76.5	81.3	73.8	70.2	77.2
2015· · · · · · · · · · · · · ·	78.9	76.4	81.4	79.5	77.1	81.8	75.0	71.4	78.2
2020· · · · · · · · · · · · · ·	79.5	77.1	81.9	80.0	77.7	82.4	76.1	72.6	79.2

[1] Life expectancies for 2000–2007 were calculated using a revised methodology and may differ from those previously published.
[2] Multiple-race data were reported by 25 states and the District of Columbia in 2006, by 21 states and the District of Columbia in 2005, by 15 states in 2004, and by 7 states in 2003. The multiple-race data for these reporting areas were bridged to the single-race categories of the 1977 OMB standards for comparability with other reporting areas.
[3] Based on middle mortality assumptions.
Source: U.S. Census Bureau, 2011, tbl. 102. Except as noted, data are from the National Center for Health Statistics, 2010.

is much higher than the 1990 number of 37,306—a 43 percent increase in only twenty years' time (HHS, Administration on Aging, 2011).

Currently, it is predicted that the population of older Americans will continue to grow significantly in coming decades (Figure 8.2). This growth did slow a bit in the 1990s due to the smaller number of infants born during the Great Depression years of the 1930s. However, the elderly population will flourish between 2010 and 2030, the period when the "baby boom" generation will reach age sixty-five. What kind of growth are we likely to see? The number of persons aged sixty-five and over increased from approximately 35 million in 2000 to 40.2 million in 2010 (a 15% increase). It is projected to rise to approximately 54.6 million by 2020 (a 36% increase for the 2010 to 2020 decade). Looking forward to the year 2030, there will be approximately 71.5 million older persons in the United States, more than twice as many as in the year 2000. Considering these projections in relation to the projections for the total U.S. population, we find that persons sixty-five and over made up 13.1 percent of the total population in 2010 but are forecast to grow to 19.3 percent of the total population by 2030. In addition, persons in the age group of eighty-five and older are projected to increase from a total of 5.5 million in 2010 to 6.6 million in 2020—a noteworthy 19 percent increase for that decade (HHS, Administration on Aging, 2011).

Although some older persons will enjoy excellent health into their later years and will have the benefit of supportive family and friends as caregivers, this country must be prepared to assist in the long-term care of its older citizens. Let's begin this preparation by reviewing the history and evolution of long-term care services in the United States.

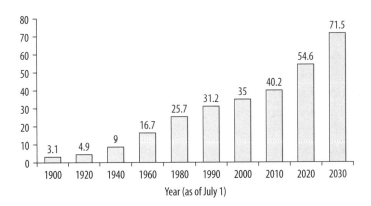

Figure 8.2 Number of People Aged Sixty-Five-Plus, 1900–2030 (in millions)

Source: HHS, Administration on Aging, 2011, p. 5.

History of Long-Term Care

The earliest models of long-term care can be traced to the first colonists who emigrated from Europe to the New World, bringing with them many of the traditional social values and ideals commonly accepted in their native countries. One of these models, the **almshouse**, was a communal living setting where the sick, the disabled, or the aged who lacked good family support and/or adequate financial means could be cared for by the community. It was relatively common for philanthropic members of the community to purchase private homes and convert them to almshouses that would serve the needs of this special segment of the population needing supportive care. Some municipalities and county governments, too, opened homes and infirmaries to care for older adults who were living in poverty (Sultz & Young, 2009). Others who were accepted into the almshouses were the mentally ill, the mentally challenged, and alcoholics—persons who were often cast off by society and had nowhere else to go. Generally, the care in the almshouses was minimal, as they were run on charity and very meager local government appropriations. Food, shelter, and clothing were provided, and those who were able to work were expected to help out in the home to defray the costs of their care (Raffel & Barsukiewicz, 2002).

almshouse
A group living setting in which the sick, disabled, and aged who lacked adequate family support and/or financial means were cared for by the community.

These early models of long-term care services that were rooted in European traditions were the basis of *elder homes*, which existed until the severe economic devastation caused by the Great Depression. The effects of the Great Depression on the economy and the financial means of people living in those times greatly affected the availability of long-term care services, particularly in the setting of the elder homes. Once the Great Depression hit, many charitable individuals and agencies could no longer afford to continue providing free care to the elderly and the poor (Sultz & Young, 2009).

As the economy continued to struggle, the difficulties in providing adequate care to impoverished older Americans led the federal government to become involved in developing, overseeing, and paying for long-term care services as part of early social welfare reforms. One example of this involvement was the passage of the **Social Security Act of 1935**, which provides financial assistance to older Americans and to persons with disabilities. The Social Security Act also created a form of old age and survivors insurance, which let working persons and their employers put money into a fund that would be set aside to supplement retirement income. This fund gave people some income stability as they aged, and the number of impoverished older persons decreased. The income from Social Security also increased the amount that older Americans could spend on the medical and assistive services that are typically needed later in life

Social Security Act of 1935
Legislation that provides financial assistance to older Americans and persons with disabilities.

(Sultz & Young, 2009). Despite this fund, many health care professionals and civic leaders were concerned about how the provision of quality care in the elder homes over time could be sustained if the homes were depending primarily on income derived from welfare recipients.

In 1948, Congress amended the Hill-Burton Act to make construction grants and lending programs available to public and nonprofit organizations to encourage the development of the more modern forms of nursing homes that we are familiar with today. For-profit proprietary facilities were slow to catch on at that time, but they grew quickly in numbers once Medicare and Medicaid came into effect in 1965. Unfortunately, even after the advent of Medicare and Medicaid, many homes when reviewing applications for admission clearly gave preference to private applicants rather than those on public assistance, regardless of an applicant's level of need for care. It was also common for facilities to have long waiting lists for the admission of Medicare and Medicaid clients, particularly those who needed the highest levels of care (and were therefore likely to be the most costly to care for) (Raffel & Barsukiewicz, 2002).

Today the steady development of the modern-day nursing home continues. The distribution of public, for-profit, and nonprofit nursing homes continues to shift, however; the numbers show that for-profit organizations are now clearly dominant. The need for additional skilled nursing beds in nursing homes has been known for some years now, and this remains a point of concern. Our population is aging and living longer, and increasing numbers of people are searching for (or soon will be searching for) higher levels of care as age-related disabilities surface. Additional related concerns are that, over time, family units have become smaller, the divorce rate has risen, and all able-bodied adults in a family are more commonly working—situations that frequently do not allow a family member to be home to care for today's elderly (Raffel & Barsukiewicz, 2002), thus sparking the need for continued expansion of residential, long-term care facilities. Of course, in cases where a family member is willing to assist in the care of an elderly or disabled person in his or her home, home health care services are another option. The ability to remain in one's home and "age in place" is now an option cherished by most elders.

Historically, the earliest home care agencies were visiting nurse agencies, which were established in the late 1800s to provide elder care in communities that did not have hospitals. Home health care services in the United States were slow to catch on through the years, but they have greatly expanded since the 1980s and now include many types of medical and social services (Raffel & Barsukiewicz, 2002). More recently, this sector of the health care industry has also gone through a period of growth as cost-effectiveness initiatives imposed by managed care organizations have led many individuals and their families to explore home care services as a less costly alternative to inpatient nursing or hospital care. In many cases home care services can minimize the need for admission to acute care or long-term care skilled nursing facilities. The cost containment pressure from payers combined with the request of many older people to age in place and enjoy their home surroundings as long as possible has made this a very popular form of long-term care. As of 2007, more than 1 million men and women sixty-five and older were receiving home health care services each day. The high demand for these services has led to an expansion of the number of home health care agencies in the United States—a number that has now surpassed the 20,000 mark, with over 80 percent of these operating on a for-profit basis, and total yearly expenditures on home health care amounting to more than $34.5 billion (Jones, Harris-Kojetin, & Valverde, 2012).

Organization of Long-Term Care

One of the most critical challenges for long-term care in the United States is that a single, organized, formal delivery system does not exist. Family members and friends of the home health care client typically provide a significant portion of the long-term care and search for additional services within the community as they are needed (Williams & Torrens, 2008). Ideally, the delivery system for long-term care services should provide its clients with access to a seamless continuum of comprehensive personal, social, and medical care services. This system should contain programs to guide and chart individual clients' needs over time, and carefully match the level of care (whether increasing or decreasing) to specific needs across the time of service. Most clients require a complex mix of services in a variety of settings, which must be expected to change over time as each client's needs and health status change.

It is hoped that the external community services in each case will be available to complement the basic caregiving services provided by the family members and friends of the client. According to Williams and Torrens (2008, p. 202), a well-organized system of long-term care does the following:

- Matches resources to the client's health and family circumstance.
- Monitors the client's condition, and changes services as needs change.
- Coordinates the care of many professionals and disciplines.
- Integrates care provided in a range of settings.
- Enhances efficiency, reduces duplication, and streamlines client flow.

- Pools or otherwise arranges financing so that services are based on need, rather than narrow eligibility criteria.

- Maintains a comprehensive record incorporating clinical, financial, and utilization data.

Some clients will have contact with the formal long-term care system for only a brief time, whereas some will need an extended level of care over a period of many years. Regardless of the length of time or the complexity of services required, the system must strive to provide all forms of needed support while fostering the independence of the client and the client's family. The cost effectiveness of care must be taken into account, too, as the costs associated with individual long-term care settings and services will vary greatly. Currently, over sixty different services are available to clients within the continuum of long-term care. These are commonly grouped into seven categories (Williams & Torrens, 2008), as displayed in Table 8.2.

When studying the overall organization of long-term care delivery, it should be noted that long-term care programs are commonly categorized in terms of the site of care delivery. The U.S. health care system currently recognizes three distinct categories of long-term care: care provided by institutional providers, care provided by community-based residential care facilities, and care provided at home and through community-based services. The remainder of this section will examine the characteristics of each of these categories and their service options more closely. As reflected here, persons needing long-term care services are typically referred to as *clients* rather than *patients*, and persons needing institutional residential care services are correctly referred to as *residents*.

Institutional providers offer long-term care services within an institution, such as a skilled care nursing home, assisted-living facility, rehabilitation hospital, intermediate care facility, long-term psychiatric hospital, or inpatient hospice facility, as well as the long-term care units of some acute care hospitals (Institute of Medicine, 2001; Sultz & Young, 2009). Although many seniors prefer to remain in their homes instead of moving to a residential care facility, some may only be able to receive proper care if they are admitted to a residential facility that can correctly manage their condition. Many skilled care nursing facilities provide a home-like environment with respectable levels of quality care while keeping the residents both socially and physically active to the best of their capabilities (Matthews, 2010).

Recent estimates indicate that over 1.6 million Americans are residing in skilled nursing facilities. This number may seem high, but it is not surprising as we know that almost one out of every three women and one out of every five men over the age of sixty-five will spend at least some time

institutional providers
Care settings such as skilled nursing homes, assisted-living facilities, rehabilitation hospitals, intermediate care facilities, long-term psychiatric hospitals, and inpatient hospice care facilities.

Table 8.2   Categories and Services in the Care Continuum

Acute care
Consultation services
Interdisciplinary assessment teams
Medical or surgical inpatient services
Psychiatric acute inpatient services
Short-term rehabilitation inpatient services

Extended care
Skilled nursing facilities
Assisted-living facilities
Adult family homes
Substance abuse or detox and care facilities
Congregate care facilities
Group homes
Step-down or transitional care units
Swing beds
Intermediate care—mental retardation
Psychiatric care—residential

Ambulatory care
Solo physician practices
Group physician practices
Hospital emergency departments
Centers for same-day surgery
Diagnostic imaging centers
Endoscopy centers
Hospital-based outpatient clinics
Community health clinics
Physical and/or occupational therapy clinics
School health services
College or university health centers
Prison health services
Family planning clinics
Women's health care centers
Childbirth centers
Renal dialysis centers
Oncology centers
Lithotripsy centers
Cosmetic surgery centers

Migrant health centers
Veterans' health system or military health
    services
Industrial clinics
Vision services
Hearing services
Dental services
Medical laboratories
Mental health services
Poison control centers
Community-sponsored hotlines
Telephone or email communications with
    providers

Home care
Home health care services (nursing, therapy)
Home hospice (adult and pediatric)
Durable medical equipment
Home visit personnel
Homemaker assistance
Personal care assistance
In-home caregivers

Outreach
Online consultations
Community information and referrals
Telephone contacts
Screenings
Emergency response systems
Transportation services
Mail-order pharmacies
Meals on Wheels
Senior services programs
Needle exchange programs
Family planning services
Substance abuse services
Support groups

in a skilled nursing home. On the brighter side, most of these residential stays are relatively short (Matthews, 2010):

- Approximately 60 percent of all stays in skilled nursing facilities are for less than three months; this figure includes people who are admitted directly from hospitals to recover from surgery or serious illness.

+ Approximately 75 percent of all stays in nursing homes are for one year or less.

+ Approximately 8 percent of residents stay in a nursing home for three years or longer.

The skilled nursing home segment of the long-term care industry in the United States clearly remains the dominant setting, with expenditures for this care being more than double those for home health care services. Nevertheless, despite the growing number of elderly Americans, the occupancy rates of skilled nursing facilities are declining, which may be attributed in part to the fact that today's elderly are generally healthier than those of past generations. Today's elderly may also be taking advantage of other options that now exist, such as assisted-living arrangements rather than residential skilled nursing care, or the option of receiving services through a community-based organization or home care agency. The majority of skilled nursing facility residents are elderly females with some degree of cognitive impairment (Sultz & Young, 2009). Some skilled nursing facilities offer specialized units to serve the particular needs of residents with a common diagnosis, such as Alzheimer's disease or dementia, or units designed to serve the postoperative or subacute therapeutic needs of residents discharged from hospitals (Institute of Medicine, 2001).

In most skilled care nursing facilities, a team of educated health care professionals come together to provide the needed services. This team commonly includes a physician (as medical director), a nursing home administrator, a nursing director, and a minimum of one registered nurse on each of the day and evening shifts, as well as several other supporting nurses on each shift. The nurses work together to provide custodial care to the residents, including distributing medications; administering medical treatments; assisting with bathing, dressing, and transferring; and also monitoring residents' overall health and social status. Most skilled care facilities also employ additional professional staff members who provide in-house physical therapy, occupational therapy, speech therapy, recreational therapy, nutritional counseling, spiritual direction, and social work services. Other supportive staff complete the picture of caring for the personal needs of the residents by preparing meals, doing housekeeping and cleaning, providing laundry services, and looking after building maintenance needs (Sultz & Young, 2009).

In contrast to the skilled care nursing facilities, **assisted-living facilities** provide long-term care for residents who are not in need of high-level skilled nursing services but rather need supportive and custodial forms of care. Residential facilities such as adult homes, board homes, and specialty

assisted-living facilities
Residential facilities for individuals who need supportive and custodial care but not high-level nursing services.

centers for persons with moderate to severe levels of mental illness or mental disability fall into this category of institutional providers. In other words, custodial care is needed, but the assisted-living residents' day-to-day medical and assistive care needs are not as great as those of the residents of skilled nursing care. The elderly residents of assisted-living facilities are generally healthy even though they have limited abilities to perform necessary self-care activities and housekeeping duties. In addition to supervisory services, these facilities commonly provide congregate meals, medication administration, and some assistance with personal care, as well as scheduled communal recreation and spiritual activities (Sultz & Young, 2009).

As mentioned earlier, recent estimates indicate that the number of assisted-living facilities in the United States is about 20,000, with over 1 million people housed in this setting. The size of assisted-living facilities varies greatly, from small buildings with only a few residents to large complexes that house several hundred residents at a time (Sultz & Young, 2009). Managers in this care setting strive to provide certain aspects of the nursing services seen in the skilled nursing facilities, while the residents live as independently as possible in a more home-like setting where many of the desirable features of home life can be preserved (Institute of Medicine, 2001).

The second long-term care category is made up of **community-based residential care facilities**. It includes a number of settings that provide varying levels of supervision and assistance: private efficiency apartments, wardlike settings containing multiple beds, both licensed and unlicensed personal care homes offering nonprofessional supervision, and licensed group homes employing professionals who are skilled in supervising and in assisting people to live as independently as possible (Institute of Medicine, 2001).

community-based residential care facilities

Settings for people who need personal supervision and assistance in living as independently as possible.

Community-based residential care homes have long been major providers of shelter as well as limited amounts of nursing and supervisory services. They may be referred to as board-and-care homes, group homes, sheltered care facilities, rest homes, or congregate living facilities. Regardless of the title used, the facilities in this category provide protective supervision to residents with functional limitations such as mental retardation, developmental disabilities, mental illness, and/or significant physical disabilities. Nearly three-quarters of persons with chronic mental illness live in these types of care facilities, where a trained staff of professionals can care for their daily needs. The other major group making use of these facilities consists of older individuals who need basic levels of custodial supervision, low levels of medical care, and light assistance with completing their activities of daily living. Compared to the residents living in skilled care nursing homes, the residents of community-based residential care homes are generally less impaired and are fairly physically functional yet are unable or unwilling to live independently in their own homes (Institute of Medicine, 2001). Residents of these homes are usually there for the long term (months or years) rather than being in residence temporarily to recover from acute conditions or surgery (Matthews, 2010).

Most community-based residential care homes provide three meals per day, medication storage and administration, organized social activities, recreational activities, transportation services, and money management assistance (Institute of Medicine, 2001). They generally do not provide skilled nursing care services, physical therapy, or other types of medical care. Depending on the design of the facility, many offer single rooms, shared rooms, and small apartment-style accommodations. On average, these homes contain about fifty-three beds, with many facilities choosing to employ and house one or more professional care providers on the property to assist with twenty-four-hour supervision of the residents. The cost of living in these homes varies greatly by region of the country, but many states offer a State Supplemental Payment in addition to the federal Supplemental Security Income that funds most of the residents (Institute of Medicine, 2001). This category of long-term care is indeed essential in supporting the guided independence of persons who would otherwise be unable to live alone safely.

The **home and community-based services** category of long-term care includes services such as home health care, hospice care, nonmedical personal care assistance, adult day care, adult night care, and **respite care** (short-term or temporary), and also includes agencies that provide durable medical equipment to home users (Institute of Medicine, 2001). The common factor is that these are all nonresidential long-term care services.

As noted previously in Chapter Five, home health care services are available to clients and their families who need assistance with maintaining or restoring a person's health and independence or at least minimizing the effects of injury, disability, or illness. Depending on the specific needs of the client, home care services can be a long-term form of care for a person who is chronically ill (thereby avoiding institutionalization) or a short-term form of care for a person discharged from a hospital following acute illness or surgery. Home care agencies are able to provide a wide range of medical, therapeutic, and also nonmedical services in the home (Jones et al., 2012), thereby allowing clients to return home much sooner than they could without these services (Jonas, 2003). If nonmedical services (nonprofessional assistance with cleaning, laundry, bill payment, meals, etc.) are required, many home health agencies can also provide staff members or local volunteers to assist with these duties. Additionally, the staff of

home and community-based services
Services such as home health care, hospice care, nonmedical personal care, adult day care, adult night care, respite care, and provision of durable medical equipment.

respite care
Temporary caregiving to give short-term relief to caregivers for family members.

home health agencies can arrange for various forms of durable medical equipment (walkers, wheelchairs, specialized beds, transfer benches, etc.) to be delivered to the home and set up for use. These devices may be either rented or purchased, depending on the expected period of need, and are important aids in preserving clients' independence and allowing them to remain in the home setting as long as possible (Williams & Torrens, 2008).

Basic medical and personal care assistance services are the core provisions of all home health care agencies; however, many agencies have now expanded their service offerings by employing professionals who are trained in collecting blood and urine specimens; taking radiographs and giving electrocardiograms; providing physical therapy, speech therapy, or occupational therapy; and offering mental health counseling and social work services. Some agencies also hire nurse practitioners, advanced practice nurses, enterostomal therapists, and clinical pharmacy consultants to increase their capability for more sophisticated levels of care. Additional advanced services such as intravenous therapies and ventilator support, which in the past were only available in an inpatient setting, may now take place in the comfort and familiar surroundings of the client's home (Fiebach, Kern, Thomas, & Ziegelstein, 2007).

When a long-term care client is terminally ill, home hospice services are the most appropriate form of care. Hospice teams are interdisciplinary and highly skilled in managing pain, alleviating emotional distress, promoting comfort and peace in the home, handling spiritual issues, and preserving the independence of the terminally ill client. Hospice care also tends to the needs of the dying client's family members, typically offering counseling services, spiritual support, respite care as needed, and finally, bereavement support (Sultz & Young, 2009). Additional information on hospice care can be found in Chapter Five.

Adult day and night care services are forms of nonresidential, short-term, supervised care. Such services can give the primary caregiver of the client (likely a spouse or child) necessary respite time or sufficient time to maintain employment, care for their own medical needs, and so forth. In these cases, the client is brought to the adult care center, where a few hours of supervised activities or rest can be provided in the absence of the primary caregiver. Some hospitals and skilled care nursing homes also provide a limited amount of temporary overnight care when caregiver relief is necessary. This type of long-term care prevents premature institutionalization of clients by giving caregivers time to attend to their own needs while the clients are protected in a setting appropriate to their level of need. It has been recently estimated that there are over 4,000 adult care centers accepting clients in the United States, with many more centers needed to meet the continuing level of demand for adult care services. Nonprofit organizations are the dominant owners of these centers, operating approximately 80 percent of them (Sultz & Young, 2009).

In-home temporary care is also an option for caregivers who need respite or other time away from the client. In the 1970s, some home care agencies began providing in-home adult care or respite care by sending a nurse or companion to supervise and assist the client in the home. In cases where extensive custodial home care is needed, it is common for families and friends to become stressed and feel overwhelmed by the burden of care over time. This form of temporary respite care allows a break from the caregiver role to tend to the needs of life. The length of the respite care varies from a few hours to overnight to a few days; however, it is meant to be short-term and intermittent care only. Although this helpful alternative form of caregiver services is available in most areas of the country, the prohibitive factor for many families is cost, as reimbursement for this type of service has been very slow to catch on. Respite caregivers may be professional staff members or nonprofessional volunteers, largely depending on the level of a client's needs. These reliable surrogate caregivers are truly helpful in facilitating home care of clients, offering a welcome benefit to both clients and family caregivers (Sultz & Young, 2009).

Considerable variation exists within these three major categories of long-term care services across the states and regions of the country. Not all clients will use every type of service, but the ideal goal is to make all services available and also accessible to any person who has a need for them. There is no set order for using these services, since clients and caregivers choose the ones that they and their physician believe are most appropriate for addressing varying needs over time. In addition, long-term care services also cover a great range in the levels of care provided, levels of staff training and certifications, facility accreditations, and costs and types of reimbursement and financing. This great variation in types of services and settings creates a considerable challenge for health care managers who work to coordinate the needed services, as well as for those who pay for the care (Williams & Torrens, 2008). Optimally, a high level of consistent communication and collaboration between care providers, clients or residents, and families will facilitate seamless transitions among the necessary services.

Payment for Long-Term Care Services

As of 2011, over 10 million Americans needed some type of long-term care services to facilitate their activities of daily living. As mentioned earlier in this chapter, the demand for long-term care services will grow significantly owing to the aging of the population and the growing number of persons, including many with chronic conditions, who are living longer. As the demand for long-term care services grows, we will see an increase in the portion of the population turning to paid care services to fulfill their medical as well as their nonmedical needs (Kaiser Commission on Medicaid and the Uninsured [KCMU], 2011). Several payers are involved in the financing of long-term care services (Figure 8.3). The source of payment has a significant influence on long-term care services, as the industry relies heavily on government funding and is thus affected by varying levels of federal and state appropriations as well as any changes in government policies regarding coverage of services (Institute of Medicine, 2001).

Surprisingly, individuals who need long-term care often pay for large portions of this care themselves. If the need for long-term care continues for months or years, services paid for out of one's pocket can easily deplete the financial resources of all but the wealthiest of persons. For example, if a person is a resident in a skilled care nursing facility, the "average annual cost per resident for private pay residents for a single room is $70,912; the average annual cost per resident for a semiprivate room totals $62,532" (Sultz & Young, 2009, p. 292). Most elderly Americans simply do not have the financial resources (such as funds in checking accounts, savings accounts, IRAs, etc.) that would afford them that level of residential skilled nursing care for more than a few weeks or months (KCMU, 2011). In fact recent statistics indicate that only about one-third of elderly persons have enough monetary resources to pay for a year or more of skilled nursing home care. Further, it is shocking to comprehend that another

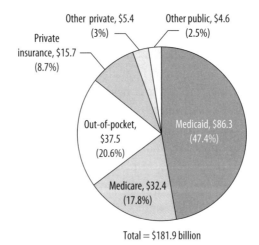

Total = $181.9 billion

Figure 8.3 National Spending on Long-Term Care, 2003 (in billions)

Source: KCMU, 2005, fig. 4. Based on Congressional Research Service analysis of data from the National Health Accounts, CMS. Includes unpublished data from CMS on Medicare and Medicaid expenditures for hospital-based nursing home and home health care, and data from Medicaid expenditures under home and community-based services waivers.

one-third of elderly persons have such severely limited financial resources (defined as savings of less than $5,000) that they could not pay for even one month of such care. If we look specifically at the group who are at highest risk of needing skilled care nursing home placement (persons over the age of eighty-five with no spouse and some functional or cognitive limitation), typical financial resources are even more limited. Two-thirds of the persons in this highest-risk group have less than $5,000 to put toward their care. If we examine a different type of consumer group, such as cases where the necessary long-term care services are for a child or a nonelderly disabled adult, the high cost of care would still impoverish most of today's middle-class American families.

Nevertheless, a large percentage of elderly skilled care nursing home residents (44%) are using their own monetary resources to pay for their long-term care. This significant financial contribution amounts to $37.5 billion paid out-of-pocket, or approximately 21 percent of the total amount of spending on long-term care services (Henry J. Kaiser Family Foundation, 2005). The reason for this is that although Medicare offers health insurance benefits to most elderly as well as some disabled persons, that insurance covers only a very limited and well-defined amount of skilled nursing services. The coverage for skilled nursing and home health care services under Medicare is closely associated with a person's need for acute care services. Currently, Medicare will pay for the first 100 days of skilled nursing facility care for a recently hospitalized person, but only if that person has a prognosis of improvement or recovery (Williams & Torrens, 2008). Home health care benefits are also strictly limited under Medicare, with personal care services being covered only when a homebound client needs skilled professional services (such as nursing and rehabilitative therapies) (KCMU, 2011). Despite these limitations, benefits paid by Medicare, Medicaid, and private insurance providers for in-home durable medical equipment are relatively good (Williams & Torrens, 2008). When it comes to respite services, however, the Medicare and Medicaid programs have offered little help. Many respite care programs have been able to offer their services only because of federal grant support for defined medical conditions; however, most payers who could choose to fund respite care have denied it, saying that the care meets a social need of the caregiver, rather than a medical need of the client. This view began to change in 2003, when work began on the **Lifespan Respite Care Act** in an effort to create and fund additional respite care programs. With clear evidence that respite care programs offer much value and significant cost savings by postponing and/or avoiding costly institutionalizations, bipartisan support helped to see this act signed into law in late 2006. This landmark piece of legislation authorized $289 million in state grant funding over a period of five years to encourage the

Lifespan Respite Care Act

Federal legislation that increases the availability and coordination of respite care services for caregivers.

development of respite programs, while making a clear public statement in support of the value of care provided by families in the home (Sultz & Young, 2009).

Returning to the issue of paying for skilled nursing home care, Medicaid, which does cover long-term care, is an option only to persons who have low incomes or who have become impoverished through paying out-of-pocket for their long-term care needs. The strict, state-defined eligibility rules of Medicaid require persons needing long-term care services to "spend down" the majority of their savings and to continue contributing the vast majority of their income (except for a small allowance to cover personal items) toward paying for care. Persons who are fortunate enough to have some financial means must first have spent their savings on their care and must fall below the state-defined resource thresholds before Medicaid coverage becomes an option for them. In light of the data regarding the financial means of most elderly persons, it is easy to see how common it is for many of them to have already spent their retirement savings supporting themselves in their retirement years and also paying for any needed community-based care services. Because of this, many seniors are or will quickly become financially destitute and likely eligible for Medicaid once admitted to a skilled care nursing home. Sadly, many elderly individuals in the United States find this requirement of spending down their assets to be both frightening and demeaning. This prospect continues to cause a considerable number of the elderly to avoid long-term care services—even when their financial means put them close to or at levels that would make them eligible for Medicaid (Henry J. Kaiser Family Foundation, 2005).

Out-of-pocket payments for skilled nursing home care are also high because most private health insurance plans currently play a very small role in paying for long-term care, and most plans' coverage options for long-term care services are extremely limited. Americans have the option to purchase private long-term care insurance; however, many of the available policies are rather expensive and are therefore unaffordable for many low- and middle-income individuals and families. Over time, the potential market of buyers has come to recognize that the available policies are largely unaffordable for many older people, and that the benefits offered under the policies do not give adequate protections against future risks and likely needs. This is an area of concern in which public health may choose to play a future role in advocating for subsidies of long-term care policies to better prepare people for this potential area of need. Yet another complicating factor is that many who apply for private long-term care insurance are turned down by insurers because of existing medical conditions that raise their risk of requiring long-term care in the future (Henry J. Kaiser Family Foundation, 2005).

Despite the barrier to qualifying for Medicaid, this program has over time developed into the central payer for long-term care services in the United States (Figure 8.4). Currently, Medicaid supports the cost of about 40 percent of the long-term care services being provided. The combined federal and state appropriations for the Medicaid program are critical for covering the broad range of services necessary for older Americans to either live independently with assistance or to be residentially cared for with dignity and respect. Medicaid remains the country's long-term care safety net for the poor as well as for those who become impoverished by spending down their assets on needed care. At least for the near future, Medicaid will remain the principal system of financing for the majority of long-term care services (KCMU, 2014). But it is also important to recognize that the annual Medicaid expenditures for long-term care continue to rise significantly, from $93 billion in 2002 to $125 billion in 2011 (Figure 8.5).

There remains the concern that the current fragmented system of financing long-term care may continue to cause a fragmented system of care, especially when eligibility criteria are strict, variable between states, and/or dependent on the variability of appropriations. Ideally, the pooling and integrating of the financial resources for long-term care should be considered in the future, so that neither the amount of care needed nor the restrictions on payments would block any individuals from getting the appropriate level of care to manage their needs across time (Williams & Torrens, 2008).

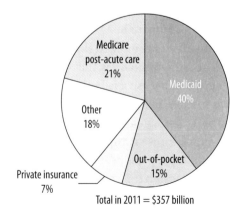

Figure 8.4 Medicaid Is the Primary Payer for Long-Term Care Services

Note: Total long-term care expenditures include spending on residential care facilities, nursing homes, home health services, and home and community-based waiver services. All home and community-based waivers are attributed to Medicaid.

Source: KCMU, 2014, fig. 1. Data are KCMU estimates based on CMS National Health Expenditure Accounts data for 2011.

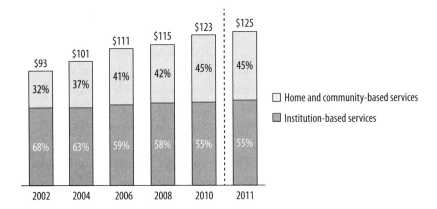

Figure 8.5 Growth in Medicaid Long-Term Care Services and Supports Expenditures, 2002–2011 (in billions)

Note: Home and community-based care includes state plan home health, state plan personal care services and §1915(c) HCBS waivers. Institutional care includes intermediate care facilities for individuals with intellectual/developmental disabilities, nursing facilities, and mental health facilities.
Source: KCMU, 2014, fig. 2. Based on KCMU and Urban Institute analysis of CMS-64 data.

Chronic Diseases and Their Complications

Recent data give us clear evidence that chronic illnesses account for 70 percent of deaths in the United States and for over 75 percent of direct health care costs. Besides high rates of mortality, chronic disease results in direct costs of over $1.5 trillion, with additional indirect costs (from lost productivity and nonreimbursed personal costs) adding several more hundreds of billions of dollars to this total each year (Thrall, 2005). Chronic diseases and their complications also increase the tendency toward frailty, falls, and delirium, the unfortunate but likely end result of many chronic diseases and age-related factors combined (Fiebach et al., 2007).

Chronic diseases and the disabilities that are inherent with them are prevalent among older persons, especially those in the higher age groups. Although older persons are generally healthier today than were older persons of decades past, the aging of the population and the extended lifespans of Americans will present the health care system with a higher number of frail and debilitated persons needing care than in past decades. Arthritic conditions, cardiac-related conditions (both cardiovascular and cerebrovascular), high blood pressure, diabetes, and osteoporosis are common among the elderly and tend to become more severe with increasing age (Olson, 1994). Population studies indicate that approximately 80 percent of older Americans have one chronic health condition, 50 percent have at least two chronic conditions (Centers for Disease Control and Prevention [CDC], 2011a), and about 33 percent suffer from four or more chronic health conditions (Berenson & Horvath, 2003). This equates to over 90 million Americans living with one chronic disease and 39 million living with more than one such condition—with 25 million Americans suffering from a chronic condition that is undoubtedly disabling (Thrall, 2005). Let's take a look at current data regarding the prevalence of some common chronic diseases and their complications.

Cardiovascular disease is one of the most widespread chronic diseases, with recent data suggesting that one or more types of cardiovascular disease currently affect 64.4 million Americans. This form of chronic disease causes about 40 percent of all deaths in the United States and is a contributing factor in another 20 percent of deaths. Specifically, if we consider the prevalence of hypertension by itself (defined as having a systolic blood pressure of over 140 mmHg and/or a diastolic blood pressure of over 90 mmHg), recent estimates indicate that 50 million people in this country fall into this disease category, including about 40 percent of those over sixty-five (Fiebach et al., 2007; Thrall, 2005). Coronary heart disease affects another 13.2 million people, and usually presents either as an acute myocardial infarction or as one of the chest pain syndromes. Further, approximately 5 million Americans are living with congestive heart failure, and each year about 4.8 million suffer at least one stroke. In addition to cardiovascular disease, pulmonary diseases and conditions have many negative effects on people's lives and activities, as well as on related health care costs. Chronic pulmonary conditions affect 15 million Americans, causing substantial levels of disability (Thrall, 2005).

Obesity and diabetes remain significant in the population of older Americans. Over one-third of U.S. adults are currently obese, and the rates of adult obesity have doubled between the years 1980 and 2008. Besides the heavy cost burden that obesity places on the health care system ($147 billion), it is associated with many comorbid diseases and health concerns, including coronary heart disease, stroke, high blood pressure, type 2 diabetes, cancers (endometrial, breast, and colon), high total cholesterol or high levels of triglycerides, liver and gallbladder disease, sleep apnea, respiratory problems, degeneration of cartilage and osteoarthritis, reproductive health complications such as infertility, and mental health conditions (CDC, 2011c, p. 2). The statistics on diabetes in the United States are just as alarming. The most recent data indicate that 10.9 million (or 26.9%) of persons aged sixty-five and over were diabetic in 2010, at a total health care cost of $174 billion. Diabetes continues to be a leading cause of kidney failure, amputations of the lower leg, and new cases of blindness in adults, and it is clearly a major cause of both heart disease and stroke (CDC, 2011b).

Osteoarthritis is another category of chronic disease that frequently has devastating effects on the lives and activities of the elderly. It is estimated that almost half of Americans over the age of sixty-five have osteoarthritis (Fiebach et al., 2007), which translates to between 50 million and 70 million people. Disability caused by osteoarthritis and back pain continues to be a significant problem, with these chronic conditions being the cause of over one-third of the nonmental illness–related disabilities in persons over the age of fifteen. With people living longer now than in past decades, it is expected that the number of Americans living with some form of documented chronic osteoarthritis will increase even further by the year 2020 (Thrall, 2005). In fact past studies of aging have found that the "incidence of dependency in the performance of basic activities of daily living, such as eating, bathing, toileting, dressing and getting out of bed doubles with each successive age group until about 75; after that, the prevalence of dependency triples" (Olson, 1994, p. 27). This well-studied and documented increase in osteoarthritis-related dependency has implications not only for the substantial number of people with osteoarthritis but also for the level of demand on the long-term care system in future years.

The next chronic diseases and conditions to consider are those that involve the loss of sight or of hearing, abilities important to living independently. Currently, over 2.9 million people in this country are dealing with visual impairments. National studies have shown that loss of vision is associated with higher rates of other chronic health conditions; of depression, falls and fall-related injuries, and social isolation (which prevents people from enjoying time with family and friends); and of death. Visual impairments cost a total of $8.3 billion per year in direct medical expenses for the over sixty-five age group alone, and are a major factor in restricting individuals' activities of daily living such as driving, watching television, reading, or the handling of bills and personal accounts (CDC, 2011d). Recent data on hearing impairments indicate that 33.9 percent of men and 20.7 percent of women in the over seventy age group have impaired hearing, which translates to approximately one in four older Americans. As people age the incidence of blindness, hearing loss, or other sensory impairments grows. Consequently, these prevalence rates will also rise in light of the longer life expectancies that Americans now experience (Dillon, Gu, Hoffman, & Ko, 2010).

The final category of common chronic diseases that affect the utilization of long-term care consists of neurodegenerative diseases. As people age the rates of chronic neurodegenerative diseases increase as well. These conditions can be difficult to diagnose correctly, but their symptoms not only affect the person with the disease but have a significant impact on his or her family and loved ones as well. Parkinson's disease (which causes tremors, difficulty with movement, and loss of balance and coordination) affects approximately 1.5 million people in the United States annually

(Thrall, 2005), and is a common cause of disability and therefore the need for long-term care services. Alzheimer's disease is another neurodegenerative disease that usually leads individuals (of varying ages) to seek out long-term care services. Alzheimer's disease is the most common form of dementia in older Americans, affecting 5.4 million people in this country. It is a disease of the brain that damages thoughts, memories, and language and thus gravely affects the ability to carry out activities of daily living. Over time, individuals with Alzheimer's disease lose the ability to remember and reason, which is confusing to them and devastating in its effects on families and friends. The number of people living with this disease has doubled since 1980 and is expected to continue to rise, to approximately 16 million by the year 2050 (Hebert, Scherr, Bienias, Bennett, & Evans, 2003). The incidence of Alzheimer's disease increases greatly in proportion to age, with rates of approximately 1 percent per year in populations aged sixty to sixty-five, and 6.5 percent per year in the eighty-five and older age group (Fiebach et al., 2007).

Regardless of the specific chronic disease or condition involved, certain well-known risk factors raise a person's likelihood of needing long-term care (National Clearinghouse for Long-Term Care Information, 2012):

- Age—the older a person gets, the more likely it is that long-term care will be needed.

- Living alone—persons who live alone are more likely to need paid care at some point than are those who are married or those who are single but living with a partner or friend.

- Gender—women tend to live longer than men (on average, 2.2 years longer), therefore women are likely to require a longer period of long-term care (on average, 3.7 years longer), compared to men.

- Lifestyle—persons who make poor choices in regard to modifiable health risk factors (lack of physical activity, poor nutrition, tobacco use, and excessive alcohol consumption) are more likely to need long-term care, as these behaviors have been shown to cause much of the chronic disease that leads to debilitation and premature death.

- Personal history—those with relevant health and family history have an increased chance of requiring long-term care services.

The prevention of chronic diseases, and thereby their complications, is truly a key component in keeping older Americans healthy. It is necessary for all individuals to become more educated about and more active in preventing chronic disease. As the Centers for Disease Control and Prevention reminds us, poor health does not have to be a direct consequence of the aging process. If we encourage and guide older adults to consistently practice healthy behaviors, regularly seek clinical preventive services, and continue to engage socially with family and friends, they are more likely to enjoy a continued state of good health and live more independently—and thus incur fewer health-related expenses (CDC, 2011a). All stakeholders in the U.S. health care system—including those who receive care, their families, health care providers, health care managers, payers, the general public, and the government—must now recognize the growing imperative of preventing the devastating human and financial consequences of chronic disease. We must come together to design better structures for accessible, lifelong continuity of care, with significant emphasis on disease preventions and evidence-based practice (Thrall, 2005).

Challenges for Long-Term Care in the Future

The complex and diverse programs and services that make up long-term care have evolved greatly throughout the years, and will continue to evolve as the demographics of the U.S. population change. It is certain that this country will need to have more long-term care services in all settings available in the near future. The long-term care delivery system is currently facing five particular challenges:

1. *The aging of the population.* Concern about the aging of the population and the forecasted number of people likely requiring long-term care cannot be understated. According to the National Clearinghouse for Long-Term Care Information, approximately 70 percent of people over the age of sixty-five will require some type of long-term care in their lifetimes. For more than 40 percent of these people, that care will occur in a skilled care nursing home setting. It is clear that the combination of an aging population and longer life expectancies will increase the demand for all forms of long-term care services in the decades to come. Additional concerns are the trends showing smaller family sizes, higher rates of divorce, and higher costs for the provision of care to a family member. These are factors with the potential to reduce the amount of informal care available to the elderly from family and friends.

2. *The staffing shortages in the health care workforce.* The demand for long-term care is predicted to exceed the supply of trained professionals who are qualified to deliver the needed services, which will lead to severe workforce shortages of 30 percent or more. This shortage of health care professionals has already begun in some areas of the country, as there are not enough qualified applicants to fill open positions for direct caregivers to the elderly. Historically, long-term care workers have been paid less than

workers in acute health care settings, and this is a factor in the shortage of workers in the long-term care system. The rapid employee turnover that is common in some long-term care settings also contributes to less than adequate staffing levels and compromises quality of care. Nurses and other long-term care professional staff members need a more competitive wage, opportunities for continuing education, and better working conditions than they have been receiving if the significant rate of turnover is to be reduced. Long-term care providers work in a difficult setting, as they must provide care for multiple clients with various medical conditions and disabilities to manage and also navigate the difficult family dynamics that often come with working in this setting. Low wages, stressful conditions due to inadequate staffing and frequent turnover, lack of benefits, lack of social support (child-care assistance, transportation), minimal job security, and high personal injury rates are the main problems that must be resolved to raise job satisfaction and increase employee retention (Sultz & Young, 2009). Additionally, long-term care facilities must begin acting now to attract additional health care personnel into their settings—possibly by offering a more competitive wage and attractive benefits, by partnering with educational institutions that train nurses and other needed professionals, or by assisting with educational scholarships and/or offering signing bonuses.

3. *The overall quality of care.* As long-term care settings have evolved, so has the need for quality care. Care for our most vulnerable population must be of the utmost quality, client-centered, responsive, efficient, accessible, and cost effective. The quality of care provided varies greatly from facility to facility at this time. Research to clearly define and update the overall outcomes that are necessary and desired in long-term care is needed. Additionally, studies should compare the quality of care and the outcomes of care across the various long-term care settings. Once clearly stated outcomes for this industry are developed, instruments to measure and benchmark the progress (or lack thereof) in long-term care can be created and put to good use. Only then can we begin to brainstorm the types of changes to the system that might lead to advances in rehabilitative care and also maintenance and custodial care. Best practices in each setting should be published and shared to promote the best types of care possible for Americans in their last phase of life. Finally, the gaps in the Medicaid long-term care safety net need to be addressed, as the quality of the safety net varies greatly from state to state. Eligibility for services and benefits is limited in many states, and not all will qualify for monetary waivers to assist with the cost of care. This, too, must be studied so that quality care is available to all, and the gaps in the safety net closed.

4. *The integration of services.* In the past few decades the long-term care delivery system has diversified its offerings and facilities have specialized in some areas of care. This kind of diversification and specialty care carries an inherent danger of fragmentation of care, duplication of services, and attempts to push clients into narrow categories of services (Sultz & Young, 2009). There is a great need to turn our attention to the coordination and better integration of services for those who receive services in one setting then move on to another setting over time. Payers and policy advocates must ensure that incentives, such as higher payments tied to faster discharges and the like, do not cause further splits in the optimal continuum of care. Pressure from competition between providers and facilities often prevents partnerships from forming that could greatly benefit the future of collaborative and seamlessly provided long-term care services. Care must be taken to create a smooth transition, in terms of both physical provisions and financial coverage, for people leaving one long-term care setting and entering another.

5. *Financing the cost of care.* It appears that state and federal governments (acting through Medicaid and, at a lesser level, Medicare programs) will continue to finance the majority of future long-term care services. In particular the burden on Medicaid will increase sharply in the next few decades, given rising health care costs, the aging of the population, and the growing demand for long-term care services. The net increase in pressure on Medicaid and other payers is going to be difficult to handle, and state budgets will carry a heavy burden of the long-term care spending that will be necessary to cover the needed services (Henry J. Kaiser Family Foundation, 2005). Public policy has a difficult question to face here: Should public funding to the states be increased to cover the services, or should more of the responsibility be transferred to private individuals, thereby lessening the burden on the government? This question is particularly concerning as a shift in the tax base is also forecast because the proportion of older individuals to working adults will change from one in five as of 2002, to one in three by the year 2025. The final part of addressing this challenge will be the consideration of policies and incentives to improve the market for purchasing private long-term care insurance and the affordability of that insurance. Incentives (such as tax credits) to purchase private long-term care insurance and/or to promote informal caregiving systems of family and friends who actively look after those close to them might alleviate some of the financial burden on the public sector as well.

SUMMARY

Long-term care refers to a broad range of medical and social service options that are available to meet the needs and compensate for the functional disabilities of persons of any age, but this care most commonly serves the elderly who can no longer function independently. The evolution and specialization of residential, community-based, and home health care services will continue. The aging of the population, rising rates of chronic disease, longer life expectancies, and advances in public health and medical technology will result in unprecedented numbers of people requiring long-term care services in the near future—even as a shortage of health care personnel is occurring. The health care industry must begin to work now to reduce the fragmentation that exists both in the continuum of long-term care services and in the system of payment for those services. Health care managers must stay current on and attentive to data trends, be prepared to quickly expand current programs, and collaborate with other care providers within their communities, and thereby be ready to serve an even greater number of people by providing seamless care that is accessible, effective, efficient, and affordable.

KEY TERMS

almshouse

assisted-living facilities

community-based residential care
    facilities

home and community-based
    services

institutional providers

Lifespan Respite Care Act

long-term care

respite care

Social Security Act of 1935

DISCUSSION QUESTIONS

1. What are the population trends in terms of life expectancies and the total number of older persons in the United States?

2. What are the categories of long-term care, and what types of services are offered in each category?

3. What are the various possibilities for public and private payment of long-term care services?

4. Which chronic diseases are likely to affect the number of persons needing long-term care in the near future?

5. What major challenges are currently facing the long-term care industry?

6. What steps could the health care industry take now to be better prepared for the increasing need for long-term care?

REFERENCES

Berenson, R. A., & Horvath, J. (2003, January–June). Confronting the barriers to chronic care management in Medicare. *Health Affairs* (Suppl. Web Exclusives), W3-37–53.

Binstock, R. H., & George, L. K. (2011). *Handbook of aging and the social sciences* (7th ed.). Burlington, MA: Elsevier/Academic Press.

Centers for Disease Control and Prevention. (2011a). *Healthy aging: Helping people to live long and productive lives and enjoy a good quality of life*. Retrieved from http://www.cdc.gov/chronicdisease/resources/publications/aag/pdf/2011 /Healthy_Aging_AAG_508.pdf

Centers for Disease Control and Prevention. (2011b). *National diabetes fact sheet: National estimates and general information on diabetes and prediabetes in the United States, 2011*. Atlanta, GA: Author.

Centers for Disease Control and Prevention. (2011c). *Obesity—halting the epidemic by making health easier*. Retrieved from http://www.cdc.gov/chronicdisease /resources/publications/aag/pdf/2011/Obesity_AAG_WEB_508.pdf

Centers for Disease Control and Prevention. (2011d). *The state of vision, aging, and public health in America*. Retrieved from http://www.cdc.gov/visionhealth /pdf/vision_brief.pdf

Dillon, C. F., Gu, Q., Hoffman, H., & Ko, C. W. (2010). *Vision, hearing, balance, and sensory impairment in Americans aged 70 years and over: United States, 1999–2006* (NCHS data brief, no 31). Hyattsville, MD: National Center for Health Statistics.

Fiebach, N. H., Kern, D. E., Thomas, P. A., & Ziegelstein, R. C. (Eds.). (2007). *Principles of ambulatory medicine* (7th ed.). Philadelphia, PA: Lippincott, Williams and Wilkins.

Hebert, L. E., Scherr, P. A., Bienias, J. L., Bennett, D. A., & Evans, D. A. (2003). Alzheimer's disease in the U.S. population: Prevalence estimates using the 2000 census. *Archives of Neurology, 60*(8), 1119–1122.

Henry J. Kaiser Family Foundation. (2005). *Long-term care: Understanding Medicaid's role for the elderly and disabled*. Retrieved from http://www.kff .org/medicaid/upload/long-term-care-understanding-medicaid-s-role-for -the-elderly-and-disabled-report.pdf

Institute of Medicine. (2001). *Improving the quality of long-term care*. Washington, DC: National Academies Press.

Jonas, S. (2003). *Introduction to the U.S. health care system* (5th ed.). New York, NY: Springer.

Jones, A. L., Harris-Kojetin, L., & Valverde, R. (2012, April 13). *Characteristics and use of home health care by men and women aged 65 and over* (National Health Statistics Reports, no. 52). Retrieved from http://www.cdc.gov/nchs/data/nhsr/nhsr052.pdf

Kaiser Commission on Medicaid and the Uninsured. (2005). *Long-term care: Understanding Medicaid's role for the elderly and disabled*. Retrieved from http://kaiserfamilyfoundation.files.wordpress.com/2013/01/long-term-care-understanding-medicaid-s-role-for-the-elderly-and-disabled-report.pdf

Kaiser Commission on Medicaid and the Uninsured. (2011). *Medicaid's long-term care users: Spending patterns across institutional and community-based settings*. Retrieved from http://www.kff.org/medicaid/upload/7576–02.pdf

Kaiser Commission on Medicaid and the Uninsured. (2012, June). *Medicaid and long-term care services and supports*. Retrieved from http://kaiserfamily foundation.files.wordpress.com/2013/01/2186-09.pdf

Kaiser Commission on Medicaid and the Uninsured. (2014). *Medicaid beneficiaries who need home and community-based services: Supporting independent living and community integration*. Retrieved from http://kff.org/medicaid/report/medicaid-beneficiaries-who-need-home-and-community-based-services-supporting-independent-living-and-community-integration

Matthews, J. L. (2010). *Long-term care: How to plan and pay for it* (8th ed.). Berkeley, CA: Nolo.

National Clearinghouse for Long-Term Care Information. (2012). Retrieved from http://www.longtermcare.gov/LTC/Main_Site/Understanding/Definition/Know.aspx

Olson, L. K. (1994). *The graying of the world: Who will care for the frail elderly?* Binghamton, NY: Haworth Press.

Raffel, M. W., & Barsukiewicz, C. K. (2002). *The U.S. health system: Origins and functions* (5th ed.). Albany, NY: Delmar.

Sultz, H. A., & Young, K. M. (2009). *Health care USA: Understanding its organization and delivery* (6th ed.). Sudbury, MA: Jones & Bartlett.

Thrall, J. H. (2005). Prevalence and costs of chronic disease in a health care system structured for treatment of acute illness. *Radiology, 235*(1), 9–12.

U.S. Census Bureau. (2011). Expectation of life at birth, 1970–2007, and projections, 2010–2020. *Statistical Abstract of the United States*. Retrieved from http://www.census.gov/compendia/statab/2011/tables/11s0103.pdf

U.S. Department of Health and Human Services, Administration on Aging. (2011). *Profile of older Americans: 2011*. Retrieved from http://www.aoa.gov/aoaroot/aging_statistics/Profile/2011/docs/2011profile.pdf

Williams, S. J., & Torrens, P. R. (2008). *Introduction to health services* (7th ed.). Clifton Park, NY: Delmar/Cengage Learning.

CHAPTER 9

MENTAL HEALTH CARE

Tina Marie Evans

The mental health care system in the United States has evolved greatly since the first recorded traces in this country of recognizing and treating the various forms of mental illness. The practice of isolating and controlling those with mental illness by institutionalizing them is largely a thing of past, and we have now come into a new age of understanding through research and advances in behavioral and pharmacological therapies. An impressive amount of progress has been made in understanding the etiologies and criteria for diagnostics as well as the best courses of treatment for many mental illnesses, but our health care system clearly still has some work to do to ensure consistent access to mental health care for all who need it.

The term *mental health* is often used to refer to *mental illness*; however, diligent research has given us the information to differentiate these two terms. Although related they represent two distinct psychological states. On the one hand mental health is "a state of well-being in which the individual realizes his or her own abilities, can cope with the normal stresses of life, can work productively and fruitfully, and is able to make a contribution to his or her community" (World Health Organization, 2001, p. 1). On the other hand mental illness is defined as "collectively all diagnosable mental disorders," or, "health conditions that are characterized by alterations in thinking, mood, or behavior (or some combination thereof) associated with distress and/or impaired functioning" (U.S. Department of Health & Human Services, 1999, p. 1).

Mental illness continues to be a central concern in public health, both alone and in conjunction with other chronic diseases and their known negative effects. Estimates are that about one-fourth of the adults in the

LEARNING OBJECTIVES

After reading this chapter you should be able to

- Understand the costs of mental illness in the United States.

- Explain the key events in the history of mental health care.

- Explain how stress can affect mental health and mental illness.

- Articulate the three categories of mental illnesses and give examples of each.

- Describe the prevalence rates of the most common mental illnesses.

- Discuss the various types of health care professionals who care for mentally ill individuals.

- Describe the problems associated with the lack of mental health parity.

United States have some type of mental illness, and nearly 50 percent of Americans will develop at least one type of mental illness at some time in their lives. These conditions, whether transient and minor or long-lasting and severe, come with a relatively high cost of care, estimated at over $300 billion in 2003 (that is, $193 billion from lost wages, $100 billion in health care expenditures, and $24 billion in disability benefits paid out). Although anxiety, depression, and mood disorders are the most commonly diagnosed mental illnesses, the health care system must be prepared to proactively diagnose and treat all forms of mental illness, as its effects can be life-altering and can range from short-term minor disruptions in day-to-day functioning to long-term total incapacitation, severe impairment, and early, untimely death (Reeves et al., 2011).

With a growing variety of mental health care service options and types of mental health care providers in the United States, much optimism surrounds the care that these specialists can now provide and the promising research that is taking place. At the same time, the fragmented system of financing mental health care services has meant that care is not accessible and consistent for all. Currently, those who have the more severe and persistent forms of mental illness still face great levels of inequality in treatment and social stigma. The following exploration of mental health care in the United States begins with a historical overview that celebrates accomplishments in mental health care but also highlights the care inequality that we must work quickly to correct.

History of Mental Health

Tracing the history of mental health care services in the United States reveals perspectives and practices that have greatly shifted over time. Documents from the 1700s show that people then were largely afraid of individuals exhibiting mental illness and wanted to keep them confined and away from the rest of society. In some instances people saw mental illness as deviant and therefore ignored it, since it appeared to be a behavioral problem. At this time care for mentally ill persons fell to their families and the parishes in which they lived. When families were unable (or were unwilling) to care for these individuals, towns or charitable groups likely assumed responsibility for their care. Mental illness was a private issue for the most part, only attracting the public's attention when an individual who could not care for himself or herself had no family support or was violent (Raffel & Barsukiewicz, 2002). If public support was needed, the town would compensate private citizens who were willing to house and care for mentally ill persons in their homes. Relatives of a mentally ill person would also receive this stipend for care if they used it to keep the person in a private home. During this time religion played a central role in the perception of mental illness, as it was a common belief that the mentally ill were possessed by the devil. Unfortunately, this perception led some communities to forcibly drive out and even kill some individuals who displayed severe symptoms of mental illness (Kemp, 2007).

As the size of towns grew throughout the 1700s, care moved away from individual homes to formally designated almshouses that were shared by the poor and the mentally ill. The Colonies passed laws that gave town councils the authority to care for mentally ill persons by referring them to the local almshouse, and to name guardians for their estates. Persons who were both mentally ill and unmanageably violent were commonly jailed (often in unheated jails), and others were placed in workhouses and houses of behavioral correction (Kemp, 2007; Raffel & Barsukiewicz, 2002). Conditions in these houses were often harsh. Some inmates were abused, others starved to death as resources were severely limited, and very little medical care was available. General hospitals came into existence in the late eighteenth century, with Pennsylvania Hospital being the first hospital in the United States to admit mentally ill patients, agreeing to house them in the basement—a choice clearly reflective of their low status in society at that time. In the nineteenth century, hospitals designated for the mentally ill were built and began to open their doors. This development allowed mentally ill persons to receive care in facilities that specialized in psychiatry, but it also marked the beginning of the separation between mental health care and physical health care, with mental health being treated as a lesser need (Kemp, 2007).

In the later part of the eighteenth century, physicians began to notice a connection between mental illness and stress and also mental illness and other diseases. A new approach of "moral treatment" for the mentally ill advocated a supportive, kind, and sympathetic environment to allow healing to take place. A related movement of reform removed many mentally ill persons from the unpleasant conditions of the almshouses and helped them find placement in the newly established state hospitals. Mentally ill persons in jails were also released and placed in more appropriate facilities. Mental health services now became available in the state hospitals for the mentally ill (referred to as *asylums*), and they attempted to insulate the mentally ill from the stresses and pressures of ordinary life in the community. States often built these facilities on rural farms that provided food for the residents and allowed some of the more functional individuals to work on the farms as well. The residents of these facilities experienced a more homelike environment, and they were encouraged to participate in education, religion, and recreation, which led to improvements in some. The focus remained on moral treatment. These state hospitals were quickly overwhelmed by the number of people who came to them needing care (Kemp, 2007).

In the later years of the nineteenth century, more and more mentally ill persons seeking care continued to arrive at the asylums. As the sheer numbers of people needing services and housing overran the system of care, the perspective on the care of mental illness shifted once again and a disappointing deterioration in the level of care occurred. Instead of providing treatment for each patient, the focus now turned to custodial care, which was a clear falling off from past moral practice. Instead of offering a supportive environment, care now mostly involved the use of mechanical restraints, drugs to sedate and calm behavior, and also surgery. Additionally, the ideas of the eugenics movement that was popular at this time led to the passing of state laws that restricted the lives and rights of mentally ill persons by prohibiting them from marrying and allowing for the involuntary sterilization of over 18,500 patients. By the end of the nineteenth century, the conditions in state hospitals were downright appalling, and these hospitals were places of last resort for the mentally ill, the alcoholic, the criminally insane, and the senile. Some smaller and better-run psychiatric treatment facilities opened, but care in those settings was cost prohibitive unless families or other charitable organizations were able to subsidize this superior form of care (Kemp, 2007).

The early 1900s saw the rise of the progressive movement, which became an important driving force of political reform and social activism in the United States. At this time, hospitals remained the central sites for mental health care, but activism by mental health advocates was succeeding in moving some mentally ill persons to cottages and other more homelike structures being built on the hospital properties. Two new treatments were studied and promoted for use at this time—music therapy and photochromatic therapy. Family care programs were started in an effort to reinvolve the loved ones of patients in the hope of moving these institutional residents back to a home setting, with supportive outpatient aftercare services provided for those returning home. Ambulatory psychiatric care was also on the rise, and short-term, assistive, inpatient psychiatric facilities were started that could temporarily care for those who had moved back into the community but then experienced temporary or transitional difficulties (Kemp, 2007).

During the years between the Great Depression of the 1930s and World War II, the numbers of mentally ill individuals needing inpatient care grew once again, yet the financial support for psychiatric institutions was limited. Some inpatient psychiatric hospitals reached record numbers of 10,000 to 15,000 patients, which may have been a reflection of the stress people were experiencing during the Depression and also a possible result of the average U.S. lifespan slowly beginning to increase. The 1930s also saw the advent of four new therapies: insulin coma therapy, Metrazol (pentylenetetrazol) shock treatment, electroshock therapy, and lobotomy. **Insulin coma therapy** attempted to alleviate psychiatric symptoms by repeatedly injecting patients with high doses of insulin to bring on brief comas; this was performed on a daily basis for approximately two months. The shock treatments used electric shocks alone or combined with the administration of Metrazol (a drug banned by the U.S. Food & Drug Administration in 1982) to either induce a coma or startle patients free of their mental illness. Although some individuals benefited, many received injuries from the therapies, including fractures, brain damage, and chemical poisoning (Kemp, 2007). **Prefrontal lobotomy** (the surgical dissection of the prefrontal cortex away from the rest of the brain) was performed on about 40,000 patients during the late 1940s and early 1950s in an effort to subdue severely ill individuals and make them less reactive to their surroundings (Kalat, 2013). Walter Freeman became known as a physician who had performed several thousand lobotomies in the United States, even though he was not a trained surgeon. In time, the recorded outcomes of the lobotomies ranged from normalization of behavior to devastating regressions to childlike conduct or zombie-like states. It became known as an unpredictable form of psychosurgery that had an uncontrollable range of consequences for the patients. Epileptic seizures were a common consequence of lobotomies, and even individuals who obtained a lessening of symptoms suffered from "some reduction in motivation to excel, capacity for insight, emotional responsiveness and social judgment" (Greenblatt, Dagi, & Epstein, 1997, p. 511).

Short-term and community care continued to be the primary sources of mental health care services during the 1940s. However, the focus of the system now turned toward the high numbers of men called up but then rejected for military service on the grounds of mental health, as well as toward the needs of soldiers who returned from war needing care for combat-related stress disorders. A series of exposés that revealed the continuing horrendous conditions in the state mental hospitals sparked some changes, and the federal government now began to take notice of the significant numbers of men rejected by the military as well as the returning soldiers in dire need of mental health care services. The **National Mental Health Act of 1946** marked the first prominent move of the federal government toward an involvement in mental health. This act funded research grants for studies of the etiologies, diagnostics, and treatments of mental illness (Kemp, 2007). At the same time, despite the many cases of harmful results, the four therapies introduced in the 1930s continued to be widely practiced. They did not come to an end until shortly after the promising release of the initial group of antipsychotic medications in the 1950s, specifically chlorpromazine (Thorazine) and reserpine (Sultz & Young, 2009).

insulin coma therapy
A former treatment that attempted to alleviate psychiatric symptoms by repeatedly injecting patients with high doses of insulin, which brought on brief comas.

prefrontal lobotomy
Surgical dissection of the prefrontal cortex away from the rest of the brain.

National Mental Health Act of 1946
Federal legislation that increased government involvement in mental health by funding research grants for the study of mental illnesses.

The 1950s saw additional encouragement of ambulatory mental health care, and in 1955, a massive deinstitutionalization began. The arrival of the new psychotropic medications suggested that many institutionalized individuals could now be either cured or reasonably well managed by medication and therefore allowed to return to their communities with an adequate level of function (Kemp, 2007). The goal, with the assistance of the new medications, became to release the patients and encourage them to function as normally as possible rather than keep them confined (a condition that encouraged passivity, dependency, and social isolation). Over one thousand state-funded, outpatient psychiatric clinics were established to provide ambulatory psychiatric care for the individuals who were released (Raffel & Barsukiewicz, 2002). In 1955, the U.S. Congress established the **Joint Commission on Mental Illness and Health**, whose findings also attacked the level of care received by patients of the large state and county psychiatric hospitals. President Kennedy took the commission's recommendations seriously, urging Congress to act prudently and pass legislation to provide federal support for community-based mental health care services. Large entitlement programs "became accessible to the mentally ill, mainly Medicaid, Medicare, Supplemental Security Income (SSI), Social Security and Disability Insurance, and housing subsidies, among others" (Sultz & Young, 2009, p. 329). The 1960s and 1970s saw increasing levels of government involvement in the financing of mental health care services. Additional community-based mental health centers opened their doors, and there was a notable influx of medical professionals training for and entering into the psychiatric disciplines. Large numbers of severely mentally ill patients who had been locked away in state or county mental institutions continued to be discharged into either the community at large, community boarding homes, or nursing homes (Sultz & Young, 2009).

Data from the 1970s indicate that 80 percent of the states' formerly hospitalized populations of mentally ill patients were released to receive outpatient or community-based services. Unfortunately, these individuals did not receive much in the way of tracking or follow-up care to assure their successful transition to outpatient life, and many fell off the states' radar, quickly becoming part of the local homeless population or landing in jail after self-medicating with illegal street drugs and excessive use of alcohol (Kemp, 2007). Those who were able to access care services contributed to the sharp rise in psychiatric-related health care costs in the late 1970s. The number of outpatient mental health care visits now greatly outnumbered inpatient mental health care visits; however, the allocation of resources was not changed to follow the shift to outpatient care. Twice as much continued to be spent on inpatient care as on

Joint Commission on Mental Illness and Health

A commission established by Congress to increase access to mental health services and revisit whether placements of mentally ill patients were appropriate.

outpatient care, and the federal government quickly became concerned with limiting mental health care costs (Kemp, 2007; Sultz & Young, 2009). States continued to provide some funding, but their allocations fell short of the amounts actually needed. Some community mental health centers were forced to reduce the services they provided, and other centers had to close. The decreasing levels of funding made it extremely difficult for communities to provide the level of consistent outpatient care clearly needed by these individuals (Raffel & Barsukiewicz, 2002). Eligibilities and subsidies gave way to cutbacks that tremendously undermined the quality of life of deinstitutionalized mentally ill individuals, who now faced a lack of housing subsidies and inadequate supportive social services and also a rising level of exclusion from SSI benefits.

During the first decade of this century, there has been disagreement over which individuals should be covered for mental health care services, and who should be responsible for covering the cost of the services (Sultz & Young, 2009). The breakdown in the provision of coverage has led to sporadic access to services and, at times, no access to services for some people. The current approach to treating mental illness centers predominantly around outpatient care, with a limited number of inpatient facilities still in existence for adults and children who require residential services. Specialized units of general hospitals are also now prepared to admit patients for short-term inpatient psychiatric care as well. Sadly, most communities in the United States still do not have a truly integrated system of care for mental illness, one that is capable of providing the necessary and consistent types of social support needed to facilitate correct treatment. In fact some reports indicate that "there are more persons with serious mental illness in street shelters and prisons than in hospitals, largely because of the failure of deinstitutionalization, which resulted in the vast majority of those discharged from mental hospitals not being cared for in the community and drifting into homelessness and destitution" (Raffel & Barsukiewicz, 2002, p. 172).

At this point in time, the system of care for mental health in the United States remained two tiered, with lower-income individuals forced to rely on the limited services of the public sector, and higher-income individuals able to access the better-quality services found in the private sector (Kemp, 2007). Just in the past few years, advances in the diagnostics and treatment of mental illnesses are giving much hope for the future, and the government has reallocated research funding in an effort to continue these advances in treatment. Yet despite this hope and the potential for helpful research discoveries to come, the unequal access to covered services allows only a small number of individuals to receive the necessary and appropriate care for their conditions (Sultz & Young, 2009).

The Role of Stress

Before discussing some specific types of mental illnesses, we must first briefly explore and understand the effects of stress. Although there are many causes of mental illness, stress and the way individuals respond to it has a lot to do with whether they maintain their mental health or whether they risk developing one or more mental illnesses. A recent study by the American Psychological Association indicates that more than half of working adults and 47 percent of all Americans are concerned about the amount of stress they are experiencing in their lives (Sutton, 2007). Early observations done many years ago showed that stress led to physical disorders and/or made existing physical conditions worse. Further research added to this knowledge and revealed that stress causes more than physical conditions—it undoubtedly has links to several mental illnesses as well. Specific follow-up studies began to highlight the interplay between stress, the development of mental illness, and the aggravation of psychiatric symptoms. Data have shown that early exposure to stressful events (usually in the childhood years) clearly sensitizes people to stress in later years. In other words, children exposed to high levels of stress (especially during certain stress-sensitive periods of their development) have a higher incidence of developing one or more mental illness as adults (Weber et al., 2008).

This knowledge is an important foundation to understanding how exposure to internal or external stress predisposes people to mental illness. Prolonged or chronic stress can have devastating consequences, as it can cause the onset of anxiety, panic attacks, depression, and many other troubling conditions. One study in particular found that people who experienced a stressful situation had almost six times the risk of developing depression within that same month, and related studies have suggested that stress might be a risk factor for suicide. In addition to mental illness, research has unmistakably linked high levels of stress with increased chances of developing heart disease, arrhythmias, hypertension, stroke, infections, gastrointestinal problems, chronic pain, poorly controlled diabetes, sleep difficulties, sexual and reproductive dysfunctions, and significant levels of emotional distress. Additionally, it is apparent that severe stress, especially over an extended period, is damaging to the immune system and our natural biological resistance to mental disorders as adults (Sutton, 2007).

People are usually experiencing some level of stress, as any factor in life that is capable of causing emotional arousal, anxiety, fear, humiliation, anger, loss, or extreme unhappiness can trigger a stress response. Other stresses can be physical (trauma, abuse, hunger, noise, and severe environmental conditions) or psychological (divorce, death of a family member, relationship difficulties, loneliness, the loss of a job, high-pressure work or schoolwork, and persistent financial worries). An individual may have a strong or weak set of coping mechanisms. These mechanisms involve personality factors, level of social support, culture, perception of the stress, spirituality and religious beliefs, dietary and exercise habits, satisfaction or lack of it with one's personal or professional life, and whether or not the person has effective ways to respond to stress (Sutton, 2007; Varcarolis & Halter, 2010).

Everyone's body responds similarly to stress, and it does not matter whether the stress is real or perceived, or positive or negative. Individuals exposed to prolonged or chronic stress are extremely vulnerable to psychological and physical responses and conditions if the stress is not mitigated as early as possible. If the effects of stress can be mitigated soon after the stress begins, the many negative effects and unhealthy coping behaviors that are unfortunately common among Americans can be lessened or halted, and the development of unhealthy coping mechanisms such as poor food choices, inactivity, drinking, smoking, or drug addiction may not occur. Conventional medicine has a variety of pharmacological and nonpharmacological methods to help people bring their stress levels under control, and additional mind-body therapies can be beneficial as well. Currently suggested mind-body therapies include relaxation exercises, meditation, acupuncture, hypnosis, massage therapy, aromatherapy, guided imagery, breathing exercises, physical exercise, biofeedback, cognitive reframing, mindfulness, journaling, and the use of humor. High-quality support systems are beneficial in minimizing long-term stress, and using one or more of the mind-body therapies can greatly improve both physical and psychological functioning (Sutton, 2007; Varcarolis & Halter, 2010).

Since the link between stress and the increased chance of developing mental illness is clear, the health care system must take steps to ensure that providers are routinely assessing stress levels as part of routine physical assessment for both adults and children. Too often providers focus on physical aspects only; it is important to question individuals about their stress level and emotional status as well. Given the findings of recent research on the likelihood of developing mental illness, the greatest concern is for persons whose family history suggests a genetic predisposition to mental illness and who additionally experience high levels of stress in their lives. In addition, everyone should be mindful of the acute and chronic effects that stress can have on otherwise healthy individuals, leading to a possible need for mental health care services. Since the data are clear on the significant health consequences of long-term stress, it is imperative that routine assessment of stress levels as well as proactive mental health screening and early interventions to reduce stress take place in the primary care setting (Sutton, 2007). The following section examines some of the more prevalent mental illnesses currently affecting Americans.

Types of Mental Illnesses

Looking back to the time when mental asylums and "nervous breakdowns" were common, we can see that we have come a long way in furthering our understanding of specific mental illnesses and of the continuum that exists between mental health and mental illness. Many health care providers now believe that a person's overall health cannot be established without specifically considering mental health status in addition to all the dimensions of physical health.

In classifying the types of mental illness, one important factor is achieving agreement about the exact behaviors that represent each particular mental illness. Currently, there are two major classification systems for defining mental illness: the *Diagnostic and Statistical Manual of Mental Disorders*, fifth edition (*DSM-5*), and the International Statistical Classification of Diseases, tenth version (ICD-10). The *DSM-5* is the most recently published source (released in May 2013), and it offers the greatest level of understanding and specific diagnostic criteria for mental illnesses, although these two classification systems are frequently used together to plan patient care and determine reimbursement levels. The updated *DSM-5* is the result of many professionals coming together to reconsider and revise the diagnostic criteria and classifications of mental illnesses; its release was much anticipated by health care providers looking for a strong resource for locating additional and more refined information with which to classify mental illnesses and thereby better match the ICD-10 classifications. The following sections will describe some of the more commonly observed mental illnesses and their effects on the population. They fall into three categories: psychotic disorders, nonpsychotic disorders, and mood disorders (Table 9.1).

Table 9.1 Common Classifications of Mental Illness

Psychotic Disorders	Nonpsychotic Disorders	Mood Disorders
Schizophrenia and related disorders	Panic disorder	Depression
	Obsessive-compulsive disorder	Bipolar disorder
	Generalized anxiety disorder	Cyclothymia
	Phobias	Dysthymia
	Posttraumatic stress disorder	

Psychotic Disorders

The first category of mental illnesses that we will review consists of the **psychotic disorders**: namely, schizophrenia and the related disorders. **Schizophrenia** is a term for a very serious group of brain disorders that "affect a person's thinking, language, emotions, social behavior, and ability to perceive reality accurately" (Varcarolis & Halter, 2010, p. 307). It affects over 3 million Americans (which translates to approximately 1 out of every 100 people), and it is one of the most disabling and disruptive mental illnesses known. The characteristic signs and symptoms include delusions, hallucinations, disorganized speech, grossly disorganized or catatonic behavior, and/or flattened affect; all of which persist for six months or more (Fiebach et al, 2007). These terrifying symptoms are more common in men than in women, and often begin in a person's mid- to late twenties. Symptoms will vary from person to person but are often so frightening and disabling for the ill person and his or her family, friends, and caregivers that all their lives are disrupted and difficult to manage.

> **psychotic disorders**
> Mental illnesses including schizophrenia and related disorders.
>
> **schizophrenia**
> A group of brain disorders that affect a person's thinking, language, emotions, social behavior, and ability to perceive reality accurately.

The exact cause of schizophrenia remains unknown at this time, but the condition currently exists in all societies around the world. There may be some interaction between genetic, environmental, and behavioral factors, and research is now finding that schizophrenia tends to run generationally in families. If a person has a close relative with the condition, he or she is more likely to develop the condition than is someone who does not have a relative with the condition. Research is continuing on chromosomes 6, 8, and 13 in an effort to obtain precise information on the etiology of schizophrenia, which will surely guide the development of the next generation of treatments (Williams & Torrens, 2008).

Because schizophrenia is considered a group of conditions instead of one single condition and because the exact cause of the condition remains unknown, current treatments are based on what has been documented in related clinical research and experience. The focus of treatment is on minimizing stress, reducing the amount of troubling symptoms, and trying to prevent such symptoms from reoccurring once they lessen. Antipsychotic medications (chosen from either conventional or atypical groupings) are the current first-line choice for the treatment of schizophrenia and have a wide range of success. Some individuals respond very well, going on to enjoy reasonably satisfying personal lives and become employed. Others suffer from breakthrough psychoses from time to time that require periods of inpatient hospital care. Although many schizophrenics find their condition well managed by medication, not all individuals will respond to drug therapy. In understanding the treatment for this group of psychotic disorders, it is important to note that the medications do not "cure" schizophrenia or ensure that a person will never have any further psychotic episodes. Schizophrenia is a lifelong illness, so there must be a stable commitment to continuing treatment at all times to control the symptoms and to reduce the intensity of any symptoms that do reoccur (Fiebach et al., 2007; Williams & Torrens, 2008).

Nonpsychotic Disorders

nonpsychotic disorders
Mental illnesses including panic disorder, obsessive-compulsive disorder, generalized anxiety disorder, phobias, and posttraumatic stress disorder.

Nonpsychotic disorders (also commonly referred to as anxiety-related disorders) include panic disorder, obsessive-compulsive disorder, generalized anxiety disorder, phobias, and posttraumatic stress disorder. As a category, these persistent and often disabling anxiety-based disorders are the most common mental illnesses in the United States, affecting approximately 19 million Americans. Persons affected by these conditions often adopt rigid, repetitive, and ineffective behaviors in attempts to control their symptoms, because the underlying feelings of anxiety are so prominent and relentless that they seriously affect personal, occupational, and social functioning (Fiebach et al., 2007; Varcarolis & Halter, 2010).

panic disorder
A condition characterized by discrete periods of extreme and disabling anxiety.

Panic disorder involves discrete periods of extreme and disabling anxiety, often termed *panic attacks*. Individuals with panic disorder may experience symptoms such as "palpitations, sweating, trembling, shortness of breath, feeling of choking, chest pain or discomfort, nausea or abdominal distress, dizziness, derealization (feelings of unreality) or depersonalization (feeling detached from oneself), paresthesias, chills or hot flushes, fear of losing control or going crazy, and fear of dying" (Fiebach et al., 2007, p. 308). For a person's experience to meet the criteria for a panic attack, at least four of the signs and symptoms listed here must be present, in addition to an intense fear or discomfort that peaks in intensity within ten minutes of the onset.

Individuals who have panic disorder are very frequent users of both inpatient and outpatient medical services, having a primary care services utilization rate three times higher than that of average persons and also higher than that of persons with other forms of mental illness. Since panic disorder is a chronic and recurring illness, treatments focus on long-term management instead of short-term symptom relief. Drug therapies involving selective serotonin reuptake inhibitors (SSRIs) or certain benzodiazepines in combination with cognitive behavioral therapy and stress management are helpful to many persons (Fiebach et al., 2007).

obsessive-compulsive disorder
A condition characterized by time-consuming ritualistic obsessions as well as recurrent, persistent, and intrusive thoughts that are upsetting to the individual.

As its name suggests, **obsessive-compulsive disorder** involves the occurrence of time-consuming ritualistic obsessions (such as repeatedly touching objects, repeatedly turning lights on and off, repeatedly washing hands, etc.) as well as recurrent, persistent, and intrusive thoughts that are upsetting to the individual. These obsessive thoughts and recurrent compulsive acts are often illogical and unreasonable, which many individuals do realize and readily admit, yet they cannot seem to control them. In most cases individuals try to rid themselves of the obsessive thoughts and lessen their high levels of anxiety by performing the compulsive behaviors; however, the relief from anxiety that the behaviors provide is only temporary. The distressing effects from this condition can range from feeling a mild annoyance in one's life up to experiencing a severely debilitating pattern of thoughts and actions throughout the day (Fiebach et al., 2007; Varcarolis & Halter, 2010).

Approximately 1 to 2 percent of people in the population have this condition, with symptoms usually starting in adolescence or early adulthood and then tending to decline with age. It is thought that obsessive-compulsive disorder has several causes: biological origins connected to personality traits, genetic factors (having a relative with the condition), head trauma, and other neurologic disorders. For most individuals this chronic and persistent condition tends to worsen a bit during times of higher than usual stress. Cognitive behavioral therapy is the primary treatment, supplemented by antidepressant medication as needed, although many people learn to control their symptoms well during short-term courses of therapy focused on blocking the obsessive thoughts, lessening anxiety, and finding healthy ways to manage stress (Fiebach et al., 2007).

Generalized anxiety disorder is another common nonpsychotic disorder, with an estimated lifetime prevalence rate of 5.1 percent. The disorder's hallmark symptom is excessive, inappropriate, unrealistic, and persistent worry on most days for a period of at least six months. Individuals with this condition experience anxiety levels that are clearly out of proportion when compared to the person's actual situation. The diagnosis of generalized anxiety disorder also involves experiencing at least three of the following six symptoms: restlessness, fatigue, difficulty concentrating, irritability, muscle tension, and sleep disturbances. Women suffer from this condition more frequently than men do. The troubling levels of anxiety for these individuals often begin in their early twenties and then persist for several decades. The cause of generalized anxiety disorder is not well understood, although it is suggested that there is a small genetic component and possible ties to trauma and stress in early childhood, especially in cases of a parent's death (Fiebach et al., 2007; Varcarolis & Halter, 2010).

In many cases, individuals with this condition use self-regulation techniques, stress-reducing techniques, and consistent avoidance of caffeine and alcohol to moderate their anxiety. If needed, one of the newer prescription antidepressant medications can bring the anxiety back down to a manageable level that supports functionality and allows enjoyment of the various

generalized anxiety disorder
A condition characterized by excessive, inappropriate, unrealistic, and persistent worry on most days for a period of at least six months.

dimensions of life. Some individuals will achieve a partial or full remission of their anxiety; however, most individuals must commit to ongoing treatment to keep the signs and symptoms in check (Fiebach et al., 2007).

Phobias are present in 13.3 percent of the population and are defined as persistent fear of harmless objects or harmless situations that causes people to avoid contact with them. There are many objects and situations known to be the subjects of phobias; for example, heights, crowded places, snakes, airplanes, spiders, blood, thunderstorms, wide-open spaces, water, germs, elevators, and needles. Even though phobic individuals often realize that their fears are unreasonable and excessive, their avoidant behavior often continues so they can also avoid the anxiety caused by exposure to the object or situation. Many people suffering from phobias do not seek treatment for their condition, as the avoidant behavior is usually effective in handling the condition. However, people whose lives are severely affected by a phobia or who cannot avoid an anxiety-provoking object or situation, for personal, social, or occupational reasons, will usually seek treatment. Treatment typically begins with systematic desensitization to the object or situation, which gradually exposes the person to the fear or anxiety-provoking object or situation through a series of increasingly vivid mental images. Relaxation techniques to control the anxiety and fear that the images produce are used to assist the person during this process. Once a person becomes desensitized enough over time and is able to encounter the actual object or situation in real life, he or she is slowly and gradually exposed to that object or situation, often accompanied by a therapist or a family member or friend for added support. Desensitization training, often accompanied by cognitive behavioral therapy and/or social skills training, is usually effective in treating the phobia and thereby releasing the individual from his or her intense fear (Fiebach et al., 2007).

The last of the common nonpsychotic disorders is **posttraumatic stress disorder**. Individuals who have this disorder frequently and persistently reexperience a highly traumatic and stressful event that involved the potential for death or serious injury to themselves or others. This intense recollection of or flashback to the horrible event often comes in the form of dreams but is also reflected in the individual's avoidant behavior toward any person, place, or thing associated with the traumatic and stressful event. Flashbacks such as these are indeed somewhat common for all persons after going through a severe trauma. However, if severe and relentless recollections and flashbacks persist for longer than one month following the traumatic event, the diagnosis of posttraumatic stress disorder is made, especially in cases where the person is showing significant difficulty in maintaining interpersonal, social, and/or occupational relationships. In any given year this persistence of symptoms occurs in approximately

phobias
Conditions characterized by a persistent fear of harmless objects or situations that causes people to avoid contact with them.

posttraumatic stress disorder
A condition characterized by persistent mental and emotional stress as a result of injury or severe psychological shock and commonly involving sleep disturbances and vivid flashbacks.

3.6 percent of adults. Many documented cases of this disorder have resulted from violent experiences during war, physical assault, rape, tornados, fires, and other severe forms of trauma. Treatment for this disorder commonly combines behavioral therapy (to desensitize the person to the trauma), psychotherapy (to address anger related to the trauma and/or the guilt that accompanies survival), and antidepressant and anxiolytic medications. The results of treatment vary, but early initiation of cognitive behavioral therapy is particularly helpful in blocking some of the persistence of symptoms (Fiebach et al., 2007).

Mood Disorders

The third category of mental illnesses consists of **mood disorders**, conditions such as depression, bipolar disorder, cyclothymia, and dysthymia. These depressive and mood disorders have a serious impact on public health in the United States, carrying an economic impact of $83.1 billion in direct medical costs, suicide-related mortality costs, and workplace productivity costs (Fiebach et al., 2007). Although the majority of people feel a bit depressed from time to time, individuals with **depression** experience an extended period of time where feelings of sadness, emptiness, worthlessness, disinterest in life's usual activities, and fatigue dominate their life and severely interfere with their ability to work, sleep, eat, and enjoy activities that were once pleasurable for them. Depression is the leading cause of disability in the United States, usually accompanied with a comorbid anxiety disorder and/or substance abuse. This condition has debilitating effects on the individual and also on his or her family and friends; however, many people do not seek treatment despite the fact that the majority of even the most severely depressed individuals can have their mood well stabilized and may even be cured. A wide range in the severity of depression exists, and it is becoming increasingly clear that this disorder runs in families, occurring generation after generation (Williams & Torrens, 2008). The expected clinical course of major depression is highly variable, as at least 60 percent of individuals will have a second episode. Of those who have experienced two major depressive episodes, 70 percent will go on to have a third episode. Finally, of those who have experienced three episodes of major depression, 90 percent will then experience continuing episodes (Varcarolis & Halter, 2010). A faithful commitment to ongoing treatment as well as practicing behaviors that support physical and emotional wellness can effectively disrupt this gloomy statistic and offer a more promising outlook.

Antidepressant medications are the first line of treatment for major depression, with effectiveness rates of about 70 percent (Fiebach et al., 2007). The newer antidepressant medications (selective serotonin reuptake

mood disorders
Mental illnesses including depression, bipolar disorder, cyclothymia, and dysthymia.

depression
A condition characterized by an extended period of feelings of sadness, emptiness, worthlessness, disinterest in life's usual activities, and fatigue, severely interfering with the ability to work, sleep, eat, and enjoy activities that were once pleasurable.

inhibitors, tricyclics, and monoamine oxidase inhibitors) offer a wide range of beneficial pharmacological options. Treatment for major depression does not come in pill form only, as various forms of psychotherapy and the teaching and encouragement of wellness activities are usually combined with antidepressant medication. For individuals suffering severe or life-threatening depression (and for those who cannot take antidepressant medications), new protocols of electroconvulsive therapy preformed under brief anesthesia may be a helpful option (Williams & Torrens, 2008).

bipolar disorder
A condition characterized by alternating periods of elation and depression.

Bipolar disorder, formerly called manic depression, is another chronic and recurrent mental illness characterized by notable shifts in mood, energy, and ability to function. The shifts are often variable and exaggerated, moving from severe mania with intense euphoria, hallucinations, or irritability to severe and hopeless feelings of depression. In many cases, individuals will experience periods of relatively normal function in between the episodes of this condition; however, most individuals with bipolar disorder experience some degree of continuing interpersonal and/or occupational difficulties even when the extreme symptoms are not present. The lifetime prevalence of bipolar disorder in the United States is 3.9 percent. Of particularly serious concern is the high mortality rate in these individuals; 25 percent to 60 percent of those with bipolar disorder will make at least one attempt at suicide during their lifetime, with 20 percent of these individuals ultimately being successful in their attempt (Varcarolis & Halter, 2010).

The treatment or management of bipolar disorder is often difficult. The wildly disruptive phase of mania is a challenge to control, as the person's behavior is extremely agitated and hyperactive. Psychiatrists usually choose a period of inpatient treatment to initially bring the condition under control, but convincing an individual with bipolar disorder to accept such treatment is often difficult. Consistent long-term management of the condition is essential, as most individuals will experience periods of remission through stabilizing maintenance medications such as lithium, anticonvulsant mood stabilizers, and/or atypical antipsychotics. These remissions may make a person decide that he or she is "fine," and some individuals may stop taking their prescribed medications—only to have the bipolar swings return in the absence of treatment. These medications must be taken daily to even out the mood swings and to protect the person from reoccurrences, even during times of remission from symptoms. It is difficult for some people to accept that they must take a combination of medications for the rest of their lives in order to get and remain well; however, this lifelong treatment is often necessary (Fiebach et al., 2007).

cyclothymic disorder
A condition characterized by alternating periods of mild elation and mild depression and lasting two years or more.

Cyclothymic disorder is a type of intermittent bipolar episode that fails to meet the diagnostic criteria for either major depression or mania because its effects are either milder or briefer than the effects of the other illnesses. Most commonly, the affected person experiences a persistent instability of mood (lasting two years or more) in which alternating periods of mild elation and mild depression take place. The alternating periods of mood may fluctuate over hours, weeks, or months, coming and going at seemingly random times. Cyclothymia occurs in 3 percent to 6 percent of the U.S. population and usually begins in the early adulthood years (Semple & Smyth, 2013). Diagnosis can be difficult, as extended periods of observation or careful subjective accounts of an individual's mood are important to document the details of the mood fluctuations over time. This disorder tends to run in families as well, and has a clinical course similar to that of bipolar disorder. Approximately 35 percent of individuals with cyclothymia will experience a full-blown manic, hypomanic, or depressive episode within two to three years of the initial onset of the condition (Fiebach et al., 2007).

Because the mood swings experienced by a person with cyclothymic disorder tend to be mild to moderate and because the periods of elevated mood are pleasurable, most individuals do not actively seek treatment for this condition. Those who do seek care are often motivated by the negative consequences the disorder has for their interpersonal relationships and/or occupational functions, or by the troubles caused by comorbid drug and/or alcohol misuse. Cyclothymia does not lessen as a person ages, and its disruptive effects usually persist throughout the person's lifespan. Fortunately, mood-stabilizing medications are effective in moderating the symptoms over time, allowing the individual a better chance for a successful and productive personal and professional life. Low-dose lithium and certain anticonvulsants (valproate, carbamazepine, or lamotrigine) have been found to be beneficial for most individuals (Semple & Smyth, 2013). Cognitive behavioral therapies, stress reduction, and an emphasis on a healthy lifestyle are excellent recommendations for people with cyclothymia as well.

Dysthymic disorder, in contrast, involves a chronic depressive state that produces symptoms that are usually milder than the symptoms required for a diagnosis of major depression. For individuals with this disorder the depressive symptoms are present on most days and for the majority of each day for at least two years. The typical age of onset for dysthymia ranges from early childhood to the teenage years and into early adulthood (Varcarolis & Halter, 2010). It is common for individuals with dysthymia to use avoidant behavioral patterns (self-imposed social isolation, physical and emotional withdrawal from others), patterns that often lead to lonely, solitary lifestyles. Drug and alcohol abuse are popular but unhealthy coping mechanisms in individuals with dysthymia, and these substances can at times mask the underlying depressive symptoms (Fiebach et al., 2007).

dysthymic disorder
A condition characterized by a mild yet chronic form of depression, often lasting two years or longer.

Most individuals with dysthymia are functional in their occupational duties; however, this chronic disorder is usually associated with noticeable impairment in social functioning, especially in close personal relationships (Fiebach et al., 2007). Because it is chronic, it can be difficult to see that the depressive disturbance of mood is different from the person's "normal" mood pattern, and thus dysthymia can be difficult to identify. Over time, many individuals with dysthymia come to think that they have always felt somewhat depressed, and a large number do not seek treatment because of this. For those who do, research indicates a strong correlation in the treatment response of individuals with dysthymia and individuals with major depression; therefore the treatment for dysthymia is now very similar to that for major depression. The selective serotonin reuptake inhibitors and tricyclic antidepressant medications are particularly helpful and are usually prescribed in conjunction with brief psychotherapies (Fiebach et al., 2007). Even though it is common for individuals with dysthymia to suffer from interpersonal, social, and occupational distress, the condition is usually not severe enough to cause hospitalization unless the person openly shares suicidal thoughts or displays suicidal tendencies (Varcarolis & Halter, 2010). It is recommended that increased attention be given to regular screening for stress levels as well as common signs and symptoms of mental illnesses during visits in the primary care setting. Many types of therapies for dysthymia and the other conditions presented here are currently available yet are underutilized, even though these therapies and medications can be dramatically beneficial and life changing for affected individuals.

Mental Health Care Providers

There is a large variety of mental health care providers in the United States who are skilled at using a substantial array of pharmacological and non-pharmacological therapies to benefit their patients' individual conditions. This section reviews the education and work of the major mental health care providers previously discussed in Chapter Three.

Psychiatrists

Psychiatrists are professionals who are fundamental in the management of mental illnesses, offering diagnostics, treatment, and social support to those with these illnesses.

Most commonly, psychiatrists treat conditions involving psychoses, nonpsychoses, mood disorders, substance abuse, adjustment reactions, developmental disabilities, and sexual dysfunctions. They may evaluate and treat patients on either a short-term or long-term basis and are legally permitted to order laboratory tests, prescribe medications, and provide various methods of psychotherapy. They may treat one patient on an individual basis, or consult with and provide care to an entire family as a group when that family is dealing with a serious situation or a period of great stress. At times psychiatrists will also offer their services as consultants to primary care physicians or to other health care professionals such as psychologists, social workers, and nurses (ABPN, 2013). Depending on their chosen subspecialty, they may use in-depth psychotherapy or medication therapy or a combination of both. Psychiatrists commonly provide outpatient services in the community and may also have admitting privileges for one or more hospitals or be employed by a hospital. It is common for those with mental illness to receive care from a team of professionals, often led by a psychiatrist, since he or she is educated as a medical doctor and has the ability to prescribe medication and write diagnostic orders (Varcarolis & Halter, 2010).

Psychologists

Psychologists universally study the interactions between a person's brain function and his or her behaviors, as well as between the environment and the person's behaviors. Using a variety of scientific methods, careful observation, creative experimentation, and thorough analysis, psychologists gather the information that allows them to diagnose and properly treat their patients. They study both normal and abnormal behaviors as they relate to human functioning, offering psychological testing and consultations and encouraging behaviors that help individuals develop physical and emotional wellness and increase their level of emotional resistance. Many psychologists are educators and researchers as well (American Psychological Association, 2013).

For the past few decades the American Psychological Association and some state psychological associations have lobbied aggressively to gain psychologists the right to legally prescribe medication, a request that is passionately opposed by the American Psychiatric Association and some other physician organizations. Psychologists have won the right to legally prescribe medication in New Mexico and Louisiana, with several other states currently considering legislation to allow this. This heated legal battle between the organizations representing psychologists on one hand and psychiatrists on the other will likely continue for years to come, as neither side is willing to back down from this legislative fight (Richard & Huprich, 2009). The lobbying efforts have created some tension between psychologists and psychiatrists, as these groups of professionals remain in disagreement over increasing the treatment privileges of psychologists.

Mental Health Clinical Nurses

Currently, two levels of psychiatric mental health nurses are recognized in the United States: the registered nurse–psychiatric mental health and the advanced practice registered nurse–psychiatric mental health. The registered nurse–psychiatric mental health (RN-PMH) is a nursing graduate who has earned an associate's or a bachelor's degree in nursing. At this basic level of training, RN-PMHs work in supervised settings and often handle multiple responsibilities such as those of a staff nurse, a case manager, a home care nurse, and so forth. They may assess symptoms of mental illness, track responses to interventional care, coordinate interdisciplinary patient care, participate in counseling, hand out prescribed medications, and educate patients. It is estimated that 4 percent of the overall population of registered nurses choose to work in the mental health care setting (Varcarolis & Halter, 2010).

A higher level of educational preparation for mental health clinical nurses is the advanced practice registered nurse–psychiatric mental health (APRN-PMH). These professionals are registered nurses who have earned either a master of science degree in nursing (MSN) or a doctor of nursing practice (DNP) degree in nursing focusing on psychiatric–mental health nursing. Almost 10 percent of these nurses choose to earn credentials in psychiatric mental health nursing, allowing them to function autonomously in this setting. These nurses are educated and skilled in diagnosing mental illnesses, prescribing psychotropic medications, and conducting psychotherapy. They frequently work in case management, consulting services, patient education, and research within the nursing profession. Currently, there is great demand for both RN-PMHs and APRN-PMHs, making the future very bright for this group of knowledgeable and valuable professionals (Varcarolis & Halter, 2010).

Psychiatric Mental Health Nurse Practitioners

Psychiatric mental health nurse practitioner (PMH-NP) are qualified to provide psychiatric services to adults, children, adolescents, and families. They may practice autonomously in a great range of settings, and commonly work in primary care settings, ambulatory mental health clinics, psychiatric emergency or crisis centers, hospitals, community health centers, and private psychiatric practices. PMH-NPs are licensed to perform psychosocial and physical assessments, make diagnoses, conduct therapy sessions, formulate treatment plans, and dispense prescription medications. In other words, they can fully manage a wide range of patient care services. The legally permitted functions and licensing requirements for PMH-NPs currently vary from state to state. In almost half of the states, PMH-NPs may open and operate their own mental health care practices, but the remaining states require that they practice collaboratively with physicians. It is best to check with the respective state licensing board regarding the exact scope of practice for PMH-NPs (American College of Nurse Practitioners, 2012).

Social Workers

Social workers are educated professionals who have earned either bachelor's or master's degrees in social work. They are essential support personnel who work in a variety of settings, including community mental health programs, hospitals and skilled nursing facilities, private psychiatric practices, military and veterans' centers, schools, and rehabilitation centers. They are often the coordinators of basic mental health services in employee assistance programs and disaster relief programs.

Case management is one of the particular strengths of social workers as they are skilled in arranging for various services that maintain or improve quality of life while meeting individuals' psychosocial needs. They often assist individuals in securing housing, employment, general medical care, and other necessary services based on the needs of each case. In addition, they are valuable consultants to other health care providers in helping people to prepare and develop a support system that will facilitate good mental health upon their discharge from an inpatient facility. Licensing requirements for social workers varies among the states; however, up-to-date information on specific state requirements is provided on the licensing board website for each state (Varcarolis & Halter, 2010, Williams & Torrens, 2008).

Mental Health Parity

Active advocacy to achieve parity in mental health care services is an ongoing effort in the United States that dates back to the 1950s (Sultz & Young, 2009). **Parity** refers to requiring insurance companies to provide mental health care coverage and benefits at the same level as medical and surgical coverage. Over the years great inequities and unnecessary limits on mental health care services in comparison to medical and surgical services have existed in most insurance plans; this lack of parity has blocked many individuals who unquestionably needed mental health services from receiving them. Strict limits on the number of visits and often higher deductibles, coinsurance rates, and copayments for mental health care services have caused, and continue to cause, serious financial barriers for individuals trying to obtain mental health care services. While these limitations may save the third-party payers some money, the result has been that either the uncovered costs have been shifted to the taxpayers as an additional tax burden or (worse) individuals simply have not received appropriate, timely, and consistent care. The continued use of these

parity
The state or condition of being equal.

Mental Health Parity Act
Federal legislation that prohibits the use of annual and lifetime limits for mental health care that are different from limits for general medical care.

cost-controlling strategies and aggressive limitations on mental health care services has angered the advocates for mentally ill persons, and their efforts have led to a series of legislative attempts to correct the lack of parity (Varcarolis & Halter, 2010; Williams & Torrens, 2008). Although some view parity as an issue of cost, it is actually a much broader issue of reducing the discrimination against those with mental illness and allowing them fair access to the care that they need and deserve.

In 1996, the **Mental Health Parity Act** was introduced into Congress and passed with an impressive amount of bipartisan support. Soon after its implementation in 1998, however, it soon became clear that the act was correcting only one part of the inequality, the catastrophic mental health care benefits. Specifically, the act prohibited the use of annual and lifetime limits for mental health care that were different from those used for general medical care. While this result was an important first step and a symbolic victory for advocates, the act's benefits were otherwise limited. It did not ban some of the commonly used cost-shifting mechanisms, such as "adjusting limits on mental illness inpatient days, prescription drugs, outpatient visits; raising coinsurance and deductibles; and modifying the definition of medical necessity" (Sultz & Young, 2009, p. 342). The act also did not compel employers to offer coverage for mental health care services, nor did it affect the amounts for coinsurance, deductibles, or inpatient care days, or the number of provider visits allowed. Additionally, it did not oblige employers to provide coverage for persons with substance use and abuse problems, which are clearly issues that continue to be of great concern in public health today (Sultz & Young, 2009; Williams & Torrens, 2008).

Mental Health Equitable Treatment Act
Federal legislation that would have expanded treatment coverage for mental illnesses to be equal to coverage for physical illnesses.

In 2001, the **Mental Health Equitable Treatment Act** was introduced in Congress in an effort to expand mental health service coverage to an additional 15 million Americans. Sadly, Congress had abandoned this proposal by 2002, even though the Congressional Budget Office estimated that the cost of a full parity mental health bill would cause premium increases of less than 1 percent. Following this failed legislation, several states began to work on mental health parity in their own ways. By 2004, thirty-four states had developed and enacted some form of parity legislation to assist in making care services more readily accessible to all. Much variation exists across the states in this legislation; for example, in the definitions of the populations included or excluded and in the level of covered services and the coverage exclusions (Levin, Petrila, & Hennessy, 2004). These state efforts have largely focused on removing the limits on benefits (which is a victory in the overall sense), but they unfortunately have not removed some of the main barriers keeping people away from mental health care services. Employers and third-party payers responded to these legislative endeavors in a variety of ways, from continuing to use some of the not specifically prohibited cost-cutting mechanisms on coinsurance, deductibles, and copayments to taking the drastic step of totally dropping mental health care benefits from their plans (Sultz & Young, 2009).

Studies by the U.S. Government Accounting Office have revealed that by the year 2000, although 86 percent of health plans were in compliance with the Mental Health Parity Act of 1996, 87 percent of those plans imposed new limits on coverage for mental health care services (Varcarolis & Halter, 2010). Other studies found a similar appalling decrease in mental health care coverage as well, likely caused by a concern that insurance premiums would rise. One study, for example, documented that in 1991, 36 percent of those working for large companies had unlimited mental health outpatient visit benefits, and by 2004, this number had declined to only 19 percent (Sultz & Young, 2009). It is disheartening that the majority of people in need of mental health care services do not seek them, yet this reluctance is well explained by the continuing service inequalities and the barriers to obtaining care that remain (Williams & Torrens, 2008). In recent years, it was found that only 25 percent of individuals suffering from mental disorders received treatment in the U.S. health care system, compared to 60 percent to 80 percent of individuals with heart disease (Kemp, 2007).

The inequalities and barriers that continue to exist today are an especially great concern for those who suffer from severe and persistent forms of mental illness. Without the appropriate mental health services and related support, these individuals are not likely to live stable, independent lives as functional members of their communities. The National Alliance on Mental Illness (NAMI) is one of the groups that continues to advocate for mental health parity, and it recently released this position statement on the continuing disparity and unfairness: "The discrimination in access to care is evidenced by limited coverage, punitive copays, and restricted access to hospitalization during acute episodes and what one would logically conclude would occur for other untreated or under-treated serious illnesses. That is to say: the outcomes for people with untreated or under-treated illnesses are disastrous and too frequently result in death or permanent disability" (NAMI, 2013).

Despite the efforts of NAMI and other mental health advocacy groups seeking corrective legislation, individuals in the United States continue to receive episodic, hit-or-miss mental health care rather than the accessible and consistent care that would effectively treat their conditions by properly aligning medication, support, and structure. The 1999 U.S. surgeon general's report on mental health further validated the distressing fact that the majority of Americans with mental illness do not seek out or receive treatment, despite the existence of many effective treatments that might lead to improved function, remission, or recovery (Levin et al., 2004). For those with severe and persistent mental illnesses, the amount of coverage needed for the proper coordination of needed resources is either underfunded or absent. To better understand the types of services that are still lacking and the significant numbers of Americans that are affected, consider the following data from a NAMI survey of families of the mentally ill:

- 59.3% needed help with illness management

- 67.9% needed help with crisis management

- 23.1% needed help with activities of daily living, including bathing, dressing and personal hygiene

- 74.3% needed help with community living skills, including shopping and managing money

- 64.7% needed help with establishing and maintaining friendships

- 72.8% needed help with gaining and maintaining productive activities [Sultz & Young, 2009, p. 343]

The National Advisory Mental Health Council (NAMHC) has studied this ongoing problem extensively, and points out that for an additional $6.5 billion, the United States could provide mental health service coverage for both adults and children with severe mental disorders. NAMHC's financial conclusions are convincing and economically attractive, as this additional investment would lead to a 10 percent drop in the use (and therefore the costs) of nonpsychiatric services. In addition, this reduction in spending would be combined with a decline in indirect costs for a savings of approximately $8.7 billion; that calculates out to an impressive net benefit of $2.2 billion per year (Sultz & Young, 2009).

Federal attempts at parity still do not require insurance plans to provide coverage for any of the categories of mental illness or substance use or abuse disorders. Future legislative efforts must compel insurance plans to provide coverage for mental health care services at the same benefit level as the covered general medical and surgical services. Without increases in consistent levels of mental health care coverage, the aforementioned needs of many Americans with mental illness will continue to go unmet as these individuals suffer the effects of a broken system of health care coverage. Intermittent care is not enough to keep these individuals from the chaos that their illnesses can cause; it will not help them to avoid unemployment, poverty, imprisonment, homelessness, and social ostracism. Clearly, we can do better than this, and there is no excuse for allowing people with the conditions described in this chapter to continue enduring the distressing effects that they do. The stigma and myths that shroud mental illness must be erased and replaced with an accurate view of this illness and its successful treatment. Access to mental health care services deserves to be one of the national health care priorities for our legislators. As a country, we have the professional, technical, and financial resources to alleviate these disparities permanently and to allow the individuals in this population to experience full and satisfying lives as valued members of our communities.

SUMMARY

Mental health is a central aspect of overall health status that is in need of a more prominent place in the primary care setting and in the mainstream of health care services. The extensive history of mental health services provision reveals that these services have come a long way, forming the mental health care system that is in place today, yet this system remains fragmented. Research has produced a wealth of information on the varied causes of mental illness, causes that commonly include genetic predisposition and exposure to acute and chronic stress. Appropriate, timely, and consistent care can alleviate and manage, if not cure, many of the common mental illnesses, thereby allowing individuals the opportunity to pursue productive and fulfilling personal and professional lives. A sickening amount of inequality continues to exist between insurance coverage for mental health services and coverage for general medical and surgical services; this lack of parity must be resolved by our legislators without delay. Parity in mental health services is a worthy goal that would remove many of the financial obstacles that currently discourage Americans from seeking treatment or from remaining in treatment for the prescribed amount of time needed to improve, stabilize, or cure their conditions.

KEY TERMS

bipolar disorder

cyclothymic disorder

depression

dysthymic disorder

generalized anxiety disorder

insulin coma therapy

Joint Commission on Mental Illness and Health

Mental Health Equitable Treatment Act

Mental Health Parity Act

mood disorders

National Mental Health Act of 1946

nonpsychotic disorders

obsessive-compulsive disorder

panic disorder

parity

phobias

posttraumatic stress disorder

prefrontal lobotomy

psychotic disorders

schizophrenia

DISCUSSION QUESTIONS

1. What are the three categories of common mental illnesses prevalent in our population today?

2. What are some of the physical and mental conditions that are caused by stress?

3. How are nonpsychotic disorders commonly treated?

4. What are some of the specific differences between psychiatrists and psychologists?

5. How do the clinical functions of the three levels of mental health nurses differ?

6. How has the lack of parity in mental health services affected accessibility and utilization of services?

REFERENCES

American Board of Psychiatry and Neurology. (2013). ABPN certification resources. Retrieved from http://www.abpn.com/what_is_abpn.html

American College of Nurse Practitioners. (2012). What is a nurse practitioner? Retrieved from http://www.acnpweb.org/i4a/pages/index.cfm?pageid=3479

American Psychological Association. (2013). What is psychology? Retrieved from http://www.apa.org/careers/resources/guides/careers.aspx?item=1

Fiebach, N. H., Kern, D. E., Thomas, P. A., & Ziegelstein, R. C. (Eds.). (2007). *Principles of ambulatory medicine* (7th ed.). Philadelphia, PA: Lippincott, Williams and Wilkins.

Greenblatt, S. H., Dagi, T. F., & Epstein, M. H. (Eds.). (1997). *A history of neurosurgery in its scientific and professional contexts*. Park Ridge, IL: American Association of Neurological Surgeons.

Kalat, J. W. (2013). *Biological psychology* (11th ed.). Belmont, CA: Wadsworth Publishing/Cengage.

Kemp, D. R. (2007). *Mental health in America: A reference handbook*. Santa Barbara, CA: ABC-CLIO.

Levin, B. L., Petrila, J., & Hennessy, K. D. (Eds.). (2004). *Mental health services: A public health perspective* (2nd ed.). New York, NY: Oxford University Press.

National Alliance on Mental Illness. (2013). NAMI's position on parity. Retrieved from http://www.nami.org/Template.cfm?Section=Issue_Spotlights& template=/ContentManagement/ContentDisplay.cfm&ContentID=8657

Raffel, M. W., & Barsukiewicz, C. K. (2002). *The U.S. health system: Origins and functions* (5th ed.). Albany, NY: Delmar.

Reeves, W. C., Strine, T. W., Pratt, L. A., Thompson, W., Ahluwalia, I., Dhingra, S. S., . . . Safran, M. A. (2011). Mental illness surveillance among adults in the United States. *Morbidity and Mortality Weekly Report, 60*(Suppl. 3), 1–32.

Richard, D. C., & Huprich, S. K. (2009). *Clinical psychology: Assessment, treatment and research*. Burlington, MA: Elsevier Academic Press.

Semple, D., & Smyth, R. (2013). *Oxford handbook of psychiatry* (3rd ed.). Oxford, UK: Oxford University Press.

Sultz, H. A., & Young, K. M. (2009). *Health care USA: Understanding its organization and delivery* (6th ed.). Sudbury, MA: Jones & Bartlett.

Sutton, A. L. (Ed.). (2007). *Stress-related disorders sourcebook* (2nd ed.). Detroit, MI: Omnigraphics.

U.S. Department of Health and Human Services. (1999). *Mental health: A report of the surgeon general*. Rockville, MD: U.S. Department of Health and Human Services; Substance Abuse and Mental Health Services Administration, Center for Mental Health Services.

Varcarolis, E. M., & Halter, M. J. (2010). *Foundations of psychiatric mental health nursing: A clinical approach* (6th ed.). St. Louis, MO: Saunders Elsevier.

Weber, K., Rockstroh, B., Borgelt, J. Awiszus, B., Popov, T., Hoffmann, K., . . . Pröpster, K. (2008). Stress load during childhood affects psychopathology in psychiatric patients. *BioMed Central Psychiatry, 8*(63). doi: 10.1186/1471-244X-8-63

Williams, S. J., & Torrens, P. R. (2008). *Introduction to health services* (7th ed.). Clifton Park, NY: Delmar/Cengage Learning.

World Health Organization. (2001). *Strengthening mental health promotion* (Fact Sheet no. 220). Geneva, Switzerland: Author.

CHAPTER 10

PUBLIC HEALTH SERVICES

Bernard J. Healey

Public health departments are an important part of the U.S. health care system. Throughout our country these health departments usually work quietly and mostly out of sight protecting the entire population from disease epidemics, and yet most Americans are not even aware of their existence. They offer many programs to the public designed to prevent disease and improve the quality of life for all age groups. We usually become aware of public health departments only when our community is faced with an outbreak of a disease that threatens the population.

The difference between public health and individual health is that public health focuses on the health of the entire population in a city, county, state, or the nation. These government-financed health agencies concentrate their resources and expertise on keeping large segments of the population free from disease and as healthy as possible. They are not in competition with anyone's family doctor or the local health care system. Indeed, they usually handle health problems and issues that have no interest for the private practitioner.

Public health involves the science of improving and protecting the health of communities through a strong focus on education and the promotion of healthy lifestyles. Public health professionals focus most of their attention on the prevention of disease rather than on treating individuals who have already become ill. Public health then is a discipline that focuses its time and resources on population-based medicine. There are many who argue that public health is one of the best-kept secrets in our entire health care system. In fact many of the greatest accomplishments in health care can be attributed to efforts by public health departments across the United States.

LEARNING OBJECTIVES

After reading this chapter you should be able to

- Identify the major health problems found in the U.S. population, and describe public health strategies to deal with these problems.

- Understand the need for leadership rather than simply management of public health services.

- Understand the value of epidemiology in the discovery of solutions to health problems.

- Discuss the reasons why public health departments need to develop health education and health promotion programs.

- Explain the importance of the public health core competencies.

public health
The organized efforts of society designed to keep populations healthy.

Johnson (2013) points out that public health activities are quite often carried out by a number of individuals schooled in different disciplines but working together to achieve public health goals to improve the health of the population. Public health professionals contribute to the prevention of disease and have developed the skills required to make a real difference in the elimination of disease throughout our country and our world. Public health departments and their employees have a long history of producing individual and community-wide prevention programs that deserve much of the credit for the increase in our life expectancy over the last hundred years, from forty-nine years in 1900 to over eighty years in 2012. This accomplishment alone should make public health one of the most cost-effective government programs in the entire United States. This list (adapted from Centers for Disease Control and Prevention [CDC], 1999) shows some of the major achievements of public health departments over a one-hundred-year history.

Ten Great Public Health Achievements—United States, 1900–1999

- Vaccination
- Motor-vehicle safety
- Safer workplaces
- Control of infectious diseases
- Decline in deaths from coronary heart disease and stroke
- Safer and healthier foods
- Healthier mothers and babies
- Family planning
- Fluoridation of drinking water
- Recognition of tobacco use as a health hazard

Often public health departments accomplish these achievements with limited funding and within larger organizations with bureaucracies that block creativity and innovation and stifle employee growth. Despite these limitations, public health department staff work together as a team to improve the health of the population. How can public health departments produce similar achievements when it comes to preventing the chronic diseases that are currently the major cause of health care cost escalation in the United States? To be successful in the battle against chronic diseases, public health departments will require additional funding along with strong, collaborative leaders who can create a compelling vision of the benefits that would result from elimination of the many chronic diseases we face today.

The new Patient Protection and Affordable Care Act offers several changes that reflect a greater interest by the government in public health initiatives. One of these changes is increased provision of immunizations at no charge to participants. It will be critical for public health leaders to prepare their staff members for such changes and for the opportunities that will be coming their way because of health care reform. Public health departments have become the primary way to deal with the major challenges that are facing our health care system over the next several years. In order to deal with these challenges successfully, public health in the United States requires increased funding, better leaders, and community collaboration. The starting point for this success needs to be a much better understanding among all Americans of the role of public health departments.

The Institute of Medicine offered numerous recommendations for public health departments in its 2002 report *The Future of the Public's Health in the 21st Century*. The most important of these recommendations included

- Utilizing a population health approach that builds on the multiple determinants of health.
- Strengthening the infrastructure of public health agencies through action at the government level.
- Creating a new generation of community partnerships that can help to create change in community health behaviors.
- Concentrating on evidence-based community prevention strategies.
- Improving communication among the partners in population health programs.

The IOM's most recent report, *Best Care at Lower Cost: The Path to Continuously Learning Health Care in America* (2013), reinforces the role of primary care in the prevention of diseases, especially chronic diseases. This report offers numerous health promotion recommendations along with strategies necessary for achieving these recommendations designed to lower the cost of health care and improve the quality of life for the population.

Recently, the *Washington Post* reported the results of the five-year Global Burden of Disease study. Involving 486 researchers at 302 institutions, this study is being called the most comprehensive look at population health ever completed. The researchers looked at changes in the world population's health from 1990 to 2010 and found great improvements in both medicine and public health over that time period. They concluded that although the risks of premature death from chronic diseases have decreased over that time, the world population is also facing a large increase in disabilities resulting from having chronic diseases over a long period of time. The researchers called this result the "expansion of morbidity" and one of the greatest challenges ever to face the health care delivery system ("How Long Will We Live—and How Well?," 2012). These disabilities are the expensive complications from chronic diseases, and they are resulting in increased health care costs along with diminished quality of life for large numbers of the world's population. The solution of course is prevention of chronic diseases and their complications, and that can be accomplished only with public health leadership.

There is a role to be played by public health departments in the reform of health care services for our population. This role will include providing community leadership in the improvement of the health of the population through the design and implementation of health promotion programs to reduce the practice of high-risk health behaviors among the population and particular population groups. Public health departments will also play a large role in the design of best practices when it comes to health education and health promotion in the community, thus increasing their current roles and responsibilities.

History of Public Health

The protection and the improvement of the health of the community has always been a function of communities, villages, cities, and nations. Unfortunately, the tools and the funding for public health in our nation have not changed very much over the years. Public health departments have never received the respect or the publicity that they deserve. In fact very few individuals recognize the many contributions of public health departments to the major improvements in the health of the population of the world over the last century. In 1920, Charles Edward A. Winslow defined public health as "the science and art of preventing disease, prolonging health through the organized efforts and informed choices of society, organizations, public and private, communities and individuals" (quoted in Turnock, 2009, p. 10). Public health departments have been instrumental in the increase in life expectancy and certainly have been successful in the prevention of many communicable diseases but are currently losing the battle with the epidemic of chronic diseases. A brief history of public health and public health departments can facilitate a much better understanding of the role that public health departments play in the modern health care system.

The concept of public health has been around a long time. Eliminating epidemics of diseases like plague, leprosy, tuberculosis, and even diarrhea has been associated with the development of the concept of public health.

Dealing with large numbers of illnesses among a population seems to define the nature of public health services for most Americans, but there is much more to public health than investigating and helping to relieve the epidemics of communicable diseases that gain a great deal of media attention. Public health departments actually spend a lot of their time developing programs designed to prevent illness from occurring.

One of the first individuals to have a significant impact on the health of the public was John Snow, who became famous for his use of epidemiology in the discovery of the cause of a significant cholera outbreak in London in 1854. This English physician was able to trace the spread of cholera to the water supply from one specific pump. His investigation demonstrated the power of epidemiology along with the role of public health during outbreaks of communicable diseases in a population.

Another notable figure in the history of public health is Edwin Chadwick, who, in effect, designed a sanitary movement in England that carved a role for public health in the protection of the population from diseases that can develop because of unsanitary conditions. Healey and Walker (2009) point out that Chadwick's *Report on an Inquiry into the Sanitary Conditions of the Labouring Population of Great Britain* led the way to a better understanding of the relationship between filthy conditions and the occurrence of disease in a population. This type of investigation and report was one of the preconditions for a much better understanding of the relationship between unsanitary conditions in the community and the occurrence of disease.

Some more recent examples of public health successes include the substantial studies published in England (Doll & Hill, 1950) and the United States (Wynder & Graham, 1950) in the 1950s that implicated the use of tobacco as a major risk factor for lung cancer. Since 1948, the Framingham Heart Study, under the direction of the National Heart, Lung, and Blood Institute (NHLBI) at the National Institutes of Health, has been committed to identifying the common factors or characteristics that contribute to cardiovascular disease. Using chronic disease epidemiology, these various studies attempted to find the causes of lung cancer and heart disease by studying large samples of the population for half a century. These prospective studies were undertaken in order to develop prevention programs to reduce the incidence of these expensive and chronic diseases.

It is important to gain an understanding of the purpose of public health in relation to the goals and objectives of the larger U.S. health care system. Baldoni (2012) believes that organizational success is obtained when an organization has purpose, understands why it has this purpose, and has successfully gained the support of its employees in the achievement of the purpose. It is the responsibility of public health leaders to articulate the purpose of public health departments to all stakeholders who have a role in the achievement of public health's purpose.

The purpose of public health in relation to the health of Americans has been a source of confusion for most Americans and also for many who work in public health agencies. In an effort to define this purpose, the **Emerson report of 1945** outlined the minimal functions to be performed by a public health department: collection of vital statistics, control of communicable diseases, environmental sanitation, laboratory services, maternal and child health services, and public health education programs. Although these functions or basic responsibilities are important, they are so general and broad that they do not provide specific goals for public health departments. This sense of a lack of real purpose is further substantiated by today's lack of funds, budget cuts, and public health positions left vacant. It is difficult for a public health department to have a sense of fulfilling a purpose when its budget is reduced on an annual basis and its staff are not replaced.

Emerson report of 1945

A landmark American Public Health Association report on local health departments that, among other things, identified six functions for a public health department: vital statistics collection, communicable disease control, environmental sanitation, public health laboratory services, maternal and child health services, and public health education.

Structure of Public Health Departments

Public health departments in the United States are usually classified by whether they operate at the federal, state, or local level. The federal government plays a big role in public health in terms of regulation and funding for local public health efforts. The frontline defense for public health is found in state and local health departments, which offer services ranging from disease investigations and health education programs to immunizations.

As Barton (2010) points out, the federal component of public health is found in the U.S. Public Health Service (PHS), which traces its beginnings back to the Marine Hospital Service established in 1798 with major responsibilities for the care of merchant seamen. Since that time the federal government has carried out a public health role addressing many aspects of population health. As Johnson (2013) notes, the U.S. Department of Health and Human Services is responsible for the eight agencies that make up the PHS. These agencies have the primary responsibility for administering public health grants to the states along with gathering national health data. Probably the most famous of these eight federal agencies is the Centers for Disease Control and Prevention (CDC), located in Atlanta, Georgia. The CDC provides funding and guidance to state and local health departments involved in communicable and chronic disease prevention and control, environmental concerns, injury prevention and control, and the gathering of statistics.

There is a functioning state health department in every state in the United States. These state health departments are structured similarly and are faced with many of the same challenges and responsibilities. They spend a great deal of their time and effort gathering health statistics concerning the population of their respective state. These state health agencies also have regulatory powers over laboratories and the licensing of health professionals and many health facilities. They also provide funding and supervision for local health departments within their state. Working with the CDC, they are also responsible for the investigation of disease outbreaks within their jurisdictions.

Local health departments (LHDs) are usually organized as county or city health agencies. These LHDs have the primary responsibility for delivering public health services to the local population. According to Healey and Lesneski (2011), the LHD is an important component for fulfilling the goal of communities to provide a healthy place to live. The services most frequently provided by LHDs in this country include

- Adult immunizations
- Childhood immunizations
- Communicable or infectious disease surveillance
- Tuberculosis screening
- Food service establishment inspection or licensing
- Environmental health surveillance
- Food safety education
- Tuberculosis treatment
- High blood pressure screening
- Tobacco use prevention
- Maternal and child health services
- Injury prevention programs
- Oral health services

According to Barton (2010), there are approximately 3,000 LHDs in the United States, with their funding coming from local taxes, permits and licenses, inspection fees, and a variety of state and federal grants. These departments are usually under the direction of a director or commissioner of health who reports to an elected political official such as a mayor or a board such as the county commissioners. LHDs collaborate on public health with other local health agencies, including hospitals and health care systems. LHDs are usually given the responsibility of implementing various public health programs for disease surveillance, disease investigations, environmental inspections, immunizations, epidemiology, and public health nursing activities.

Determinants of Health

Public health departments are continuously working on gaining a better understanding of what determines good or bad health. These departments have concentrated a great deal of research on identifying the many basic factors that determine and influence personal and population health. Even though the vast majority of Americans believe that our private health care system has the largest influence on achieving good health, it has become clear over the years that numerous other components contribute to an individual's wellness. Public health departments have long recognized many components that may result in good or bad health for the individual and the population. In fact, according to Schimpff (2012), individual health behaviors have been shown to be the cause of over 70 percent of premature deaths in our country.

A large number of those concerned with the development of health policy on both the national and local level seem convinced that the most important determinant of good health is the actual receipt of health services. Schimpff (2012) argues that poor health is a direct result of being without health insurance coverage for a period of time. This belief in the power of the adequate receipt of health care services helps to explain our national interest in making health care insurance available to everyone. According to this line of reasoning, all that needs to be done to improve the health of Americans is to make health insurance available to the population. However, health insurance alone does not guarantee good health. There are many other determinants of health that need to be considered if we are serious about improving the health of the population.

According to Healey and Lesneski (2011), the "determinants of health are the factors in the personal, social, economic, and environmental areas of life that affect the health status of individuals and populations" (p. 3). When public health departments focus on all the determinants of health, they must move beyond the normal bits of data gleaned from surveillance statistics like morbidity, mortality, and disease occurrence. For example, poor health behaviors like an unhealthy diet, smoking, and alcohol abuse can have an enormous effect on the future individual and population health of a given community. Understanding the role of these high-risk health behaviors is critical if we are ever going to design an appropriate approach to deal with the epidemic of chronic diseases affecting our population. It is important to understand that merely providing health insurance to the majority of the population in 2014 does absolutely nothing, by itself, to deal with the vast majority of other health determinants that have a direct effect on the health of the population.

Health Disparities

According to Cohen, Chavez, and Chehimi (2007), a **health disparity** is a difference in health among individuals that is avoidable, unjust, and unfair. The key word in this definition is *avoidable*, because that means these disparities are socially structured. Some of the determinants of this inequitable treatment are gender, race, and socioeconomic status. Figure 10.1 outlines the major elements that produce the poor health outcomes often found in low-income communities throughout the United States. As we saw in Chapter One, this figure tells us to look backward from the problem of disparities in order to determine the root causes of the disparate health problem. Cohen et al. (2007) argue that this trajectory can be prevented through primary prevention efforts that seek to remove the root causes before illnesses occur.

health disparity
A difference in health among individuals, particularly one that is avoidable, unjust, and unfair.

Our country has yet to grasp the value of preventing illness among all Americans, no matter their gender, race, or economic or educational status. There is an old saying that you can pay now or pay later. If we allow any individuals, rich or poor, male or female, of any race, to become ill as a result of our not providing health education, we are going to pay more for their illness than we would have paid for their wellness.

Communicable and Chronic Disease Control

The most important function of the early public health departments in the United States was the control of communicable disease outbreaks. In fact, in 1900, the leading causes of mortality were communicable diseases spread by close personal contact, like tuberculosis, influenza, measles, and polio, along with diseases spread by food and water. These communicable diseases often became epidemic, resulting in large numbers of cases of illness and deaths along with mass hysteria among the general public. This required a response from government through the public health departments. Early public health agencies were given the responsibility of protecting the health of a given population from epidemics of communicable diseases.

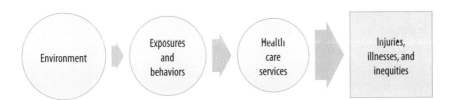

Figure 10.1 Trajectory of Health Disparities
Source: Cohen et al., 2007, p. 31.

These epidemics led to the development of specialized programs in public health departments that were frequently labeled communicable disease control programs. Professionals working in these programs usually were well versed in the principles of epidemiology, which they used to discover the source of each disease outbreak and limit the numbers of cases resulting from an epidemic. Their mandate was never to eliminate communicable diseases but rather to control the numbers of people who were exposed and consequently infected. Since resources for these communicable disease programs were scarce, health departments never really focused on prevention of these diseases but rather emphasized cleaning up epidemics after they occurred. In fact only one communicable disease has ever been eradicated from the world—smallpox.

As public health departments gained control over communicable diseases in the United States, they also noted a slow increase in the numbers of individuals developing and dying from chronic diseases. Public health leaders attempted to use the same model of disease control with the chronic diseases. However, this effort was doomed to fail from the beginning because there was no treatment for the chronic diseases. This lack of treatment led public health agencies to abandon the control process and work instead on surveillance activities in order to determine the true incidence and cost of chronic diseases in our country. The money appropriated for these new chronic disease programs was never enough to really make a dent in the chronic disease epidemic that we were about to face. In fact some diseases, like tuberculosis and the human immunodeficiency virus (HIV) that causes acquired immunodeficiency syndrome (AIDS), became both communicable and chronic diseases at the same time. Therefore the epidemic of chronic diseases escalated and began to affect younger age groups.

Public health disease intervention specialists' initial response to the HIV epidemic was to treat this new infection like a sexually transmitted disease. Their strategy became prevention of new infections through contact tracing, as if this disease were similar to syphilis or gonorrhea, and attempting to discover all sexual contacts of the individual infected with HIV. This strategy was doomed to fail because discovering sexual contacts did very little to prevent or control the epidemic because there was no treatment and the incubation period for this disease is relatively long. Unfortunately, public health departments still practice this same strategy. That the strategy has failed is shown by the fact that we have recently experienced an increase in a number of communicable diseases, including tuberculosis, many of the sexually transmitted diseases, severe acute respiratory syndrome (SARS), influenza, and Legionnaires' disease, and even a pandemic of bird flu. So although chronic diseases have surpassed communicable diseases as the major cause of morbidity and mortality in the United States we must also be prepared to deal with the occurrence of a number of difficult communicable diseases.

Core Functions of Public Health

In 1988, the Institute of Medicine (IOM) defined the **core functions of public health** as assessment, policy development, and assurance. Figure 10.2 displays ten essential public health services in relation to these core functions. Assessment involves investigations and identification of community health needs; policy development involves establishment of community health needs along with availability of required resources; and finally, assurance entails managing required resources and implementation and evaluation of necessary health-related programs (Mays, Miller, & Halverson, 2000). Healey and Lesneski (2011) have described assessment more fully as follows: "Assessment involves the monitoring of health status and the investigation of health problems. The development of policy includes informing, educating and empowering individuals about actions they can take in order to remain healthy. Finally, assurance requires regulatory powers utilized to protect the health of the public along with evaluating the effectiveness and quality of various public health programs that were designed to improve the public's health" (p. 217).

core functions of public health
Assessment, policy development, and assurance.

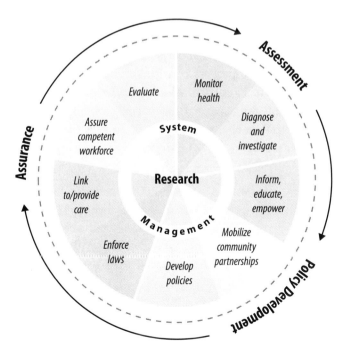

Figure 10.2 Core Functions and the Ten Essential Public Health Services
Source: CDC, 2014b.

Epidemiology and Public Health

epidemiology

A sound methodology used to investigate hypotheses about disease causation.

surveillance system

A means of collecting data that may contribute to knowledge about the occurrence of disease.

epidemiologist

A disease detective who gathers medical evidence on the occurrence, determinants, and cause of disease.

triad of disease

The agent, the host, and the environment related to the occurrence of a disease.

One of the most important activities of public health agencies is the use of sophisticated surveillance systems guided by the science of epidemiology. The cornerstone of public health, **epidemiology** focuses on the distribution and causes of disease in populations and the development and testing of ways to prevent and control disease. Epidemiological methods are used to track the origin of disease, how it spreads, and how to control it. A key element in epidemiology is the **surveillance system**, a means of systematically collecting, recording, analyzing, interpreting, and disseminating data about the health status of a population. Raw health data gathered from public health surveillance systems are used to look for statistical relationships, and conclusions drawn from those relationships are disseminated to relevant organizations. A well-developed surveillance system is a necessary prerequisite for defining a health problem and determining appropriate strategies for its elimination. Public health surveillance systems work so well because public health departments have the authority to make certain diseases reportable by health care providers, including physicians, hospitals, and laboratories. Figure 10.3 illustrates the flow of surveillance data.

A person who practices epidemiology is called an **epidemiologist**. Epidemiologists are disease detectives who conduct intense investigations to discover disease causes and effects. The principles of epidemiology, which had their origins in outbreaks of communicable diseases, are now being used for understanding chronic diseases and occupational health problems and even for managerial decision making.

The epidemiological process consists of a series of steps designed to discover why an event happened. Along the way to the discovery of this cause, multiple tools are used that have been developed over time in the solution of other public health outbreaks of disease. One of these tools is the **triad of disease** (Figure 10.4). Epidemiologists look for the components

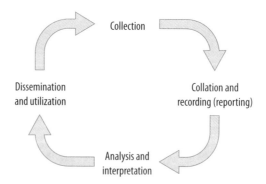

Collection

Collation and recording (reporting)

Analysis and interpretation

Dissemination and utilization

Figure 10.3   Flow of Surveillance Data

Source: California Department of Public Health, 2013, p.12.

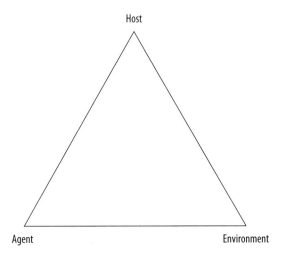

Figure 10.4 Triad of Disease
Source: CDC, 2006, updated 2012, p. I-52.

of this triad—the host, the agent, and the environment—because their intersection is usually involved in the occurrence of a disease. The host in most cases is an individual, the agent is the organism causing the disease, and the environment is where the disease actually occurs. For example, salmonella is a bacterial agent, the host can be human or animal, and the environment is improperly cooked or refrigerated food. When searching for causal relationships, epidemiologists must look at all three components to find effective prevention and control measures.

Epidemiologists use the concept of the **chain of infection** as their frame of reference when investigating clusters of disease (Figure 10.5). Following the chain of infection consists of investigating each link in the chain: pathogen, reservoir, mode of transmission, and host. For an infection to develop, there cannot be a break in this chain. Public health epidemiologists investigate these links in order to find the cause of the disease outbreak and immediately implement control measures. With the discovery of vaccines for many communicable diseases, public health departments are now capable of holding mass immunization campaigns in order to reduce the number of individuals who are susceptible to infectious diseases. This allows public health departments to virtually eliminate many communicable diseases as a threat to the health of the general population in their communities.

chain of infection
A series of stages in the development of a disease outbreak.

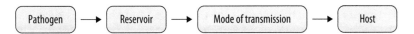

Figure 10.5 Chain of Infection for Disease
Source: Healey & Walker, 2009, p. 29.

The epidemiological process can be divided into descriptive epidemiology and analytical epidemiology. **Descriptive epidemiology** is the starting point for a public health investigation and involves looking at the time, place, and person involved in the event under consideration. It is done first in order to develop a case definition of the problem being investigated by the epidemiologist. Analytical epidemiology is usually completed after descriptive epidemiology has defined the problem. **Analytical epidemiology** seeks to identify risk factors for the disease under investigation. This type of study, whether a case-control or a cohort study, is an attempt to prove causation through statistical analysis. The results of descriptive epidemiology studies are usually further analyzed and proven by the analytical study.

Although epidemiology has gained its importance in public health through its success in managing outbreaks of communicable diseases, it is now becoming a source of information about chronic diseases as well. Numerous chronic disease epidemiological studies conducted in the last several decades have revealed the causes of many chronic diseases. Many of these chronic disease epidemiological studies are large cohort studies that follow individuals over time in an attempt to discover why they develop various chronic diseases. The best example of this type of study is the famous Framingham Heart Study. This large study, started in 1948, tracked the residents of Framingham, Massachusetts, over a fifty-year period and identified many heart disease factors. There is also a great deal of epidemiological interest in what causes individuals to develop the various complications seen among those who live with chronic diseases for long periods of time.

descriptive epidemiology
The examination of time, place, and person in relation to a disease occurrence in order to define the problem.

analytical epidemiology
The use of statistical methods to attempt to prove the cause of a given disease.

Population-Based Health

The major characteristic that separates public health departments from the rest of the medical care system is their focus on the health of the population rather than the individual. On the one hand our health care system is for the most part concerned with individual health. Physicians see individual patients, and hospitals admit a patient at a time, not an entire population. Apart from public health departments, our system of health care services has a focus on delivering health care services to individuals who present themselves to providers for services, usually when they become ill.

On the other hand public health departments have the responsibility for the health of a given population such as a community. Public health departments spend the majority of their time and resources developing, implementing, and evaluating community-wide prevention programs. They have a mission statement that calls for health care delivery that concentrates on large numbers of well individuals rather than on individual patients who are already ill. This is the opposite of the rest of the health care system, which waits for individuals to become ill and then treats the illnesses, attempting to bring them back to health.

Interventions designed to affect the determinants of disease for a population rather than an individual patient are labeled **population-based interventions**. These interventions focus on health promotion efforts designed to prevent disease rather than treat it. According to the Association of American Medical Colleges (1998), population-based medicine usually involves

- An assessment of the health of the entire population of a given area

- Implementation and evaluation of specific interventions to improve the health of the entire population in a given area

- The provision of care to individual patients while also considering the characteristics (culture, health status, and needs) of the population under consideration

This approach to health care delivery employed by public health departments encourages a strong focus on prevention, also called **primary prevention**. There are three levels of prevention, as shown in Exhibit 10.1, which uses a childhood lead poisoning program as an example.

population-based interventions
Control measures designed to abate a given problem for the entire at-risk population.

primary prevention
An effort to prevent a disease from occurring in the first place.

EXHIBIT 10.1. RECOGNIZING THE DIFFERENCES BETWEEN PRIMARY, SECONDARY, AND TERTIARY PREVENTION: CHILDHOOD LEAD POISONING

Lead poisoning occurs when the body absorbs too much lead by breathing it in or swallowing it. Children are exposed to lead primarily through the lead-based paint that is frequently found in older homes and through soil that has been previously contaminated by lead-based paint. Lead affects nearly every system in the body and in high enough quantities can cause irreversible neurocognitive damage in developing children under six years old.

Primary Prevention

According to the CDC (2014c), data from the National Health and Nutrition Examination Survey (NHANES) show that blood lead levels in children younger than thirteen years of age declined nearly 90 percent from 1976 to 2014. This dramatic decrease is attributed to population-based environmental policies that banned the use of lead in gasoline, paint, drinking-water pipes, and food and beverage containers. The decrease in blood lead level from 1990 to 2000 is also associated with trends in housing demolition and substantial housing rehabilitation. Such primary prevention is the only way to reduce the neurocognitive effects of lead poisoning.

Secondary Prevention

Lead-level screening programs for at-risk children are followed by the treatment of children with high levels and by removal of lead paint from households. Screening can prevent recurrent exposures and the exposure of other children to lead by triggering the identification and remediation of sources of lead in children's environments.

Tertiary Prevention

At the tertiary prevention level, there is treatment, support, and rehabilitation of children with lead poisoning who manifest complications of the disease. Lead chelation of the blood and soft tissues of exposed individuals can reduce morbidity associated with lead poisoning. Chelation can reduce the immediate toxicity associated with acute ingestion of lead but has limited ability to reverse the neurocognitive effects of chronic exposure.

Primary prevention programs have always been part of the public health mission and are now starting to gain the attention of more and more health policy experts as a way to keep our health care system sustainable for future generations. These public health programs that prevent disease are hard to evaluate because it is difficult to place a monetary value on that which did not happen. In other words, how do we provide evidence that a particular intervention was the only reason a population remained well rather than becoming ill? This is the major reason why it is so hard to convince those who fund public health programs of the need to increase rather than reduce annual budget outlays. There is also the political side of the equation, found in the fact that health care providers, including physician groups, are frightened by the thought of a reduction in ill patients. Improved population health will negatively affect their income stream.

Healthy People 2020

Public health departments have always had a focus on preventing disease but have never had a guiding vision on how to accomplish this goal. The closest that this nation has come to developing solid principles for the prevention of disease can be found in *Healthy People: The Surgeon General's Report on Health Promotion and Disease Prevention*. This 1979 report offered the nation a series of goals and objectives designed to prevent many health behaviors that usually lead to the development of disease. This report was intended to start a national discussion regarding community involvement in the health of the population, and it began the Healthy People initiative. The next Healthy People report appeared in 1990, and reports are now being produced every ten years. They address the progress made in the health of the population and set new topics, goals, and objectives for the next ten-year time period.

The fourth and latest report, released in 2010, is titled **Healthy People 2020**. These reports have become a management tool designed to help communities deal with various population health issues. Healthy People 2020 offers communities a number of prevention and wellness activities backed up by a strong model that can be used to measure the progress of communities toward achievement of the goals and objectives put forth by the report (U.S. Department of Health and Human Services, 2010).

This new report pays more attention to health equity and addresses the social determinants of health throughout the various stages of life. It can be accessed from an interactive website along with improved technology that is designed to disseminate the report to communities throughout the United States. An important new addition in Healthy People 2020 is a list of the leading health indicators. According to the U.S. Department of Health and Human Services, Office of Disease Prevention and Health (2010; also see CDC 2014a), these leading health indicators will assist communities to assess population health in key areas. Table 10.1 displays these leading health indicators, which are organized under twelve topic areas.

Koh (2010) observes that Healthy People 2010 (published in 2000) focused on two major goals: increased life expectancy and the elimination of health disparities. While life expectancy increased during the 2000 to 2010 time period, the goal of eliminating health disparities remains unmet. These health indicators can serve as a road map for the improvement of the health of the entire population through community collaboration. The health problems underlying these indicators are great, but by creating national objectives for population health and evaluating our progress on a periodic basis, we are better able to see which interventions work and which need to be improved.

Healthy People 2020
The most recent report in the series of Healthy People reports; a new report is issued every ten years.

Health Promotion Programs

Most individuals worry about poor health after they become ill and then spend a great deal of time trying to discover how to return to wellness. However, if that illness is a chronic disease, there is no cure. Moreover, because chronic diseases may be asymptomatic, individuals may develop life-threatening complications before they realize they are ill, and these may permanently reduce their quality of life. Chronic diseases can be prevented when people become educated about the unhealthy behaviors that are responsible for the development of most chronic diseases and their later complications.

For the most part, children do not think about their health. Why would they waste their time thinking about poor health when they are young

Table 10.1   Healthy People 2020: The Leading Health Indicators

12 Topic Areas	26 Leading Health Indicators
Access to Health Services	• Persons with medical insurance
	• Persons with a usual primary care provider
Clinical Preventive Services	• Adults who receive a colorectal cancer screening based on the most recent guidelines
	• Adults with hypertension whose blood pressure is under control
	• Adult diabetic population with an A1c value greater than 9 percent
	• Children aged 19 to 35 months who receive the recommended doses of diphtheria, tetanus, and pertussis (DTaP); polio; measles, mumps, and rubella (MMR); Haemophilus influenza type b (Hib); hepatitis B; varicella; and pneumococcal conjugate (PCV) vaccines
Environmental Quality	• Air Quality Index (AQI) exceeding 100
	• Children aged 3 to 11 years exposed to secondhand smoke
Injury and Violence	• Fatal injuries
	• Homicides
Maternal, Infant, and Child Health	• Infant deaths
	• Preterm births
Mental Health	• Suicides
	• Adolescents who experience major depressive episodes (MDEs)
Nutrition, Physical Activity, and Obesity	• Adults who meet current Federal physical activity guidelines for aerobic physical activity and muscle-strengthening activity
	• Adults who are obese
	• Children and adolescents who are considered obese
	• Total vegetable intake for persons aged 2 years and older
Oral Health	• Persons aged 2 years and older who used the oral health care system in the past 12 months
Reproductive and Sexual Health	• Sexually active females aged 15–44 years who received reproductive health services in the past 12 months
	• Persons living with HIV who know their serostatus
Social Determinants	• Students who graduate with a regular diploma 4 years after starting ninth grade
Substance Abuse	• Adolescents using alcohol or any illicit drugs during the past 30 days
	• Adults engaging in binge drinking during the past 30 days
Tobacco	• Adults who are current cigarette smokers
	• Adolescents who smoked cigarettes in the past 30 days

Source: U.S. Department of Health and Human Services, Office of Disease Prevention and Health Promotion, 2010.

and healthy and when there is little health education in their schools? Unfortunately, most Americans begin to concern themselves with the possibility of poor health only when they are older adults or when they experience a health problem. This lack of early intervention places our children at a distinct disadvantage because many will begin practicing unhealthy behaviors while they are young, yet they are currently unaware of the true cost of these high-risk behaviors.

Among the most important tools for the improvement of the health of the population are health education and health promotion programs, which are quite often developed by public health departments. These programs have been designed to educate the population about the disease processes for both communicable and chronic diseases. The most important goal of these health education efforts is to prevent disease from occurring in the first place. This goal is much different from the goal of treatment and cure found elsewhere in the current health care delivery system, which makes profits only when people become ill. In fact, if health education and health promotion programs are successful, our current health care system will lose a substantial portion of its profits.

The starting point for the development of a health education initiative or a community-wide health promotion program is a **needs assessment** of the population designated to receive the health education. In fact most individuals working in health promotion programs in public health departments believe that the needs assessment is the most important component of health promotion efforts at the population level. A needs assessment is a discovery, evaluation, and prioritizing of the health-related needs of a distinct population. This important step in the development of health promotion programs requires population data from secondary sources and primary data about the problem under consideration. A needs assessment helps the health educator assigned to the program to decide on the focus of the effort.

needs assessment
A method of discovering, evaluating, and prioritizing the needs of a population.

The next important step is the creation of specific health promotion projects designed to abate the public health threat uncovered during the needs assessment. The starting point for this step is a review of the literature that can help public health workers uncover model programs that have been successfully implemented.

Public Health Leadership

The United States failed to meet 85 percent of the goals set out in Healthy People 2000, largely due to insufficient resources and poor public health leadership in getting community support for this project. Public health departments operate in a bureaucratic environment that relies heavily on rules and regulations and this environment often blocks ingenuity and inventiveness. Bureaucratic organizations do not work well in times of rapid change, and this is especially true in government-run public health departments. Public health agencies are often faced with annual budget cuts along with political appointees placed in charge of their operations. Often these bureaucratic organizations block change because it threatens the power of the manager. Public health departments in the United States have a very important role to play in reforming the health care system in our country. That role requires excellent leadership and the use of creativity and innovation, along with collaboration with the private health care sector, so that these departments can develop and implement health education initiatives designed to improve the health of the population. To be successful, public health departments need transformational leaders skilled in empowerment of public health employees and collaboration with other health-related agencies.

As stated previously in this chapter, public health departments are very political because they usually receive their funding from the government and their directors usually report to a city mayor or a board of county commissioners. Public health directors usually have very short tenures and are well aware that they can lose their coveted appointment and the power that goes with it if they anger anyone with political power. This makes them very reluctant to innovate in their approaches to disease prevention, for fear of political risk. At the same time, the current epidemic of chronic diseases that this country faces requires creativity and innovation from the leaders of public health departments and therefore a willingness on their part to take great political risks.

The entire U.S. health care system, including public health, is facing monumental change that must be led to success through community-level collaboration. The important thing to remember about major change is that it forces organizations to adapt. Strong leadership is the skill that allows the organization to adapt, look for change, and grow. The successful public health leader will use adaptation to empower public health workers and community collaborators to concentrate on the accomplishment of the vision.

One of the most important attributes of a successful leader is the ability to gain the trust of his or her followers. Such trust is an absolute necessity for those leading a bureaucratic agency in the attempt to adapt to a rapidly changing environment where bureaucracies are unable to achieve their goals. Public health departments face a lack of trust because they usually represent the government. It is the public health leader's job to regain the trust of public health employees and of the community where they work. According to Horsager (2009) no matter who you are or what your position entails, trust affects your ability to influence the people you are attempting to lead. In short, in order to be an effective public health leader, you must first gain the trust of your followers.

Public health departments have experienced a great deal of success in their various programs to reduce the numbers of communicable diseases affecting our population. These same departments have a less than stellar performance in their attempt to reduce the epidemic of chronic diseases and their complications that is responsible for the escalating costs of health care. Our failures with this epidemic are evidence that public health departments are in need of innovative solutions to the increasing numbers of Americans acquiring one or more chronic diseases as they age.

Echeverria (2013) argues that there is great tension for the leader who attempts to promote organizational creativity and innovation and who must then also be successful at getting these new ways of doing things actually implemented. This is an especially difficult task for public health departments operating under a stifling government bureaucratic structure, but it can be done with leadership.

Public health leaders need to produce a work environment of trust that allows employees the freedom and resources that are so necessary to make new ideas realities. According to Diamandis and Kotler (2012), individuals, by their very nature, will always attempt to block breakthrough ideas until these ideas become reality. Public health leaders not only need to encourage innovation but also must lead their followers in adopting a strategy of innovation for developing and implementing public health programs. In their new book *Abundance: The Future Is Better Than You Think*, Diamandis and Kotler (2012) identify four motivators that push innovation along: curiosity, fear, a desire to create wealth, and a desire for significance. These motivators can easily be promoted by public health leaders to their followers in the development of strategies designed to reduce the incidence of chronic diseases in our country.

Most individuals who work in public health departments desire to improve the health of the population and have a number of ideas on how to develop new programs and a curiosity about how to make these new programs work. This curiosity is an excellent motivator to become innovative in the development of new programs to improve the health of a given population. Fear is also a motivator for innovation in that public health employees are afraid of the consequences of a failure to deal with the challenge of chronic diseases. The last two motivators discussed by Diamandis and Kotler can also be present in the development of public health prevention programs. The increased wealth can be found in an increased public health budget that is critical for new program development. The desire for significance is a widespread human desire and requires only that the leader listens to the employees' thoughts and desires concerning the improvement of the health of the population.

Public health departments are likely to assume a new role in the improvement of the health of the population in the next several years. These departments have the skills and the knowledge necessary to develop, implement, and evaluate prevention programs that can reduce the incidence of chronic diseases and prevent many chronic disease complications. In order to assume these new responsibilities these agencies require leadership training for all their employees, with an emphasis on collaborating with communities in the implementation of community-based programs designed to improve the health of the population of every community in our nation. Health care reform efforts have produced an enormous opportunity for public health departments to make yet one more major contribution to the good health of Americans. The starting point for this new public health leadership can be found in the challenge produced by the chronic disease epidemic.

Future of Public Health

All Americans are demanding an answer to the rising costs of health care that are leading to health insurance payments that the government, businesses, and individuals can no longer afford. According to Milistein (2013), there is an annual gap of 2 to 3 percent between the increase in health care spending and the growth of our gross domestic product. What this means is that we have to reduce spending on things like education, infrastructure maintenance, and a whole host of other essential government programs to pay for health care. This is clearly an unsustainable situation. The only answer to reducing costs while improving the health of the population is effective prevention programs brought to life through public health departments.

U.S. public health departments are facing numerous challenges in the future, and their approach to disease prevention is exactly what our current health care system needs in order to deal with the chronic disease epidemic. In order to be successful in all their challenges, public health departments require effective leadership from top to bottom and also better funding sources in order to accomplish their vision for a healthy

America. Public health departments also need to empower the members of their workforce, in order to gain employee creativity and innovation in discovering solutions to the most pressing problems with population health. Public health leaders and their empowered followers also require the support of their communities, including the health care providers, in order to be successful in finding solutions to the major public health problems like the chronic disease epidemic.

The Affordable Care Act is about to be fully implemented, making health care reform in our country a reality. The prevention programs brought about by this new law will produce numerous opportunities for the development and implementation of various health promotion programs. Thanks to health care reform, the United States is finally realizing the necessity of keeping people free from illness and disease as long as possible. The problem seems to be how to get the entire population to better understand the importance of the chronic disease epidemic. Public health departments in America are about to assume new responsibilities in keeping the population healthy and seeking the required funding to make this vision of a healthy population a reality. This opportunity should not be squandered because of poor leadership in public health departments and lack of collaboration with other community health agencies. The core functions of public health departments—namely, assessment, policy development, and assurance—are going to assume a new importance in our reforming health care system. There will be a much greater focus on the health of the population rather than the current pattern of providing too much health care to those with insurance coverage. There will also be a greater demand for the use of epidemiology in the development of evidence-based medicine along with best practices in medicine, including health education initiatives.

Public health departments have many other responsibilities that will only grow in number and intensity as our entire health care system moves into the future. Healey and Lesneski (2011) argue that public health departments also face dealing with such significant threats as the effects of climate change on human health, the epidemic of violence facing this nation and the world, the threat of bioterrorism, and many other community and national threats to the health of the population that are just emerging. Two other areas where public health departments should play a major role are reducing medical errors, including nosocomial (hospital-acquired) outbreaks of disease, and developing evidence-based medicine, including the development of best practice models of care. The development and use of sophisticated surveillance systems should be a necessary adjunct to reducing the incidence of medical errors and nosocomial infections in health care facilities. Epidemiological studies conducted by public health departments will be very useful in helping develop evidence-based medicine along with best practices.

Many of these threats to health are producing opportunities to show leadership in the development of the collaborative, evidence-based, and population-based responses that are so very necessary for the survival and growth of our population. Our nation and in fact the world cannot afford to allow these many health threats to continue without a well-developed community response that is led by knowledgeable public health professionals.

SUMMARY

Public health departments are responsible for the health of the entire population rather than for individual health, which is the responsibility of the rest of our health care delivery system. The U.S. system of public health is financed through tax revenues and is charged with the prevention of disease. Public health departments are classified as federal, state, or local, with public health services actually delivered at the state or local levels.

These public health departments develop, implement, and evaluate a number of community efforts designed to prevent disease. Their history contains numerous programs that have been successful in extending the length of life for most Americans along with reducing the number of cases of communicable diseases throughout the country.

Healthy People 2020 offers the nation a vision that includes numerous goals and objectives designed to increase both the length and quality of life for the population. In order to achieve these very important goals, public health departments require transformational leadership, empowered followers, community collaboration, and increased funding. The chronic disease epidemic faced by our nation requires public health departments to develop, implement, and evaluate the success of community-based health education and health promotion programs. This epidemic is providing opportunities for public health departments to lead the way to a sustainable health care delivery system for all Americans.

The future of public health in the United States is filled with many challenges, with the chronic disease epidemic gaining the most attention. These challenges can be successfully met only with strong public health departments that are enabled to use the skills they have developed over many years of population health success stories. These departments have the answers to our health problems and deserve the opportunity to improve the health of our entire population.

KEY TERMS

analytical epidemiology

chain of infection

core functions of public health

descriptive epidemiology

Emerson report of 1945

epidemiologist

epidemiology

health disparity

Healthy People 2020

needs assessment

population-based interventions

primary prevention

public health

surveillance system

triad of disease

DISCUSSION QUESTIONS

1. What are the core functions of public health departments, and how would you explain each function?

2. What role does epidemiology play in the improvement of public health, and how would you explain the workings of this role?

3. Why is leadership such an important component of a successful public health department?

4. What are the necessary steps for conducting a successful health promotion program?

REFERENCES

Association of American Medical Colleges. (1998, June). *Contemporary issues in medicine: Medical informatics and population health* (Medical School Objectives Project, Report II). Washington, DC: Author.

Baldoni, J. (2012). *Lead with purpose: Giving your organization a reason to believe in itself*. New York, NY: American Management Association.

Barton, P. L. (2010). *Understanding the U.S. health services system* (4th ed.). Chicago, IL: Health Administration Press.

California Department of Public Health. (2013). *Basics of infection prevention.* Retrieved from http://www.cdph.ca.gov/programs/hai/Documents/Slide-Set -6-Basics-of-Epidemiology-and-Surveillance.pdf

Centers for Disease Control and Prevention. (1999). Ten great public health achievements—United States, 1990–1999. *Morbidity and Mortality Weekly Report, 48*(12), 241–243.

Centers for Disease Control and Prevention. (2006, updated 2012). *Principles of epidemiology in public health practice: An introduction to applied epidemiology and biostatistics* (3rd ed.). Retrieved from http://www.cdc.gov/OPHSS/CSELS/DSEPD/SS1978/SS1978.pdf

Centers for Disease Control and Prevention. (2014a). *Healthy People 2020: Leading indicators.* Retrieved from http://www.healthypeople.gov/2020/LHI/default.aspx

Centers for Disease Control and Prevention. (2014b). *The public health system and the 10 essential public health services.* Retrieved from http://www.cdc.gov/nphpsp/essentialservices.html

Centers for Disease Control and Prevention. (2014c). *What parents need to know to protect their children.* Retrieved from http://www.cdc.gov/nceh/lead/ACCLPP/blood_lead_levels.htm

Cohen, L., Chavez, V., & Chehimi, S. (2007). *Prevention is primary: Strategies for community well-being.* San Francisco, CA: Jossey-Bass.

Diamandis, P. H., & Kotler, S. (2012). *Abundance: The future is better than you think.* New York, NY: Simon & Schuster.

Doll, R., & Hill, A. B. (1950). Smoking and carcinoma of the lungs: Preliminary report. *British Medical Journal, 2*(4682), 739–748.

Echeverria, L. M. (2013). *Idea agent: Leadership that liberates creativity and accelerates innovation.* New York, NY: American Management Association.

Healey, B. J., & Lesneski, C. D. (2011). *Transforming public health practice: Leadership and management essentials.* San Francisco, CA: Jossey-Bass.

Healey, B. J., & Walker, K. T. (2009). *Introduction to occupational health in public health practice.* San Francisco, CA: Jossey-Bass.

Horsager, D. (2009). *The trust edge: How top leaders gain faster results, deeper relationships, and a stronger bottom line.* New York, NY: Free Press.

How long will we live—and how well? (2012, December 13). *Washington Post.* Retrieved from http://www.washingtonpost.com/wp-srv/special/health/healthy-life-expectancy

Institute of Medicine. (2002). *The future of the public's health in the 21st century.* Retrieved from http://www.iom.edu/Reports/2002/The-Future-of-the-Publics-Health-in-the-21st-Century.aspx

Institute of Medicine. (2013). *Best care at lower cost: The path to continuously learning health care in America.* Washington, DC: National Academies Press.

Johnson, J. A. (2013). *Introduction to public health management, organizations, and policy.* Clifton Park, NY: Delmar/Cengage Learning.

Koh, H. (2010). A 2020 vision for Healthy People 2010. *New England Journal of Medicine, 362*(18), 1653–1656.

Mays, G. P., Miller, C. A., & Halverson, P. K. (2000). *Local public health practice: Trends & models.* Washington, DC: American Public Health Association.

Milistein, A. (2013). Code red and blue: Safely limiting health care's GDP footprint. *New England Journal of Medicine, 368*(1), 1–3.

Schimpff, S. C. (2012). *The future of health-care delivery: Why it must change and how it will affect you*. Washington, DC: Potomac Books.

Turnock, B. J. (2009). *Public health: What it is and how it works* (4th ed.). Sudbury, MA: Jones & Bartlett Learning.

U.S. Department of Health and Human Services, Office of Disease Prevention and Health Promotion. (2010). *Healthy People 2020* (ODPHP Publication No. B0132). Retrieved from http://healthypeople.gov/2020/TopicsObjectives2020/pdfs/HP2020_brochure_with_LHI_508.pdf

Wynder, E. L., & Graham, E. A. (1950). Tobacco smoking as a possible etiologic factor in bronchiogenic carcinoma: A study of six-hundred and eighty four proved cases. *Journal of the American Medical Association, 143*(4), 329–336.

CHAPTER 11

THE PURSUIT OF QUALITY CARE

Tina Marie Evans

One of the greatest challenges continuing to face the U.S. health care system today is closing the gap between evidence-based diagnostic and treatment practices and the actual practices taking place in clinical settings. Ensuring the quality and safety of the care provided in inpatient and ambulatory settings is central to saving lives as well as unnecessary costs. We frequently hear discussions about the quality and safety of care in every part of the health care delivery system, and we are well aware that the struggle to close the quality gap continues. The enhancement of quality has been at the center of health care research, reports, and policy for several years now, but many organizations still find the features of this intangible "quality" focus difficult to define, measure, and implement effectively.

A good starting place for this discussion of quality care then is to establish a baseline definition of the term *quality* as it applies to health care settings. **Quality** is "the degree to which health services for individuals and patient populations increase the likelihood of desirable health outcomes and are consistent with current professional knowledge" (Williams & Torrens, 2008, p. 311). A **quality gap** is the area between what research tells us are the optimal processes and outcomes for each portion of health care delivery and the processes and outcomes actually in place.

One would hope that quality of care has always been the point of highest concern for all who have any role in or interaction with the provision of health care; however, it seems that quality was not first on everyone's list until pressures for cost containment as well as efficiency of care began and then steadily increased. The fee-for-service environment of the past cultivated a health care delivery system that did not pay much attention to the efficiency of care. Today we know that spending more money does

LEARNING OBJECTIVES

After reading this chapter you should be able to

- Define quality as it applies to the U.S. health care system.

- Understand the history of quality care in the United States.

- Explain the major findings and suggestions of the Institute of Medicine reports.

- Identify the nine categories of quality improvement strategies for correcting deficiencies in the quality and safety of care.

quality
The degree to which health services for individuals and patient populations increase the likelihood of desirable health outcomes and are consistent with current professional knowledge.

quality gap
The area between what research tells us are the optimal processes and outcomes for each portion of health care delivery and the processes and outcomes actually in place.

not necessarily lead to a better quality of care provided and received. Many payers now demand a greater level of quality care than ever before, and they look carefully for the most efficient care possible at the most reasonable price. Consumers have begun to speak up in anger as well, demanding better treatment outcomes and a higher level of provider accountability in cases where outcomes are less than expected.

Although the health care system in the United States continues to improve, it still faces many quality-related obstacles and criticisms, specifically in the areas of reducing medical errors and improving patient safety, patient centeredness, effectiveness of care, timeliness of care, efficiency of care, and equitability of care resources. The continuous evolution and frequent technological updating of the health care delivery system poses serious challenges for managers and clinicians alike. The demands for quality care will certainly not go away in the upcoming years, nor will the pressures for cost containment and efficiency. Let's review the origins of the quality movement in health care, and see what is known now compared to a few decades ago.

Origins of the Quality Movement

Many individuals have contributed their thoughts and theories, many systems and models have been implemented and then modified, and much research has been undertaken to bring the quality movement to where it is today. The roots of the movement are diverse and colorful, extending back to remains from Babylonian society in 2000 B.C. that identify billing guidelines for physicians as well as suggested penalties for physician incompetence and patient injury. Thus we know that even in ancient times, people had a solid interest in obtaining the best possible medical care that they could.

As we review the history of quality in health care, keep in mind that in the early 1900s, hospitals were more or less almshouses with no safety or cleanliness standards in place and conditions that were poor at best. The famous Flexner report of 1910 not only shed light on the inadequacies of medical education but also provided a detailed description of the horrid conditions. Patients were not given proper examinations, diagnostic and treatment records were not always kept, equipment was lacking, hygiene was awful, no one verified the qualifications of physicians, and no data on patient care outcomes were kept. Provider accountability at this time was all but nonexistent (Gassiot, Searcy, & Giles, 2011).

It was also in 1910 that Ernest A. Codman proposed a new method of evaluating patient care (Taylor & Taylor, 1994). Codman (1869–1940) was a Boston surgeon who had developed a way to examine care delivery that he referred to as the "end result system of hospital standardization." He carefully abstracted the case history of each of his patients and then evaluated patient outcomes over a period of time to determine the effectiveness of his care. He classified the outcomes as either satisfactory or unsatisfactory and studied the likely causes behind the unsatisfactory outcomes (Ostrow, 1983). His method of tracking the surgical outcomes of all patients long enough to determine whether treatments were effective and his work to improve methods of surgical practice were both integral to the development of early standards for the surgical setting. Codman believed that hospitals needed three standards to bring quality to a higher level: (1) hospital physicians must be appropriately trained and licensed; (2) staff meetings and clinical reviews must occur regularly; and (3) medical histories, physical exam data, and laboratory data should always be collected and kept (Luce, Bindman, & Lee, 1994). His friend and colleague, Franklin H. Martin, who went on to found the American College of Surgeons (ACS) in 1913, also used Codman's system as the basis for improving quality (Taylor & Taylor, 1994).

The ACS soon joined the quality movement as well, by launching a project of its own aimed at improving hospital care. ACS members worked together to develop criteria for quality, then promoted these criteria as goals that hospitals should strive to attain. These goals addressed the definition of practicing staff members, the competence and character of physicians and surgeons, the need for periodic review of all records, the adequacy of facilities used for care, and the regulation of practice. These goals were then refined (with support from a Carnegie Foundation Grant), and were released in 1917 as the Minimum Standard for Hospitals. This one-page document continues to be recognized as the forerunner of standards in place today. For example, one criterion suggested by the ACS involved the examination of tissues removed during surgery. It proposed that all surgically removed tissues be sent to a lab for further study as well as for comparison with the patient's preoperative diagnosis, which is similar to the regulations in place today (The Joint Commission [TJC], 2012; Taylor & Taylor, 1994). The ACS began its first onsite quality inspections of hospitals in 1918, with only 89 of the 692 hospitals surveyed meeting the ACS criteria. Additional information and criteria were added to the Minimum Standard in the following years, and an updated, eighteen-page version was published in 1926 (TJC, 2012).

The Minimum Standard of the American College of Surgeons' Hospital Standardization Program, 1918

- Physicians and surgeons privileged to practice in the hospital should be convened organized medical staff.

- Membership in the medical staff is restricted to physicians and surgeons who are both competent in their field and worthy in character and professional ethics.

- The medical staff, with the approval of the governing board, adopts rules, regulations, and policies concerning their work in the hospital. Included in these rules, regulations, and policies are requirements for staff meetings and review and analysis of the different medical departments based upon the information in the clinical records of patients.

- Accurate and complete clinical records for all patients are to be developed and maintained by the hospital. These records need to contain history and a physical, working diagnosis, treatment, medical progress, condition on discharge with final diagnosis, and autopsy findings when appropriate.

- Clinical laboratory facilities must be available to facilitate the treatment of patients. These laboratory facilities should include chemical, bacteriological, serological, histological, radiographic, and fluoroscopic services with trained technicians present [Bowman, 1919].

After World War II the focus on improving hospital quality strengthened with the passing of the Hill-Burton Act. During this time of great hospital expansion, this act was effective in strengthening regulations and hospital licensure laws because meeting these requirements was now a prerequisite for receiving hospital construction project funding from the government. There was a notable improvement in the standard of care at some hospitals by this time, especially at the 3,200 hospitals that had earned ACS approval for meeting its standards. The ACS's hospital standardization program continued to grow, and eventually it became so large and its management so time consuming that it became clear that a governing body to oversee hospital standardization was needed. In 1951, the American College of Physicians, the American Hospital Association, the American Medical Association, the Canadian Medical Association, and the ACS joined together to found the Joint Commission on Accreditation of Hospitals (JCAH). The JCAH, formed as an independent and nonprofit organization, was organized to guide and direct hospital standardization as well as to provide voluntary accreditation services. This allowed the ACS to transfer the oversight of administrating the hospital quality standards program to JCAH, which offered its first hospital accreditations in January 1953 (TJC, 2012). Many believe that this early system of standards to quantify objective care outcomes signaled the coming end of the days of anecdotal evidence, subjective impressions, and non-evidence-based policy in medicine. The importance of carefully tracking objective data over time as well as keeping accurate data became increasingly imperative as the movement toward improved treatment practices continued.

The JCAH continued its work of developing and refining criteria that would increase quality of care in the hospital settings, and in 1953 published updated Standards for Hospital Accreditation. The Social Security Act Amendments of 1965 and 1972 continued to reinforce the prominent place that quality was taking in health care settings, which led the JCAH to move closer to using peer reviews, clinical reviews, and patient chart audits to better examine care outcomes and carefully study any negative issues that arose during such reviews. The establishment of Medicare and Medicaid in 1965 also brought with it the concept and practice of the **utilization review**, which allows health insurance companies to examine the medical necessity for care. It also brought the government into the realm of health care reimbursement in a substantial way. Utilization review is a safeguard against unnecessary and inappropriate medical care. With the government now involved through these programs, the impact of the JCAH standards increased, as compliance with these standards was the preferred method for hospitals to show that they indeed provided quality care services and were thus eligible for reimbursement. The utilization review boards attempted to control the expenditure of taxpayers' money on health care, trying to prevent misuse of the funds by ensuring that the services provided were of high quality and necessary (Ostrow, 1983). In addition, this was the point at which quality of care and reimbursements (or lack thereof) became tied together. Cost and quality were now viewed a bit differently as a new payment versus sanction system was now in place (Taylor & Taylor, 1994). This perspective remains in place today, as payers from this point in history forward began to demand accountability and quality of care if payment for services was to be made.

> **utilization review**
> A case-by-case assessment of the appropriateness of care prior to its provision, used by or on behalf of health care purchasers to influence care decisions and thus manage costs.

The 1953 JCAH standards were in effect until 1970, when they were updated once again to codify "optimal achievable levels of quality, instead of minimum essential levels of quality" (TJC, 2012, p. 2). The Social Security Act Amendments of 1972 further strengthened the ties between cost and quality by establishing **professional standards review organizations (PSROs)**, external agencies for additional peer review. The PSROs and the associated supporting legislation highlighted retrospective audits and medical care evaluations as popular supplementary methods of reviewing patient care and identifying specific ways to improve quality. Once the PSROs were in place, many researchers jumped at the chance to provide input on the best way to review and suggest best practices for medical care. Avedis Donabedian (1919–2000), whom many now consider the "father of quality assurance" (Best & Neuhauser, 2004), published a great amount of research during this time and proposed a conceptual model for understanding the interactions behind quality of care. Donabedian's model, which related the concepts of structure, process, and outcome,

> **professional standards review organizations (PSROs)**
> External agencies that provide peer reviews of health care quality and supply suggestions for improvement.

became widely used—and is still in use today. This model, combined with his research findings, formed a solid foundation for quality care and put a visual framework in place so managers and clinicians alike could better grasp the concept of quality and the relationship between the components of the model (Taylor & Taylor, 1994).

As time progressed the JCAH also expanded its accreditation services beyond the hospital setting, adding similar services for long-term care settings, organizations caring for developmentally disabled persons, psychiatric facilities, substance abuse programs, ambulatory care facilities, and community mental health programs. This expansion led to the decision to change the name of the organization from the Joint Commission on Accreditation of Hospitals (JCAH) to the Joint Commission on Accreditation of Healthcare Organizations (JCAHO) in 1987 (TJC, 2012). (Later the name would be changed again, to The Joint Commission.) The standards were updated once again to be even more rigorous than previously, drawing on Donabedian's classic and still widely respected structure-process-outcome model as well as adding in some elements of organizational system change from the works of management theorists W. Edwards Deming (1900–1993) and Joseph M. Juran (1904–2008) (Donabedian, 2003).

Even with some improvement in the quality of care as a result of the improved voluntary accreditation process, some remained doubtful that the quality improvement efforts of these initiatives were actually working. The mid-1980s were a time of growing public interest in and outcry for a better quality of care, and this had clearly become a popular health care consumer concern. A turning point occurred in December 1986, when the Health Care Finance Administration (HCFA) publicly released the data from its study on the mortality statistics in hospitals (Taylor & Taylor, 1994). This study found that many hospital services were indeed inadequate, which caused HCFA to move forward in implementing several of its own corrective initiatives (Lohr, 1990). With the HCFA study's information readily available in newspapers, magazines and widely covered by local television news channels, the American public received an unprecedented inside look into how Medicare patients were being treated in hospitals. Once these data were released, people began to demand even higher levels of study and provider accountability for any unacceptable findings or harms, and they pushed to have future data released publicly (Taylor & Taylor, 1994). The increasing level of concern, complaints, and vocal awareness led Congress to commission a full study on the quality of care from the Institute of Medicine (IOM).

Although the data from the HCFA study surprised many, they did not surprise those performing similar research, since they were already well aware that, up to this point, quality (much like beauty) was in the eye of the beholder and that individual health care organizations measured quality as they saw fit. Peer reviews had their limitations too, as physicians were hesitant to criticize the work of their colleagues (and to have their colleagues comment on their own work). The practice of examining quality only when cases of exceptionally poor care, patient harm, or patient death were brought to light was common during this time. Quality assurance checks commonly occurred only after a serious mishap or breach of standards, and in the absence of such problems the status quo continued. The use of this hit-or-miss corrective practice was predicated on the idea that the best way to assure quality of care was "picking the bad apples," that is, removing them. This practice of examining quality of care only after mistakes led many health care providers to develop a somewhat twisted view of the definition of quality—in this case it appeared to be defined as the absence of critical mistakes (Sultz & Young, 2009).

The 1990s saw greatly increased research into quality of care initiatives, activities, outcomes, and methods of provider accountability. Advances in technology in such areas as cardiac surgery and transplantation piqued the interest of all, and led to questions on how such new (and therefore expensive) technologies would affect the quality of care, patient safety, and patient outcomes. Additional studies by JCAHO focused on assessment processes and the many types of systematic monitoring of quality that could be chosen for use. Periodic reviews of care were now replaced by ongoing assessment reviews of care.

The explosion of research interest in quality of care projects led to many additional studies and subsequent attempts at fixing particular quality issues in a wide variety of ways (Taylor & Taylor, 1994). For example, in the 1960s, only about 100 clinical studies of quality of care were published each year, but by the early 1990s, over 10,000 studies were published and shared annually (Williams & Torrens, 2008). Many groups became involved—hospitals, hospital associations, accrediting bodies, universities, foundations, businesses, advocacy groups, and government agencies (Taylor & Taylor, 1994). Much concern was also being expressed about the quickly rising costs of health care and the tremendous amount of economic resources going toward that care. The consumers of health care services continued to take notice of the research data made available to them, and became less willing to simply trust health care providers to act in their best interest—especially when the pressures of managed care were noticeably increasing. Despite this, although varied attempts at quality assurance continued throughout the decade, the priority status quality had achieved several years previously was slipping away. The quality movement seemed to fall off the national radar for a few years; however, that did not last long. Two unprecedented reports released by the IOM in 1999 and 2001 sent shockwaves throughout the American health care system and put quality in health care under the national microscope, highlighting critical statistics and an immediate need to correct deficiencies. To better understand the results of each of these reports, let's examine summaries of their findings and consider their main points and implications.

IOM Report on Medical Errors

The results of Congress's request that the Institute of Medicine conduct a study on the quality of care were published in two reports. The first report completed by the IOM Committee on Quality of Health Care in America was released in November 1999, and it focused on medical errors. Titled *To Err Is Human: Building a Safer Health System,* the report established a baseline of information on the current state of the system and made a shocking yet convincing case for high levels of concern for the safety of patients seeking care within that system. Focused primarily on medical errors, the report presented these errors as a serious health threat, one that could be compared with the lethality of breast cancer, motor vehicle accidents, and acquired immunodeficiency syndrome. The report asserted that the old systems of quality care were unreliable, and that varied hit-or-miss attempts to fix the broken portions of the system were simply not enough to correct the overall problem—an overhaul of the health care system itself was called for (Shaw, Elliott, Isaacson, & Murphy, 2007).

This 1999 IOM report found that at least 44,000 Americans, and possibly as many as 98,000, die each year in hospitals because of serious medical errors that could have been prevented. In addition to the patients who lose their lives, this report documented how tens of thousands of patients "suffer or barely escape from nonfatal injuries that a truly high-quality care system would largely prevent" (p. 2). As a clinician myself I believe that although these numbers were indeed alarming, they barely began to evaluate the true situation. The errors that were tracked and analyzed in this report were mostly those that occurred in the hospital setting; the report did not account for errors that occurred in the many ambulatory care settings that provide the majority of health care services to Americans.

The Committee on Quality of Health Care in America concluded that it was not acceptable for patients to be harmed in any way by the system of medical care intended to provide healing in time of illness and comfort to the sick, especially given that American health care was expected to be premised on the concept that a provider should "first, do no harm" (translating the Latin phrase *primum non nocere*). After spotlighting the appalling number of medical errors, the committee went on to present a comprehensive four-tiered strategy (outlined below) for government agencies, health care providers, and health care industry stakeholders, as well as patients themselves, to come together to reduce preventable medical errors. The report concluded that many methods of prevention for these errors already existed but were not being used consistently (IOM, 1999).

The report also explained that the majority of the medical errors identified were not due to the recklessness of individual providers or the actions of a particular group of providers—thus thoroughly refuting the bad apple picking approach. Instead, large numbers of errors were found to be the end result of flawed systems and flawed processes and conditions that either led health care providers to make mistakes or failed to prevent those mistakes. Therefore specific areas of redesign of the system itself could greatly improve safety at many levels. In many cases the alterations suggested by the committee would make it more difficult for providers to do something wrong while making it easier for them to do what is correct.

After the committee's extensive examination of the data and current practices, it proposed the following four-tiered approach to enhance safety and reduce error (IOM, 1999).

Tier 1. "Establishing a national focus to create leadership, research, tools, and protocols to enhance the knowledge base about safety" (IOM, 1999, p. 6). This portion of the report brought to people's attention that health care is at least a decade behind many other high-risk industries in attaining good outcomes with regard to safety practices. This might be the result of not having one government agency named to take charge of consistently assessing and working to enhance safety practices in all parts of the health care delivery system. The report recommended that Congress establish a Center for Patient Safety (under the Agency for Healthcare Research and Quality). This proposed center would "set the national goals for patient safety, track progress in meeting these goals, and issue an annual report to the President and Congress on patient safety; and develop knowledge and understanding of errors in health care by developing a research agenda, funding Centers of Excellence, evaluating methods for identifying and preventing errors, and funding dissemination and communication activities to improve patient safety" (IOM, 1999, p. 7).

Of course, the responsibilities of this center would need appropriate and secure funding to support the suggested activities. An initial funding level of $30 to $35 million per year was recommended, with steady increases over time, to eventually reach $100 million. These costs were justified in the report as a small price to pay in light of the costs that were the consequences of medical errors. In addition, this suggested budget was comparable to the funding already earmarked for other public safety issues.

Tier 2. "Identifying and learning from errors by developing a nationwide public mandatory reporting system and by encouraging health care organizations and practitioners to develop and participate in voluntary reporting systems" (IOM, 1999, p. 6). This recommendation for a uniform mandatory reporting system for medical errors would require state governments to consistently gather information about adverse medical events, those that led either to patient harm or patient death. The hospitals would be the first facilities required to report, with mandatory reporting then phased in over time for all other types of health care organizations.

It was hoped that a mandatory reporting system would guarantee that patient injuries and patient deaths would not be taken lightly or go unexamined. Health care providers would now be held more accountable for vigilance to safety. Additionally, health care organizations would be motivated via incentives to create and put internal safety systems into practice to lessen the possibility of medical errors, as well as to respond to the larger public's desire for more information about patient safety and prevention practices used to minimize medical errors. A voluntary reporting system (for minor errors that do either no harm or minimal harm to the patient) was another Tier 2 recommendation. The intention behind this second level of reporting was to cast the net more broadly and thereby catch even the smaller errors in order to gain more information. These smaller errors could show areas of weakness in the health care system that could, if found in time, be corrected before serious or lethal harm was done. Between these two reporting systems, health care organizations would receive a wealth of information to use in evaluating their system of care and making positive changes toward enhancing quality and reducing preventable medical errors. The report also recognized that providers would likely and understandably be concerned about reported error information being subpoenaed and used against them in malpractice cases, so this recommendation included a request that Congress create and enact legislation to protect the confidentiality of the information collected.

Tier 3. "Raising performance standards and expectations for improvements in safety through the actions of oversight organizations, professional groups, and group purchasers of health care" (IOM, 1999, p. 6). This recommendation was intended to put very specific performance standards in place through several mechanisms. Patient safety would be enhanced via consistent attention to meeting licensing, certification, and accreditation requirements. In addition, health care organizations would clearly list the minimum levels of performance expected from employees in fulfilling care-related duties and in using equipment and pharmaceuticals to care for patients. The publication and promotion of such standards would illustrate to both the health care professionals and the larger community that the organizations have made a firm commitment to ensuring patient safety and minimizing harm from medical errors.

Suggestions were also aimed at those who educate health care professionals, because attention to safety must be an innate part of the training and education process. Professional societies were encouraged to step up and support this movement by leading the way in demanding improvements in safety. Professional societies could accomplish this through the development and publication of their own performance standards for their members, by providing educational sessions and other communications about safety practices, and by sponsoring and encouraging interprofessional collaboration on safety enhancement research and efforts.

The last portion of the Tier 3 recommendation addressed those who pay for health care costs. These large purchasers of health care services could readily influence behavior and affect change by making patient safety a priority issue in contracting decisions with health care organizations. This would effectively create additional financial incentives for health care managers and providers to do all that is possible to find the areas where improvement in safety processes are needed and then actually make the changes.

Tier 4. "Implementing safety systems in health care organizations to ensure safe practices at the delivery level" (IOM, 1999, p. 6). This last recommendation suggested ways to make patient safety part of an overall organizational culture. Hit-or-miss mentions and efforts are no longer good enough; safety must now be stated as an explicit goal of each health care organization, and firmly backed by strong leadership from the managers, the care providers, and the governing bodies that help to regulate the provision of care services. Specifically, the most appropriate safety policies and principles should be matched to each setting of care, and then implemented. Some examples of this are taking safety into account when jobs are created and working conditions are reviewed; standardizing and simplifying equipment, supplies, and processes in the best ways possible; and putting assistive aids in place so clinicians are relying less on memory alone. In addition to implementing these and other forms of safety initiatives, a system for monitoring ongoing patient safety efforts must be designed and consistently supported by the budget of each organization.

In summary, *To Err Is Human: Building a Safer Health System* offers an inclusive and thorough strategy for starting to address the critical level of preventable medical errors. The time to ignore this issue or use hit-or-miss corrective strategies has now passed, and health care providers, as well as all other stakeholders, must step up their levels of awareness and do all that is possible to eliminate the risk of these errors to which we are *all* vulnerable.

Clearly, much change is needed to better align reimbursement systems with liability systems so that they encourage safety improvements instead of overlooking them or causing errors to be hidden. Appropriate programs of training and subsequent updating of knowledge regarding patient and care provider safety are undoubtedly needed for health care managers and the trustees of all health care facilities and organizations. Learning this information is crucial. However, these individuals must then put the knowledge into practice if they are to successfully create an organizational culture of safety and error prevention. Regular communications and actions to reinforce solid support of such a culture are necessary.

No one single activity or program can give us the entire solution for preventing medical errors; however, the IOM report highlights a series of activities that can certainly be incorporated into planning as facilities and organizations move toward enhanced levels of safety and the minimization of preventable errors. Though error may be inherent in humans, it is also within the nature of humans to study errors, to carefully devise solutions to them to provide the safest care possible, and to proudly raise the bar for future generations of health care providers (IOM, 1999).

IOM Report on the Quality Chasm

On March 1, 2001, the second report containing the IOM's findings on the quality of care was released. The first report, which described the frequency of medical errors and the need for much better safety practices, set the stage for this second report to act as an official call to action for the improvement of all quality dimensions across the entire U.S. health care system. Called *Crossing the Quality Chasm: A New Health System for the 21st Century*, this report described how the health care delivery system is in need of major changes—not small incremental changes but rather a complete overhaul of the system as a whole. The IOM Committee on Quality of Health Care in America asserted, "In its current form, habits, and environment, American health care is incapable of providing the public with the quality health care it expects and deserves" (IOM, 2001, p. 43). Such stunning assertions continued, strongly backed by recent data illustrating that people were not being provided consistent levels of high-quality services based on sound scientific knowledge. In many cases what the committee found from the studies behind this report and a review of the relevant published literature was that health care harms too many patients, and does not consistently deliver the benefits it is capable of giving to best meet patient needs. Because of these findings, the IOM committee believed that what lies between the existing health care system and the optimal health care system is not just a gap but rather a chasm.

Americans should certainly not have to worry about the quality of the health care services they receive, and they should be able to trust that providers will take correct actions on their behalf in a timely manner. There should not be a gap, let alone a chasm, between the health care that people deserve and the health care they actually receive. The IOM committee points out several of the factors that collectively led to this chasm. To begin with, the advances in new technology and research discoveries in the past fifty years or so have given clinicians many new diagnostic and treatment tools. These new options came into play as the health care system itself was becoming increasingly more complex in terms of the amount of knowledge needed to provide care, the number of items to be simultaneously managed, and the numbers of people involved in interdisciplinary care. These changes, combined with the already multifaceted nature of care, strained the system, causing it to fall far short in its capacity to convert rapidly advancing new technology into actual practices that are both safe and correct. As the IOM was preparing this report, it found over seventy other studies, published in highly respected peer-reviewed journals, that documented serious quality shortcomings in the health care system. This was particularly concerning, because if the health care system was not handling the past and more recent changes well, just imagine the problems it would be likely to have once the technological advances of the future arrived.

In addition, the report made it clear that the health care needs of Americans have changed greatly as well. People are now enjoying longer life expectancies than ever before (partly due to technological advances coupled with better public health practices), but with living longer comes a higher incidence and prevalence of chronic health issues such as diabetes, heart disease, and asthma. Despite the rising rates of chronic conditions (along with the fact that over 40 percent of the population has more than one chronic condition), the IOM study found that the health care system continues to be focused mainly on caring for acute and intermittent needs, rather than coordinating multidisciplinary care to best meet the needs of the many patients who suffer from chronic conditions.

To that end, the report identified the overall organization of the health care delivery system to be a problem in itself. It asserted that the provision of care in America is routinely overly complex and sometimes lacking in coordination—which obviously does not lead to success in meeting the challenges the system is up against. This complexity and lack of coordination raises the potential risk for breaches of safety and also slows the process of care by requiring extra steps—and we know that the conditions of many patients do not allow for wasted time. Every second counts in many health care settings, and this lack of coordination is a risk to human lives, and also a clear waste of personnel and fiscal resources wherever it occurs.

As a data-driven assessment of the health care system, the IOM report frightened many people and overwhelmed others. However, the IOM committee did not stop with an assessment of the current state of the system. It proceeded to provide a specific listing of aims for improving and strengthening the system, and suggested some guiding rules for redesigning it. This strategy for redesigning the system would bring fundamental, sweeping changes to the entirety of the system, with the intended result of bringing quality state-of-the art care to Americans in all areas of the country. Massive change of the kind suggested by this report is intimidating, but the IOM committee was clear in pointing out that small and incremental changes in the current system of care would not be nearly enough to fix the existing problems. Therefore, this report presented a broadly focused and comprehensive redesign strategy as well as an action plan that organizations could adapt to their settings for promoting innovation and improving the delivery of health care services in the years to come.

The IOM's vision for its redesign strategy began with an "agenda for the future and road map for the report" (IOM, 2001, p. 33), which listed some general principles for creating a new system of care. Basing its suggestions on relevant data and information on likely trends in the near future, the IOM committee shared its beliefs in an organized and systematic fashion. It believes that the redesigned health care system's framework needs to be constructed of components capable of organizing themselves to accomplish shared purposes. By following a few well-prescribed general rules and modifying those rules as needed to address local circumstances, they could then honestly analyze their own successes and failures. With such a framework in place, the full measure of medical science and technology benefits can be offered to all. This would then lessen pain, suffering, and disability while promoting even greater longevity in patients and increased productivity and morale in health care providers. The necessary ingredients for this include local adaptation, innovation, commitment, and initiative. With that said, the IOM committee offered the following five-point agenda for crossing the quality chasm and subsequently bridging the quality gap:

- That all health care constituencies, including policymakers, pur-chasers, regulators, health professionals, health care trustees and management, and consumers, commit to a national statement of purpose for the health care system as a whole and to a shared agenda of six aims for improvement that can raise the quality of care to unprecedented levels.

- That clinicians and patients, and the health care organizations that support care delivery, adopt a new set of principles to guide the redesign of care processes.

- That the Department of Health and Human Services identify a set of priority conditions upon which to focus initial efforts, provide resources to stimulate innovation, and initiate the change process.

- That health care organizations design and implement more effective organizational support processes to make change in the delivery of care possible.

- That purchasers, regulators, health professions, educational institutions, and the Department of Health and Human Services create an environment that fosters and rewards improvement by (1) creating an infrastructure to support evidence-based practice, (2) facilitating the use of information technology, (3) aligning payment incentives, and (4) preparing the workforce to better serve patients in a world of expanding knowledge and rapid change [IOM, 2001, p. 34].

In addition to this agenda, the IOM committee identified six specific aims for improvement. These aims consisted of performance characteristics that (if focused on and refined as much as possible) would lead to improved quality of care. These specific aims were meant to serve as a common vision that could be shared by all who are involved in the health care system in any way. As you read them below, you will find that ideas behind these aims are not new. They are recognizable tenets of quality that have been well respected for many years, but they are also areas where the system has been known to fail much too often. In explaining how the aims were chosen, the report says, "The ultimate test of the quality of a health care system is whether it helps the people it intends to help" (IOM, 2001, p. 44). Thus, after much careful consideration, the six aims were written to emphasize the results for the patient, as follows:

- *Safe*: avoiding injuries to patients from the care that is intended to help them.

- *Effective*: providing services based on scientific knowledge to all who could benefit, and refraining from providing services to those not likely to benefit (avoiding underuse and overuse).

- *Patient-centered*: providing care that is respectful of and responsive to individual patient preferences, needs, and values and ensuring that patient values guide all clinical decisions.

- *Timely*: reducing waits and sometimes harmful delays for both those who receive and those who give care.

- *Efficient*: avoiding waste, in particular waste of equipment, supplies, ideas, and energy.

* *Equitable*: providing care that does not vary in quality because of personal characteristics such as gender, ethnicity, geographic location, and socioeconomic status [IOM, 2001, pp. 39–40].

The six aims are for the most part complementary, producing a positive synergy to guide us to a better level of quality care. They can be viewed as goals to work toward in constructing the path to take in creating the changes needed in management and in clinical practice. Because these aims are focused on patients as the recipients of care, it is understandable how a health care system that is focused on excellence in these six areas would be successful in meeting the needs of its patients. Those who receive care from such a system are likely to enjoy care that is safer, more reliable, responsive to their needs and requests, more integrated, and more readily accessible. Patients could then be more at ease (and possibly more trusting) in knowing that they have a full array of beneficial services available to them—from preventive care to acute and chronic services—all that would best meet their needs over their entire lifespan.

The IOM report assists us even further in offering ways that we can reach the six aims and transition to a health care system that does a better job of meeting patients' needs. Even though the committee recognized that it would not be very useful (or possible for that matter) to hand out a specific blueprint for exactly how the redesigned health care delivery system should look, it provided a helpful listing of generalized guiding principles—otherwise known as the **ten rules of redesign**. Organizations could use these rules as a foundation, and then adapt them to fit their individual settings. The ten rules for redesigning health care processes call for the following:

ten rules of redesign

A set of guiding principles from the Institute of Medicine to assist in redesigning health care delivery systems.

1. *Care based on continuous healing relationships.* Patients should receive care whenever they need it and in many forms, not just face-to-face visits. This rule implies that the health care system should be responsive at all times (24 hours a day, every day) and that access to care should be provided over the Internet, by telephone, and by other means in addition to face-to-face visits.

2. *Customization based on patient needs and values.* The system of care should be designed to meet the most common types of needs, but have the capability to respond to individual patient choices and preferences.

3. *The patient as the source of control.* Patients should be given the necessary information and the opportunity to exercise the degree of control they choose over health care decisions that affect them. The health system should be able to accommodate differences in patient preferences and encourage shared decision-making.

4. *Shared knowledge and the free flow of information.* Patients should have unfettered access to their own medical information and to clinical knowledge. Clinicians and patients should communicate effectively and share information.

5. *Evidence-based decision making.* Patients should receive care based on the best available scientific knowledge. Care should not vary illogically from clinician to clinician or from place to place.

6. *Safety as a system property.* Patients should be safe from injury caused by the care system. Reducing risk and ensuring safety require greater attention to systems that help prevent and mitigate errors.

7. *The need for transparency.* The health care system should make information available to patients and their families that allows them to make informed decisions when selecting a health plan, hospital, or clinical practice, or choosing among alternative treatments. This should include information describing the system's performance on safety, evidence-based practice, and patient satisfaction.

8. *Anticipation of needs.* The health system should anticipate patient needs, rather than simply reacting to events.

9. *Continuous decrease in waste.* The health system should not waste resources or patient time.

10. *Cooperation among clinicians.* Clinicians and institutions should actively collaborate and communicate to ensure an appropriate exchange of information and coordination of care [IOM, 2001, pp. 61–62].

The IOM committee also intended these rules to be a behavioral guide for the years ahead, key tasks for developing a health care system capable of spectacular changes in quality. In the IOM report each of the ten rules is compared and contrasted to an approach being taken at the time of the study. The broad latitude given by these rules allows us to apply them in the most appropriate way for individual settings as we work toward increases in safety, effectiveness, patient centeredness, timeliness, efficiency, and equity in care. The rules and the descriptive statements attached to them are excellent starting points, but innovation as well as common sense must guide their interpretation and application to our settings.

Beyond supplying the ten rules to guide our behavior as we make the necessary changes, the IOM recognized that the suggested changes would likely involve altering the structures and processes used in health care as well. Four areas of infrastructure were pointed out in the report as areas where alterations would certainly be required. First, we must apply evidence-based practices to the delivery of health care. The IOM committee found that research showed that scientific knowledge regarding optimal care practices was not being systematically applied in a consistent and effective way to guide clinical practice. It was upsetting for many researchers and clinicians to hear that it was taking an average of seventeen years for new information gained from randomized controlled trials to be fully incorporated into clinical practice—and even after that many years the application of the information was not consistent. Therefore stakeholders should work together to build a comprehensive program to increase the usability and quick dissemination of new scientific knowledge and should get the latest data and information into the hands of the clinicians who can make effective care decisions with it.

Second, we are called to examine our use of information technology, including the use of Internet and email. The automation of patient-specific health care information is called for as a means of improving care. Patient information was found to be located in the paper records of one or more health care providers, records that were often lacking in organization, illegible at times, and not easy to recover quickly if needed in a medical emergency. This decentralization of patient records detracts from quality care and makes it extremely difficult for clinicians to receive complete medical information on a patient, making proper care nearly impossible from the start—especially for patients with chronic conditions that require frequent visits and ongoing intervention by multiple types of care providers. Email is suggested as a valid mode of quick and inexpensive contact between patients and providers that could increase the level of communication while meeting patients' needs at the same time. In addition to the automation of patient records, the automation of systems for ordering prescription medications was recommended, to decrease the number of medication errors arising from the process of prescribing. Computerized systems could track prescriptions, dosages, and quantities dispensed and also check for interactions, as well as send reminders to both providers and patients when refills are needed. Of course it was also noted by the IOM that these suggestions come with a considerable financial investment and the need for an openness to new computer-based programs.

Third, we need to better align payment policies with quality of care. Payment is one of many factors that play into the behavior of both care providers and patients, and it carries a good amount of motivation with it. The IOM committee recommended that all payers (whether public or private) take the time to reevaluate the payment policies they use, giving careful attention to removing any and all barriers to improving quality. As barriers are located and removed, strong incentives and rewards for quality-enhancing efforts leading to better patient outcomes could be built into the policies. For example, compensation should be fair for clinicians who care for a wide range of patients, from those with mild conditions to those who are gravely ill; there should not be a specific financial gain or loss for caring for sicker patients or ones with conditions that are more complicated to manage. The IOM suggests that reimbursement methods should give providers opportunities to share in the benefits of enhancing quality, and that financial incentives for good care should align with the use of research-identified best practices. Changes to policies and explaining positive incentives would give both the purchasers and the consumers of health care enough information to discern differences in health care quality and make better choices according to such information.

The study of and subsequent redesign of payment policies is another task that was recognized as likely to be time consuming. To lessen the burden on personnel, the report recommends that the federal government (after receiving input from the private sector) create a program that would identify, pilot-test, and examine the many existing options for creating alignment between reimbursement and specific and measurable goals for quality care. Several ways of aligning these factors are available, so a careful examination of the options by one government committee is a sound starting place for narrowing the possibilities. Some suggested options to be studied include using hybrid methods of payment that would counter the negatives of one particular payment method with the positives of another particular method, multiple-year contracts, financial incentives to encourage use of electronic communications between providers as well as between providers and patients, and the bundling of payments made for caring for priority conditions.

Fourth and finally, a recommendation was made to better prepare the health care workforce for the redesign and its inherent changes. Health care is a profession that relies on successfully building stable provider-patient relationships as well as building and maintaining of trust. This is necessary for successfully treating illness and properly managing conditions that cannot be cured. All health care providers must be prepared for and understand their role in our changing health care system so that the stress created by recommended changes does not affect the trusting clinical relationships that must be in place. Managers could play a central role here by helping to evaluate the correct steps to take to ensure the smoothest transition possible in their setting as changes occur.

The IOM offers three ideas for helping organizations and health care professionals during the transition period. First, a shift in training to emphasize the six aims for improvement would effectively place more attention on using proven, evidence-based practices that are associated with improvements in patient care outcomes, and would make it more likely that the six aims will shape providers' clinical practice in a constructive way. Second, accrediting bodies and state boards should consider changes to their policies for certifying or licensing health care personnel in order to support the provision of quality care and deter practices that would detract from this goal. Third, the liability system must be made supportive of the changes called for in the report, and take steps to ensure accountability for quality care (or lack thereof) among health care organizations and their providers. Applying all of these ideas will likely lead to the best outcomes, which further underscores the need to first study various options and their possible outcomes before one particular path for redesign is chosen.

In summary, *Crossing the Quality Chasm* calls for immediate attention to the state of the health care system and asserts that now is the time to reevaluate health care delivery policies and processes. With the aging of the population, the longer life expectancies of Americans, and the foreseeable advances in technology, steps must be taken to enhance quality before an increased patient load combines with new diagnostic and treatment possibilities to make the provision of quality care more difficult. Health care providers, patients, managers, policymakers, and payers have long been aware of the system's issues; now these issues can no longer be ignored or minimized. The IOM's call to action is clear, and systematic change is necessary to correct the shortcomings that have been identified. Although *Crossing the Quality Chasm* does not present a specific prescription for organizations, managers, payers, and accreditors to follow, it does provide a vision of the possibilities for the health care system of the future as well as the six aims for improvement, the ten rules for design, and an agenda for closing the quality chasm to help us get the process started.

Quality Improvement Strategies

Managers and clinicians who have searched for information on quality improvement (QI) techniques have probably been overwhelmed by the number of ideas, strategies, and competing models that exist in books, journals, and websites. Some of these ideas, strategies, and models have been developed in health care settings and others in business industries that value quality. Some theories—many of which draw upon the work of Juran and Deming—have already been applied in clinical medicine, with varying degrees of success. The lesson that success is not guaranteed is now causing health care managers to be careful about assuming that QI models borrowed from other industries (such as total quality management and continuous quality improvement) will lead to advances in health care quality. After much searching and poring over comprehensive reviews, the Agency for Healthcare Research and Quality engaged the Stanford-UCSF Evidence-Based Practice Center to study and then refine nine QI strategies that closely relate to the priorities found in the IOM reports. Those strategies are discussed in the remainder of this section.

Quality improvement (QI) strategies in health care are defined as "any intervention(s) aimed at reducing the quality gap for a group of patients representative of those encountered in routine practice" (Shojania, McDonald, Wachter, & Owens, 2004, p. 21). Many classification systems for QI strategies and other intervention methods exist, which can be very confusing to those trying to decide which ones best fit their organization or specific problem needing correction. The taxonomy used to classify the following nine strategic categories combines the QI strategy with the intended target for improvement (Table 11.1); this should make it easier to choose particular QI strategies and substrategies that best fit your organization's needs. Some categories may seem a bit broad, but it is common to implement multiple QI techniques simultaneously in health care to achieve the results that are desired. Let's review each of the categories and some examples of the techniques that best fit into them.

quality improvement (QI) strategies
Any intervention(s) aimed at reducing the quality gap for a group of patients representative of those encountered in routine practice.

1. *Provider reminder systems.* Reminder systems can help health care providers to maintain quality as they navigate through the management of multiple patients and the distractions of other simultaneous aspects of their work. Reminders can be given in charts, by phone, by email, or by an electronic system to prompt clinicians on any aspect of care. Computer-based reminders are a common QI technique, as are computer-based systems that aid in decision support. Providers can also receive a prompt or reminder to finish an incomplete chart, report required data, order a colonoscopy for a patient who hasn't had one in eleven years, or view updated recommendations from an evidence-based study just published in their discipline. These are just a few examples of how reminder systems can be readily adapted to all clinical situations and settings to improve care.

2. *Facilitated relay of clinical data to providers.* This strategy involves examining the transfer rate of patients' clinical information that is not directly collected during an in-person visit to the care provider. QI is commonly needed in this area as relay times in receiving results from off-site locations or from a provider using a different medical record system can be slow. A careful examination of the overall information relay process is called for with this strategy. Are phone calls or faxes received in a timely manner so as to support rather than disrupt quality care outcomes? Where are the greatest lags in time between the collection of information and the provider receiving it? Which relays are most critical to successful patient care, and can the relay time for those pieces of information be shortened?

Table 11.1 Taxonomy of QI Strategies with Examples of Substrategies

QI Strategy	Examples
Provider reminder systems	• Reminders in charts for providers • Computer-based reminders for providers • Computer-based decision support
Facilitated relay of clinical data to providers	• Transmission of clinical data from outpatient specialty clinic to primary care provider by means other than medical record (e.g., phone call or fax)
Audits and feedbacks	• Feedback of performance to individual providers • Quality indicators and reports • National/state quality report cards • Publicly released performance data • Benchmarking—provision of outcomes data from top performers for comparison with provider's own data
Provider education	• Workshops and conferences • Educational outreach visits (e.g., academic detailing) • Distributed educational materials
Patient education	• Classes • Parent and family education • Patient pamphlets • Intensive education strategies promoting self-management of chronic conditions
Promotion of self-management	• Materials and devices promoting self-management
Patient reminder systems	• Postcards or calls to patients
Organizational change	• Case management, disease management • TQM, CQI techniques • Multidisciplinary teams • Change from paper to computer-based records • Increased staffing • Skill mix changes

Table 11.1 *Continued*

QI Strategy	Examples
Financial incentives, regulation, and policy	*Provider-directed*
	• Financial incentives based on achievement of performance goals
	• Alternative reimbursement systems (e.g., fee-for-service, capitated payments)
	• Licensure requirements
	Patient-directed
	• Copayments for certain visit types
	• Health insurance premiums, user fees
	Health system-directed
	• Initiatives by accreditation bodies (e.g., residency work hour limits)
	• Changes in reimbursement schemes (e.g., capitation, prospective payment, salaried providers)

Source: Walsh, McDonald, & Shojania, 2005.

3. *Audits and feedback.* Audits and feedback are summaries of information that can be collected on any aspect of clinical performance (outcomes, error rates, etc.) for individual care providers, departments, or organizations as whole systems of care. The results of the summaries can be discussed confidentially with a single care provider whose performance was studied or a group of providers and can be reported to the internal organization only or externally as well. In addition, other quality-related data from health care organizations can be reported internally or externally via report cards and at varying levels of specificity, from detailed to aggregated. Benchmarking and setting clinical targets are also useful in this strategy. For example, your facility may want to study the percentages of care providers who do and do not achieve a particular clinical target, such as having 75 percent of established patients return for a preventive well-adult exam within fourteen months of their last exam. The success rates of the top performers in a specialty could be shared and rewarded, and comparable providers encouraged to work toward achieving such success rates. The benchmarks or clinical targets should be made well known to the providers and to the organization as a whole, as well as to the community. This establishes them as goals everyone is aware of.

4. *Provider education.* This strategy supports QI by advancing care providers' knowledge of the latest and greatest clinical information through providers' attendance at educational workshops, conferences, meetings, or

online lectures and coursework, or through their traveling to research and educational settings to learn new technologies. Raising the level of care provider expertise on new evidence-based care practices and innovations increases the likelihood of quality care. Provider education can also take the form of internally distributed materials (print or electronic) that put useful information directly into the hands of the clinicians.

5. *Patient education.* Educating patients, especially during in-person, one-on-one encounters or in a class aimed at a target group or community of interested persons can be an excellent QI strategy by itself or in combination with one of the other eight strategies discussed in this chapter. The weak areas of patient knowledge can be identified by a formal survey and study or by asking providers familiar with a particular patient base to identify a few topical areas where information seems to be needed and could readily be disseminated to achieve better outcomes in care. This strategy may be particularly useful in educating parents, helping those with chronic disease to better self-manage their condition, or assisting postoperative patients in understanding important aftercare instructions to achieve the best possible outcome of care. Ideally, patient education is done in person; however, many patients prefer to receive printed materials to take home, review, and refer to as needed. To be effective, printed educational materials must be written at a level the average person can understand and must be free of the medical terms that clinicians take for granted in their everyday language.

6. *Promotion of self-management.* Helping patients with self-management may overlap with the strategies of patient education and patient reminder systems, and it may be beneficial at times to combine all these strategies. This category of QI initiatives includes the distribution of any materials, resources, or equipment that improves patients' abilities to self-manage their condition(s). For example, care providers could share recent blood work results with patients, explaining trends in the values and comparing the values to optimal ranges that the patients can work toward in reaching a better state of health. In addition, some organizations lend or give self-monitoring equipment such as glucose or blood pressure monitors to patients to encourage self-management of easily measurable disease factors and proactive behaviors on the part of patients to achieve more desirable outcomes.

7. *Patient reminder systems.* Similar to the strategy of provider reminder systems, this strategy supplies patients with care-related prompts via phone calls, text messages, mailed postcards, or emails. Any efforts that providers implement to direct their patients to come in for appointments, understand the necessity of screenings, or better manage aspects of self-care in times of wellness, injury, or illness are appropriate to this QI

category. For example, reminders can be given to patients about their next appointment or the date of their next test or screening. This strategy can easily be customized to fit any clinical setting and adapted to address the particular outcomes that are most in need of improvement or are deserving of support for continued success.

8. *Organizational change.* This category of QI strategies houses many of the familiar methods used in health care; for example, adopting specific techniques for case management and disease management and total quality management or continuous quality improvement techniques. Some health care organizations choose to implement multidisciplinary teams (led by primary care providers) to collaborate on patients' care. This approach facilitates communication among providers and may foster improved outcomes through combining the thoughts and skills of many professionals. A recent requirement that fits into this category is the changeover from paper-based medical record systems to electronic systems (computer-based records and patient tracking systems), which is forecast to be mandatory in 2015 for those who are interested in the possibility of federally funded bonuses or wish to avoid the noncompliance penalties that are likely to follow. Staffing increases are also considered organizational change strategies, as adding new members to existing treatment teams or creating new roles for care providers can increase the quality of care outcomes in areas that are deserving of more focus.

9. *Financial incentives, regulation, and policy.* In this final strategic category, the QI incentives can be either positive or negative and can be directed at the care providers, the patients, or the health care organization itself. For example, incentives directed toward care providers include bonuses for meeting clinical targets or benchmarks that have been set, changes to reimbursement systems to encourage or discourage behaviors, or changes to licensure requirements. Incentives directed toward patients may include raising or lowering the copayments and fees charged for certain types of office visits or altering premium rates based on proactive and healthy behaviors. Lastly, incentives directed at the health care organization itself may include those put in place by accreditation bodies, state licensing boards, or the payment systems. For example, work hours for residents are now limited to allow those providers to rest between shifts, and organizations can be penalized for overrunning the limit, which is expected to improve the quality of care these residents give (Shojania et al., 2004).

When working with strategies in any of these QI categories, it is important to remember that any QI efforts chosen and put into practice must be followed by periodic examination of the relevant quality indicators or targets to see if the strategy is indeed beneficial or if it needs to be altered in some way. Quality must be defined within the structure of each care setting, and standards and goals must be put in place so that the success or failure of any QI effort that is implemented can be measured. These standards and goals that are set for increasing the quality of patient care outcomes must be specific as well as measurable. It is essential to protect the accuracy and reliability of data, as valid conclusions on QI outcomes cannot be drawn from incomplete, inaccurate, or poorly collected data.

Medical Errors

medical error
The failure of a planned action to be completed as intended or the use of a wrong plan to achieve an aim.

Even in this current age the American health care system is not as safe as it should be—or has the potential to be. A **medical error** can result from the failure of a planned action to work as it was intended or the selection of an incorrect action to reach a particular outcome. Common medical errors include misdiagnoses, adverse drug events, incorrect transfusions, injuries during surgical procedures, wrong-site surgical procedures, retained surgical instruments, patient restraint-related injuries or deaths, burns, falls, bedsores, charting inaccuracies, and cases of mistaken patient identity. These errors can occur in any setting; however, the ones that carry the most serious consequences to patients are more likely to take place in intensive care units, operating rooms, and the emergency departments of hospitals.

The effects of medical errors reach far beyond the individual patient and the patient's family, causing estimated financial losses of between $17 billion and $29 billion per year (inclusive of the costs of additional care needed by the patient, lost income and household productivity, and disability costs). Mistakes by health care providers are also costly because they destroy patients' trust in providers and in the health care system itself. Errors that lead to necessary and time-consuming follow-up services cause additional physical and psychological consequences for the patient as well. From the provider side, it is common to see health care providers respond to cases of medical error with a loss of morale and frustration at not being able to give patients the best care possible—the care that is deserved (IOM, 1999).

Many factors continue to come together to cause the epidemic of errors in today's health care system. The fragmented and decentralized system of care sits at the top of the list. It is common for many patients to receive care from multiple providers, and this leaves much room for error since most providers will not have access to their patients' complete medical information before care is given. This predisposes patients to medical errors right from the start—especially in emergency settings where time is precious. In addition, the processes used to certify and license health care professionals give only a small amount of attention to individuals' histories of medical errors—with even this small amount causing confrontations with and opposition from some health care organizations and individual care providers. The ongoing perception held by some health care professionals is that the medical liability system is a clear obstacle to efforts to find, document, and learn from various types of medical errors; the possibilities of litigation and intimidating sanctions cause errors to be swept under the rug instead of reported and studied for the greater good. Finally, there is much ongoing discussion about the fact that many third-party payers do not provide any financial incentives for either the health care organizations or the health care providers to enhance safety practices and raise the bar on quality of care.

Since the 1999 publication of *To Err Is Human,* follow-up studies on medical errors across the U.S. health care system have been few and far between—likely because of one or more of the factors mentioned in the preceding paragraph. Some facility-specific and defined geographic area studies are available; however, it is not possible to extrapolate a full and accurate picture of the national system of care from these limited studies. One national study that specifically assessed medication errors (inclusive of prescription medications, over-the-counter medications, vitamins, minerals, and herbals) found a rather frequent rate of error in every phase of the process—from prescription to administration to postadministration monitoring of the patient. In this study, although error rates varied across facilities (IOM, 2006), additional data indicated that there was at least one medication error per hospital patient per day (IOM, 2006). Overall, there are approximately 400,000 errors per year in hospitals, 800,000 errors in long-term care settings, and another 530,000 errors in Medicare patients visiting outpatient clinics for care (IOM, 2006). Thankfully, not all medication errors lead to patient injury or death, but knowledge of the over 1.5 million preventable injuries per year resulting from medication errors alone is enough to illustrate the point that our work to correct this serious issue is not yet complete.

Health Care–Associated Infections

A **health care–associated infection (HAI)**, also previously known as a nosocomial infection or hospital-acquired infection, is a potentially deadly infection that was not clinically present in a patient (nor showed clinical evidence of incubation) at the time the patient was admitted to a hospital or health care facility (Coffin & Zaoutis, 2008). Within only a few hours after admission, a patient's natural flora can begin to acquire the traits of the surrounding bacterial pool. Most HAIs become clinically evident at approximately forty-eight hours postadmission (Sadeghzadeh, 2010), and

health care–associated infection (HAI)
A potentially deadly infection that was not clinically present in a patient (nor showed clinical evidence of incubation) at the time the patient was admitted to a hospital or health care facility.

so the possibility of an HAI must be carefully evaluated in patients who are febrile or who are displaying signs and symptoms that are inconsistent with their admitting diagnosis. HAIs may be caused by bacterial, viral, or fungal pathogens, and commonly take the form of bloodstream infections, pneumonia, urinary tract infections, or surgical site infections.

Whether HAIs are localized or systemic, they are a common cause of longer inpatient stays, higher mortality rates, and a notable increase in associated health care costs. Despite some studies that note incremental decreases in HAIs at some facilities, other studies continue to document unfortunate HAI numbers. Recent studies estimate that there were 722,000 HAIs in U.S. acute health care facilities in 2011 (Centers for Disease Control and Prevention [CDC], 2014). In March of 2009, the CDC published a report stating that the overall direct medical expenditures for HAIs ranged from $28 billion to $45 billion per year. In addition, in 2001, it was estimated that at any given time, one out of twenty admitted hospital patients had an HAI while undergoing treatment. These numbers are disastrous, especially considering that these infections are extremely preventable when correct precautions and procedures are followed (CDC & Association of State and Territorial Health Officials, 2011).

Despite the call to action by the IOM report and the attempts to put mandatory reporting practices in place for every state, we currently do not have uniformly collected data from facilities around the country that would enable us to track the progress (or lack thereof) in preventing HAIs in each of their forms. Without this consistent information, it is impossible to tell which regions of the country are doing better or worse, which hospitals are doing better or worse, and whether or not our health care system as a whole is headed in the right direction with respect to infection rates. As of 2011, only thirty-two states and the District of Columbia had passed laws regarding HAI prevention and reporting, and sadly, not all of these states have made reporting mandatory (Figure 11.1).

Even without uniformly collected data, we have reason to believe that the current situation is unacceptable, especially given the preventable nature and devastating consequences to the patients of HAIs and also the costs of the additional care for treating the infections and any related disabilities. There is no infection rate that has been identified as "acceptable" in this situation, but it is known that other industries would not accept a failure rate as high as the HAI rate is estimated to be in health care. In fact other industries would likely set goals as close to zero as possible when faced with preventable issues that are as costly and as high risk for mortality. It is also surprising that rates seem to be remaining high in light of the fact that the Centers for Medicare & Medicaid Services implemented a no-pay rule

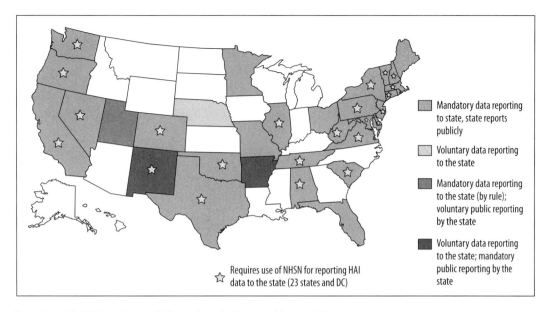

Figure 11.1   Health Care–Associated Infection Reporting Laws, as of January 2011

Note: NHSN = National Healthcare Safety Network, a function of the CDC.
Source: CDC & Association of State and Territorial Health Officials, 2011, p. 7.

in 2008, which now denies additional payments to hospitals when patients develop bloodstream and urinary tract infections associated with central lines or catheters.

Currently, it appears that there are two major reasons why infection control is failing in the clinical health care system. First, the existing infection control guidelines, based on thousands of clinical studies and case examinations, are not being implemented correctly. The research on this topic is clear: when infection control guidelines are explained well, are used consistently by every level of care provider, and are enforced by those in positions of authority, HAI rates drop in a dramatic fashion—in some cases close to zero. Second, it seems that some health care providers believe that HAIs are not always preventable even with adherence to infection control practices. This incorrect viewpoint persists despite current research that shows that infection control practices are well worth their cost, training time, and implementation and ongoing monitoring efforts. Because infection control requirements may be viewed as bothersome or not fully effective by some providers who are already dealing with competing priorities for time and productivity in patient care, strong oversight by managers and accreditors is a necessity.

Moving forward, states must implement reporting programs and be uniform in their tracking of progress toward eliminating these deadly and preventable infections. Strict infection control programs based on the latest clinical recommendations need to be enforced with regard to prevention, detection, and treatment of all infections. Only with consistent infection control programs and practices as well as nationwide mandatory reporting will we be able to correctly track the trends related to HAIs, which will in turn allow us to fine-tune our approach to eliminating them.

SUMMARY

The history of quality assurance in the U.S. health care system comprises many diverse efforts to improve care for the good of all, yet we still have much work to do in optimizing the system of health care and removing the persistent quality and safety problems. Better methods of mandatory reporting are needed to facilitate data and trend analysis for all acute and chronic care settings. Professional standards, licensure requirements, accreditation requirements, and payment system policies must be revisited to remove barriers to quality and replace them with incentives for achieving quality. More work is needed on reducing medical errors and HAIs, which in turn would reduce patient harm and patient deaths, as well as generate significant savings in financial expenditures. Quality of care indicators should be more accessible to patients and payers as a matter of transparency to allow informed consumer choices and incentivize providers to raise their standards. Systemwide change is indeed necessary, and the suggestions made by the IOM reports of 1999 and 2001 provide us with a clear vision as well as suggestions that are adaptable to all care settings.

As disturbing as the IOM reports were for many, we needed to be confronted with these alarming facts, and needed to recognize that the information contained in them represents only a small portion of the overall story to be told on the state of quality of the health care system. As health care organizations attempt to improve the quality of their care and safety of their patients, some will be more successful than others. Redesigning the system and correcting its faults will not be an easy task, but it is a necessary one that can bring about remarkable benefits. Strong leadership, careful study of best practices, thorough review of policies and procedures, an openness to change, and the consistent dedication of professional staff as well as health care providers have never been more important than they are right now. As we work to bring about the changes that are needed, we must look for solutions that are truly patient centered, safe, and equitable. It is time for all stakeholders to come together to rebuild the U.S. health care system into what it is capable of being—a system of high quality that serves the medical needs of all, while carefully protecting our safety, functioning, individual preferences, dignity, comfort, and resources.

KEY TERMS

health care–associated infection
(HAI)

medical error

professional standards review
organizations (PSROs)

quality

quality gap

quality improvement (QI) strategies

ten rules of redesign

utilization review

DISCUSSION QUESTIONS

1. What are some specific ways in which the IOM's error prevention tiers could be implemented in your current or future health care setting?

2. What are the IOM's six aims for improvement in health care quality? Choose one, and discuss specific examples of how it can be achieved.

3. Which of the IOM's ten rules for redesign do you think would be the easiest to implement in most health care settings? Which would be the most difficult to implement? Why?

4. What are some specific barriers that need to be removed to improve the quality of health care services in the United States?

REFERENCES

Best, M., & Neuhauser, D. (2004). Avedis Donabedian: Father of quality assurance and poet. *Quality and Safety in Health Care, 13,* 472–473.

Bowman, J. (1919). Hospital standardization series: General hospitals of 100 or more beds. *Bulletin of the American College of Surgeons, 4*(4). Chicago, IL: American College of Surgeons.

Centers for Disease Control and Prevention. (2014). HAI prevalence survey. Retrieved from http://www.cdc.gov/hai/surveillance

Centers for Disease Control and Prevention & Association of State and Territorial Health Officials. (2011). *Eliminating healthcare-associated infections: State policy options.* Retrieved from http://www.cdc.gov/hai/pdfs/toolkits/toolkit -hai-policy-final_01-2012.pdf

Coffin, S. E., & Zaoutis, T. E. (2008). Health care–associated infections. In S. S. Long, L. K. Pickering, & C. G. Prober (Eds.), *Principles and practice of pediatric infectious diseases* (3rd ed.). Philadelphia, PA: Elsevier.

Donabedian, A. (2003). *An introduction to quality assurance in health care.* New York, NY: Oxford University Press.

Gassiot, C., Searcy, V., & Giles, C. (2011). *The medical staff services handbook: Fundamentals and beyond.* Sudbury, MA: Jones & Bartlett.

Institute of Medicine. (1999). *To err is human: Building a safer health system.* Washington, DC: National Academies Press, 1999.

Institute of Medicine. (2001). *Crossing the quality chasm: A new health system for the 21st century.* Washington, DC: National Academies Press.

Institute of Medicine. (2006, July 20). Medication errors injure 1.5 million people and cost billions of dollars annually. News from the National Academies. Retrieved from http://www8.nationalacademies.org/onpinews/newsitem.aspx?RecordID=11623

The Joint Commission. (2012). *The Joint Commission history.* Retrieved from http://www.jointcommission.org/assets/1/6/Joint_Commission_History.pdf

Lohr, K. N. (1990). *Medicare: A strategy for quality assurance.* Washington, DC: National Academies Press.

Luce, J. M., Bindman, A. B., & Lee, P. R. (1994). A brief history of health care quality assessment and improvement in the United States. *Western Journal of Medicine, 160*(3), 263–268.

Ostrow, P. C. (1983). The historical precedents for quality assurance in health care. *American Journal of Occupational Therapy, 37*(1), 23–26.

Sadeghzadeh, V. (2010). The frequency rate of nosocomial urinary tract infections in intensive care unit patients. *Retrovirology, 7*(Suppl. 1), 93.

Shaw, P., Elliott, C., Isaacson, P., & Murphy, E. (2007). *Quality and performance improvement in healthcare: A tool for programmed learning* (3rd ed.). Chicago, IL: American Health Information Management Association.

Shojania, K. G., McDonald, K. M., Wachter, R. M., & Owens, D. K. (2004). *Closing the quality gap: A critical analysis of quality improvement strategies: Vol. 1. Series overview and methodology* (AHRQ Publication No. 04-0051-1). Rockville, MD: Agency for Healthcare Research and Quality.

Sultz, H. A., & Young, K. M. (2009). *Health care USA: Understanding its organization and delivery* (6th ed.). Sudbury, MA: Jones & Bartlett.

Taylor, R. J., & Taylor, S. B. (1994). *The AUPHA manual of health services management.* Gaithersburg, MD: Aspen.

Walsh, J., McDonald, K. M., & Shojania, K. G. (2005). *Closing the quality gap: A critical analysis of quality improvement strategies: Vol. 3. Hypertension care.* Rockville, MD: Agency for Healthcare Research and Quality.

Williams, S. J., & Torrens, P. R. (2008). *Introduction to health services* (7th ed.). Clifton Park, NY: Delmar/Cengage Learning.

CHAPTER 12

THE CHRONIC DISEASE EPIDEMIC

Bernard J. Healey

Thanks to efforts by public health departments along with the improvement of medical care, Americans can expect increasing life expectancy. This increase in longevity has resulted in both good and bad news for the most important component of people's lives: their health. The good news, of course, involves having more time to spend with one's family and friends and on fulfilling one's dreams. The bad news involves quality of life, which may deteriorate along with the development of chronic diseases and their complications. The longer one lives, the greater the chance of developing one or more chronic diseases.

According to the National Center for Health Statistics in the U.S. Department of Health and Human Services, a **chronic disease** is one that lasts for three months or more. Chronic diseases generally cannot be prevented by vaccines or cured by medication, nor do they just run their course and disappear. The leading chronic diseases in developed countries are arthritis, cardiovascular disease such as heart attacks and strokes, cancers such as breast and colon cancer, diabetes, epilepsy and seizures, obesity, and oral health problems. Chronic diseases place a tremendous burden on all segments of our society and are by far the greatest medical threat that we have ever faced. A chronic disease can begin early in life and progress at a very slow pace over many years. Affected individuals usually feel well in the beginning and are unaware that they have a dangerous disease that will manifest itself with time. These diseases are for the most part caused by individual health behaviors, such as lack of physical activity, poor nutrition, tobacco use, and excessive alcohol consumption, and they can be prevented only by eliminating these behaviors from the population. The majority of the chronic diseases result in many complications; they do not have an

LEARNING OBJECTIVES

After reading this chapter you should be able to

- Explain the extent of the epidemic of chronic diseases in the United States.

- Understand how chronic diseases are changing the U.S. health care delivery system.

- Understand the costs of chronic diseases in the United States.

- Understand the value of health education and health promotion programs in the reduction of chronic diseases and their complications.

chronic disease
A disease that cannot be cured and never disappears.

easy resolution, and will usually result in limited functioning and reduced quality of life, as one grows older.

These chronic diseases have replaced communicable diseases as the major threat to the health of the U.S. population and the global population as well. They are silent killers, taking decades to inflict damage on a very large proportion of the population. They result in 75 percent of total U.S. health care costs, and yet our health policy experts seem more concerned with the issues of health care financing and access than they do with dealing with this costly epidemic. According to Schimpff (2012), "there are about 465,000 preventable deaths per year from smoking, 395,000 from high blood pressure, 216,000 from obesity, 191,000 from inactivity, 190,000 from high blood sugar levels, and 113,000 from high cholesterol" (p. 14). These medical issues caused by personal behaviors all lead to the development of one or more chronic diseases. These behaviors usually begin when we are young and become more pronounced as we grow older. The diseases are all preventable through health education programs that could be offered by the family, school, workplace, medical care providers, or a combination of all of these potential sources of medical education. Of course the effectiveness of these programs depends upon how well the program participants follow through on what they learn.

High rates of chronic disease development and of subsequent complications are occurring because the paradigm the current system of medicine is following for dealing with diseases is now outdated. This system of medical care developed and grew as antibiotics were discovered in the 1930s, and people came to believe in curing disease through the use of prescription drugs. The acute diseases, many of them communicable from person to person, were for the most part treatable through medications or immunizations that would prevent spread of the disease. Communicable diseases are usually severe in the beginning of the disease process but usually respond very well to appropriate treatment so that the patient has a complete recovery. The system of **quarantining**, the separating of individuals with a given communicable disease from those who are well, also proved to be an excellent mechanism for preventing large-scale epidemics of disease. Deaths could often be limited to relatively small numbers of those afflicted with an acute disease, and when deaths did occur, age and underlying medical conditions were often factors.

quarantining
Separating individuals with a given communicable disease from those who do not have the disease.

Modern health care providers, in concert with public health departments, have done an excellent job of controlling epidemics of communicable diseases and treating patients with acute disease by utilizing an ever-growing choice of available drugs. Unfortunately, during that same period when antibiotics and other life-saving drugs were being developed, our lifestyles changed in ways that ushered in a whole host of new diseases caused not by pathogens but by our own health behaviors. As our society moved from agricultural and blue-collar employment involving physical labor to service and information-processing employment that required less physical exertion, the stage was set for a new epidemic of diseases caused primarily by bad habits. These changes along with the reluctance of medical systems to change from a "cure" to a prevention mentality allowed an alarming rise in chronic diseases.

The chronic disease epidemic has caught the entire U.S. health care sector unprepared for its ramifications. This has happened because of the failure of the health care system to recognize the possibility that disease etiologies were changing and that the old system of caring for disease needed to change with them. The acute care model of disease care was not designed for individuals who have acquired one or more chronic diseases. Chronic diseases are far too complex to be handled by a model that allows disease to occur and then provides treatment and cure for that disease after the fact.

Chronic Diseases and Their Complications

The chronic disease epidemic has been expanding in the United States at an alarming rate and shows no signs of slowing down. According to Wennberg, Fisher, Goodman, and Skinner (2008), the number of individuals in the United States with at least one chronic disease has risen to over 90 million and these diseases result in 70 percent of the deaths among Americans on an annual basis. Many of these chronic diseases are contributors to the premature death of individuals. The epidemiology of chronic diseases shows a large increase in the number of reported cases because the population is growing older and a large proportion of individuals have practiced high-risk health behaviors for long periods of time. Consequently, there is very little that can be done now to prevent the current epidemic from becoming even larger over the next several years. This is the reason why we have to improve the management of these diseases immediately in order to avoid an epidemic of further complications from these diseases.

The incubation period of a chronic disease is quite long, often taking decades to fully manifest as a diagnosed chronic disease and then taking more time to present complications from this chronic condition. According to Harris (2012), the process of aging produces a heightened susceptibility to disease. The epidemiology of chronic diseases has also shown that the causes of these diseases are usually high-risk health behaviors that are practiced over long periods of time and usually began very early in life. Moreover, the high-risk health behaviors that cause chronic diseases quite often result in multiple chronic diseases and multiple complications that limit function, hinder quality of life, and cost billions of dollars to address across the population.

Our system of medical delivery has been reluctant to understand the differences between communicable diseases and chronic disease and has attempted to treat both types with the same formula, waiting until individuals exhibit symptoms before attempting medical treatment. This approach is doomed to failure with chronic diseases because once the patient develops symptoms, it is too late for successful intervention in the disease process. Sultz and Young (2011) believe that our system of health care delivery is finally beginning to understand that the traditional way of delivering medical care is not appropriate for those who have developed multiple chronic diseases. Individuals are taking too many medications with too little monitoring and often have a single physician who has the responsibility for their overall health care even though that care is getting more and more complex. Fuchs (2009) also points out that in order to improve quality and reduce the costs of health care there needs to be better coordination of care, especially for those who have chronic diseases.

Figure 12.1 shows the number of people reporting selected chronic diseases in 2003. The Milken Institute (DeVol & Bedroussian, 2007) reports that the cost of treatment and lost output for these seven diseases totaled $1.3 trillion in 2003, representing more than 50 percent of U.S. total health care costs in that year. The costs of the epidemic of chronic diseases have continued to rise, reaching 75 percent of the $2.7 trillion expended on health care costs in 2011. Figure 12.1 also reveals a large number of reported cases of hypertension; hypertension is associated with the development of heart disease and diabetes. According to Morewitz (2006), hypertension is one of the most diagnosed medical conditions in the United States and a leading contributor to other chronic diseases, which are then known as comorbidities. **Comorbidity** occurs when two or more medical conditions coexist in an individual—the initial disease and one or more additional diseases. Comorbidities are the leading causes of poor health and high medical bills as people grow older.

comorbidity
The occurrence of one or more medical disorders along with a primary disease.

We will look at four of the most numerous and dangerous chronic diseases to explain their etiology, epidemiology, and dangers and to demonstrate that a new paradigm of disease intervention is the only hope for successful intervention. These diseases are heart disease, cancer, stroke, and diabetes.

Heart Disease

Cardiovascular disease (CVD) still remains the leading cause of death in the United States, despite enormous progress in preventing this chronic disease. Heart disease encompasses numerous problems with the heart

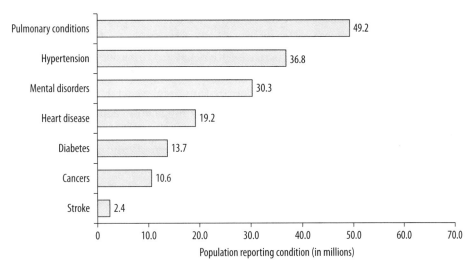

Figure 12.1 Number of People Reporting Selected Chronic Diseases, 2003
Source: DeVol & Bedroussian, 2007. Data from the Medical Expenditure Panel Survey.

that are usually the result of **atherosclerosis**. This condition is the result of plaque accumulation in the walls of the arteries. This plaque buildup blocks the flow of blood, which can result in a heart attack or stroke. The risk factors for heart disease include family history, hypertension, elevated cholesterol, use of tobacco, elevated glucose, overweight and obesity, and chronic inflammation. Many of these risk factors are preventable.

atherosclerosis
A disease in which plaque builds up in the arteries and can eventually lead to a heart attack or stroke.

Cancer

The Centers for Disease Control and Prevention (CDC) (2012a) defines **cancer** as a disease in which abnormal cells divide without control and then invade other tissues. The term *cancer* encompasses a collection of many diseases that originate within the patient's own body rather than from some external pathogen, and are capable of spreading to distant sites in the body through the blood and lymph systems. Most medical experts tend to agree that progress against this chronic disease has been slow and that we may never succeed in obtaining a cure for many of the forms of cancer. This makes prevention of cancer the most important goal.

cancer
A group of diseases that result in abnormal growth of cells and that may spread from an original site to other parts of the body.

A diagnosis of cancer is probably the most feared health occurrence for most Americans as they grow older and become more concerned about their health status. Agus (2011) argues that we fear cancer because it has touched all of us, if not personally then through relatives and friends, and because it represents our own body turning against us. It can also evoke uncertainty about our happiness, our quality of life, and our future, because even when the disease is beaten back it can return.

Prevention of cancer can be enhanced through screening tests, regular medical examinations, and use of certain vaccines, and also through avoiding certain high-risk health behaviors. In order to help prevent cancer individuals need to remain tobacco-free, limit alcohol use, eat the right foods including a diet rich in fruits and vegetables, avoid exposure to ultraviolet rays from the sun and tanning beds, keep off excess weight, and remain physically active.

Skin cancer is the most common form of cancer and melanoma is the most deadly type of skin cancer. It has been known for some time that ultraviolet radiation from the sun and from indoor tanning is the most prevalent risk factor for this very preventable form of cancer. Despite this knowledge the CDC (2012c) has reported one recent study that showed half of adults younger than thirty had had a sunburn in the previous year. A second report revealed that indoor tanning is common among young adults, with the highest rates found in white women aged eighteen to twenty-one.

Stroke

stroke
A stoppage of the flow of blood to the brain.

A **stroke**, which is also called a brain attack or cerebral infarction, occurs when the flow of blood to the brain is stopped. When an individual has a stroke, the brain is deprived of blood and oxygen, and this may cause brain cells to die, resulting in permanent damage. Strokes are classified into two major categories: ischemic strokes and hemorrhagic strokes. The **ischemic stroke** represents almost 90 percent of all strokes and occurs when arteries to the brain are blocked, reducing blood flow to the brain. The **hemorrhagic stroke** results from a rupture of a blood vessel in the brain. This type of stroke can result from uncontrolled hypertension or from an aneurysm. Behavioral risk factors associated with a stroke include uncontrolled hypertension, cigarette smoking, obesity, poor diet, and abuse of alcohol.

ischemic stroke
A stroke resulting from a blockage of the arteries to the brain.

hemorrhagic stroke
A stroke resulting from a weakened blood vessel that ruptures and bleeds into the brain.

Diabetes

diabetes
A group of metabolic diseases in which an individual's blood sugar remains elevated.

The prevalence rate for diabetes mellitus in the United States continues to rise every year, and diabetes is now being diagnosed in increasingly younger individuals. According to the CDC (2011), **diabetes** results from defects in insulin production and can lead to serious complications and premature death. This chronic disease affects 25.8 million people in the United States, representing 8.3 percent of the population. Diabetes is the leading cause of kidney failure, nontraumatic lower limb amputation, and new cases of blindness among adults. These long-term complications from poorly controlled diabetes pose tremendous physical and economic threats to an ever-growing segment of the population.

Diabetes is the sixth most common cause of death from disease in the United States, and approximately one-third of those with diabetes are unaware that they have it. The most common form of diabetes is **type 2 diabetes**, formerly called non-insulin-dependent or adult-onset diabetes, which represents over 90 percent of the reported cases. Type 2 diabetes is normally associated with aging and being overweight. These individuals usually exhibit insulin resistance or relative insulin deficiency.

type 2 diabetes
A chronic condition that affects the way the body metabolizes glucose.

The most alarming fact about type 2 diabetes is how rapidly it is increasing in younger age groups. According to research conducted by The Today Study Group (2012), this severe metabolic disease, which prior to the 1990s was not seen in children, is becoming a very serious epidemic. Type 2 diabetes is much harder to treat in children than in adults, probably due to hormonal changes occurring with puberty. The obesity epidemic among children seems to be the catalyst for this alarming increase in diabetes among young men and women. Grady (2012) indicates that youth face a different threat from type 2 diabetes than adults do because the disease progresses much more rapidly in young people than in adults. The American Diabetes Association (2011) points out that a large number of individuals with type 2 diabetes are obese or have an increased amount of body fat around their abdomen. This risk factor is becoming very prevalent in adolescents due to poor diet, weight gain, and sedentary lifestyles. According to Akinci, Healey, and Coyne (2003), diabetes can be managed properly, reducing the long-term complications that may result from this disease over time.

This short description of four of the leading chronic diseases illustrates some of the dangers as the numbers of disease cases increase over time, and also offers an argument for the need to reduce the high-risk health behaviors that are most certainly responsible for the increased occurrence of these diseases. Two of these behaviors, tobacco use and overeating that leads to obesity, have each resulted in more disability, reduced quality of life, economic costs, and premature deaths on an annual basis than all of the communicable diseases combined. The sad fact remains that even though these high-risk health behaviors can be prevented, they have been allowed to become epidemic. Let's take a closer look at one of the most common results of poor health behavior that then goes on to cause disease: obesity.

Obesity as a Common Element in Chronic Disease

obesity
A medical problem in which excess fat accumulates to the point where health is negatively affected.

Harris (2012) observes that there is a global epidemic of **obesity** that is primarily the result of excess calories consumed combined with reduced physical activity. In other words, a large and growing proportion of the world population is consuming large amounts of foods high in fat, salt, and sugar while performing less physical activity because of more sedentary work. According to the CDC, over one-third of U.S. adults and 17 percent of U.S. children are obese. Brown (2012) cites a new study recently published in the *Journal of Preventive Medicine* that says by 2030, 42 percent of U.S. individuals will be obese, with a body mass index (BMI) of 30 or more. The obesity epidemic in America has become a much larger public health problem than the use of tobacco.

According to Graham (2012), obesity costs our country $147 billion to $190 billion, compared to $96 billion for tobacco use. Despite this enormous cost in terms of money, morbidity, and mortality, the obesity epidemic has been allowed to grow without a great deal of concern or response from our health services delivery system. Just like tobacco use, obesity often has its origins in childhood from numerous forces that, in the case of obesity, come together to produce overweight and obese adolescents and then adults. Graham (2012) points out that these forces include the food and beverages we consume, the amount of television we watch, the unlimited use of video games we allow ourselves, and the resulting sedentary lifestyles we lead.

The most common way of determining whether a person is overweight or obese is the **body mass index (BMI),** which is based on height and weight and can be determined for both adults and children by this formula.

body mass index (BMI)

A calculation based on weight and height that is a good indicator of body fatness.

$$BMI = \text{weight (lb.)}/[\text{height (in.)}]^2 \times 703.$$

For adults a value of less than 18.5 means the person is underweight, a value between 18.5 and 24.9 indicates normal weight, 25 to 29.9 indicates overweight, and a value over 30 indicates obesity. The more body fat a person has, the more likely he or she is to develop type 2 diabetes, heart disease, high blood pressure, stroke, fatty liver disease, and some cancers.

The increase in the weight of vast numbers of Americans is alarming, especially over the last few decades. "If we don't take the obesity epidemic seriously as individuals and as a nation, we will pay a serious price," says National Institutes of Health director Francis S. Collins. "It's going to take diverse and rigorous research to understand the causes of obesity and to identify interventions that work in the real world" (May 15, 2012, personal communication with the author). We already know many of the reasons for weight gain among most Americans. Weight gain is a result of environment, family history, genetics, metabolism, and poor lifestyle choices, including the eating of unhealthy foods coupled with a desire to be sedentary. Obesity causes lower productivity, reduced quality of life, higher health care costs, and massive increases in premature deaths due to chronic disease complications.

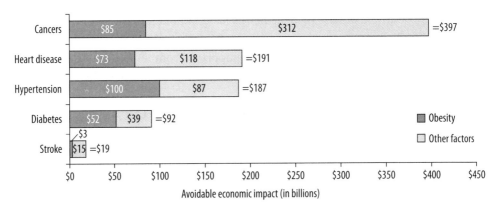

Figure 12.2 Avoidable Economic Costs Attributable to Decline in Obesity, 2023
Source: DeVol & Bedroussian, 2007.

Figure 12.2 shows the economic costs that could be avoided in 2023 if the United States could achieve a return to the lower 1998 levels of obesity by that year. The Milken Institute (DeVol & Bedroussian, 2007) believes that the most important component to lessening the burden and cost of chronic diseases is to reduce the number of obese individuals. Weight increase in Americans is the key contributor to many of the chronic diseases and is certainly the major determinant of the complications that can result from having a chronic disease for a long period of time. The Milken Institute (DeVol & Bedroussian, 2007) points out that "if the country could reverse the growth rate of obesity and return to 1998 levels in 2023, the impact would be close to 15 million fewer reported cases compared to baseline (a reduction of 14 percent) of the seven chronic diseases studied. This would translate to a reduction in health-care spending of $60 billion and an increase in productivity of $254 billion, and account for a large proportion of the overall economic impact" (p. 22). The potential monetary costs avoided more than justify current investment in disease prevention programs.

Costs of Chronic Diseases

Chronic diseases are very expensive in both monetary and nonmonetary ways. Because most of these diseases cannot be cured, they tend to increase in number and severity as the body ages, allowing more physical damage to accumulate over time and resulting in serious complications later in life. As chronic diseases ravage the body, disability becomes the norm, resulting in increased sick days, lower productivity, decreased quality of life, increased medical costs, and for some, premature death. Many of these outcomes can be eliminated or at the very least reduced with proper chronic disease management. Healey and Lesneski (2011) argue that these diseases are going to force our health care system to change by making disease prevention the most important component of our new system of health care. Figures 12.3 through 12.6, from the Milken Institute, reveal the true costs of chronic disease.

Figure 12.3 shows the lost productivity that resulted in 2003 from seven important chronic diseases. This lost productivity of American workers owing to various chronic diseases has been translated into dollar amounts to help policymakers understand just how costly the chronic disease epidemic has become. These monetary figures for lost productivity will only increase as numerous chronic diseases start showing up earlier in life due to tobacco use, weight gain, poor diet, and physical inactivity. This loss of productivity due to the complications that result from chronic diseases over time affects the ability of the United States to compete and sell products and services in the global economy.

Figure 12.4 shows the economic impact of seven of the chronic diseases in 2003. This figure looks at both total treatment costs and total lost economic output due to these diseases. In 2003, these costs and losses amounted to over $1.3 trillion. This leads to a relatively simple conclusion. In order to avoid this enormous loss we have to begin preventing chronic diseases from ever developing and pay much greater attention to better management of the chronic diseases that have already occurred.

Figure 12.5 shows the projected rise in cases of chronic diseases from 2003 through 2023. The alarming increases in these seven chronic diseases

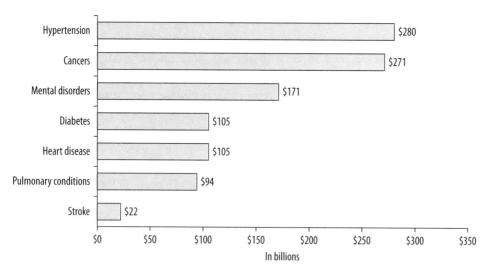

Figure 12.3 Lost Productivity by Chronic Disease, 2003
Source: DeVol & Bedroussian, 2007. Data from the National Health Interview Survey.

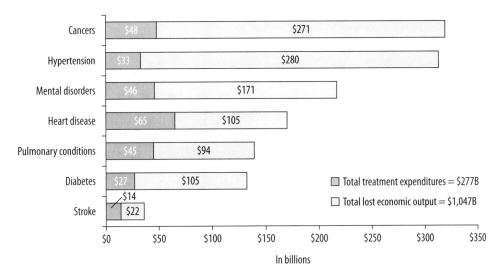

Figure 12.4 Economic Impact of Chronic Disease, 2003

Note: Treatment expenditures for individuals in nursing homes, prisons, or under other institutional care are not included. Treatment expenditures for comorbidities and secondary effects of listed diseases are also excluded.

Source: DeVol & Bedroussian, 2007. Data from the Medical Expenditure Panel Survey and the National Health Interview Survey.

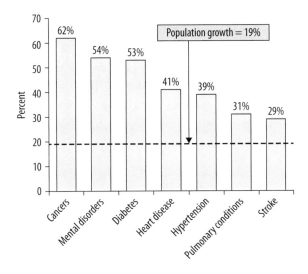

Figure 12.5 Projected Rise in Cases of Chronic Disease, 2003–2023

Source: DeVol & Bedroussian, 2007. Data from the Medical Expenditure Panel Survey.

in such a short time period offer a clear indication of the cost of the chronic disease epidemic well into the future. The Milken Institute (DeVol & Bedroussian, 2007) found that "the indirect impacts of the seven chronic diseases total $3.4 trillion annually, more than four times the cost of treatment" (p. 11). If we add the cost of disease treatment, which is $790 billion, the total cost rises to $4.2 trillion in 2023. These projected cost

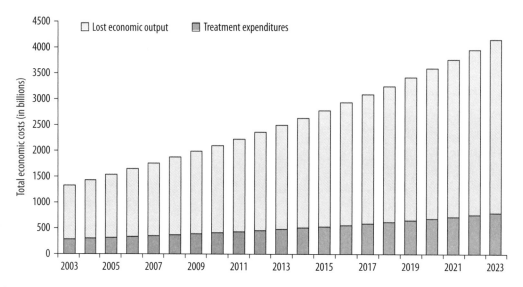

Figure 12.6 Current Path: Combined Value of Treatment Expenditures and Productivity Losses, 2003–2023
Source: DeVol & Bedroussian, 2007.

increases should be a wake-up call about the need to immediately begin preventing chronic disease development.

Figure 12.6 shows the projected current path of treatment expenditures and productivity losses resulting from chronic diseases during the time period from 2003 to 2023 in billions of dollars. This estimate does not even consider premature death and loss of quality of life due to the occurrence of one or more chronic diseases and their complications during this time period.

Chronic Disease Prevention and Behavioral Changes

Healey and Lesneski (2011) point out that prevention and change in behavioral patterns of the population should be a major goal of U.S. public health departments. In order to be successful in this goal these departments require an increase in resources so they can help communities to reduce high-risk health behaviors through the development, implementation, and evaluation of health education programs. Turnock (2009) argues that health education programs represent a long-term investment in the health of the population that will reduce health care expenditures for chronic diseases in the future.

The tremendous costs of chronic disease should provide enough incentive to increase expenditures on preventing these diseases from developing in the first place. There are, however, numerous problems with our current efforts to prevent and/or control the chronic disease epidemic. For example, often government agencies, employers, and health insurance companies do not focus on population health care when diseases are in their incubation phase, beginning with children and carrying on into young adulthood.

Because high-risk behaviors usually begin in individuals' childhood and adolescent years, the health education process must start very early in the young child's life. Currently, there is very little quality health education being offered to young children in the home, in the school, or by the family physician about the dangers associated with the practice of high-risk health behaviors. Instead, our children are allowed to learn poor health behaviors from the media, their peers, and even from family members. The result has been the development of an epidemic of high-risk health behaviors among children, and these behaviors are already contributing to an increase in overweight and obesity leading to early development of type 2 diabetes among adolescents.

It stands to reason that if high-risk behaviors begin at an earlier age, resulting in earlier onset of chronic diseases, then complications from these diseases will also begin at much earlier ages. It must be understood that the chronic disease is not as important as the complications that arise from having the chronic disease over time. If the complications from chronic diseases begin early in life, health care costs increase more rapidly along with disability, diminished quality of life, and premature death. Prevention of these chronic diseases must be looked at as an investment that will only pay dividends in the long-term. The Milken Institute cites the following areas in prevention and behavioral patterns as ones we should be working on to improve the future of chronic disease outcomes:

- A reduction in number of obese persons
- Continued reduction in smoking
- Reduced alcohol consumption
- Increased physical activity
- A reduction in high cholesterol
- A gradual decline in illicit drug use
- An improvement in early intervention and treatment
- Lower health care cost growth

Applying Business and Other Models to Chronic Disease Prevention

In order to solve complicated problems, it is often helpful to draw on other disciplines that may provide alternative solutions. The chronic disease epidemic is certainly a problem that asks us to consider the use of new and different models, including successful business models used by the private sector of the economy. Remington, Brownson, and Wegner (2010) argue that to achieve success in the battle against chronic diseases, any effort must consider the multiple determinants of the development of these diseases. The determinants of a chronic disease include personal health behaviors, the physical environment, social and economic factors, and the system of health care delivery available to the individual. In consideration of these multiple complex determinants, successful intervention to reverse the growth of the chronic disease epidemic can best be achieved by a collaborative, community-based population strategy.

The Chronic Care Model

chronic care model
A collaboration between an informed patient and a health care team that is proactive in preventing chronic disease complications.

Bernstein (2008) points to a model that represents a major change in the care of patients with chronic diseases, dubbed the **chronic care model**. This new method of treating patients with chronic diseases entails collaboration between an informed patient and a health care team that is proactive in preventing complications from the patient's chronic disease(s). This is an **evidence-based system** of health care delivery, where disease is handled proactively by health care providers who actively measure and track patient outcomes.

evidence-based system
A system in which health care decisions are made through the conscientious, explicit, and judicious use of current best evidence from relevant and valid research.

According to Glasgow, Orleans, and Wagner (2001), the chronic care model offers a template for the care of chronic diseases that is evidence-based, population-based, and patient-centered. The health system that applies this model will know the value of best practices from population and clinical studies, be concerned about the health of the patient, and be very aware of what the patient wants and needs to know about his or her health. This is a tall order for a health care system that has trained providers of care to deal with individual patients and not to be very concerned about population health. These same providers of care may also be unaware of the recommended best practices for preventing chronic diseases and their complications.

These components of care found in the chronic care model entail both the prevention of these devastating diseases and the management of chronic diseases if and when they do occur. Glasgow et al. (2001) discuss the important parts of the chronic care model, which include "making chronic illness care a key goal of the organization, ensuring that leadership is committed and visibly involved, instilling support for change and quality-improvement trials, and realigning or creating incentives for providers and patients to improve care and adhere to evidence-based guidelines (including both financial and nonfinancial incentives, such as recognition and status)" (p. 585). The key words here are *leadership* and *incentives*. The other areas of concern put forth in this template for the care of chronic diseases are self-management support and the utilization of community resources. These components are very important in dealing with the current epidemic of chronic diseases and their many potential complications.

According to Glasgow et al. (2001) **self-management support** involves preparing patients and their family members to face the challenges that will occur in taking control of their wellness despite the occurrence of one or multiple chronic diseases. The patients and their families who take on this responsibility require the availability of tailored educational resources designed to prevent the potential complications that may result from having a chronic disease for a period of time. It seems obvious that if this use of educational resources could only begin earlier in life, the chronic diseases and other comorbidities could be prevented, avoiding the use of expensive medical resources later in life.

self-management support
Helping the individual to take a supporting role in the management of his or her disease.

The other result of using the chronic care model is that one gains a much better understanding of the need to use community resources in the improvement of the health of a given population. This need to work with the community is where the leadership component of this model becomes so necessary. The importance of these environmental community resources cannot be overstated.

Business Models

Remington et al. (2010) point out that 80 percent of heart disease and type 2 diabetes cases could be prevented through individuals increasing their exercising on a daily basis. This fact alone should encourage all schools and workplaces to increase health education and promotion activities since these programs offer a tremendous return on investment. But lack of exercise is only one of the reasons that the chronic disease epidemic is growing so rapidly. There are many other high-risk health behaviors that are all working together to produce chronic diseases and their complications. It is time to look outside our health care and public health systems for components of a model that can work collaboratively to solve this national epidemic.

Zook and Allen (2012) argue that programs of change must focus energy on the most critical routines that need to change and then concentrate on changing those routines. Although this advice comes from business authors it is very applicable to changing high-risk health behaviors. There are many proven business theories and models that might help us to address the chronic disease epidemic. McChesney, Covey, and Huling (2012) point out that in order to be successful in goal achievement, we need to focus our maximum effort on one or two important goals, rather than giving minimum effort to a larger number of goals. In *The 4 Disciplines of Execution*, these authors outline a step-by-step procedure for the achievement of major goals: focus on the wildly important, act on the lead measures, keep a compelling scoreboard, and create a cadence of accountability. Although this procedure was developed for business applications, it offers great potential for dealing with chronic diseases on both an individual and population basis.

The process of execution begins with success. Gallo (2011) points out that Steve Jobs, one of the most successful innovators of all time, stated that his successful innovations involved nothing more than keeping them simple to understand and simple to use. In order to deal with the change required to reduce the epidemic of chronic diseases, we need to look at a change model that has been successful in business in recent years.

Figure 12.7 provides a diagram of a process of change that could be very useful in improving the health of the population. The outer core of this diagram calls for those involved in bringing about change to be resolute and to complete an evaluation in order to know the impact of the change process. The inner core of the change process, as proposed by Fullan (2011), involves motivating the masses, which surely needs to be a goal of population-based health education programs. Another inner process in this particular model is collaboration, which is also necessary to make community-based health education and promotion programs successful. This diagram of the components of the change process is helpful for the individual attempting to change high-risk health behaviors.

These business models are also applicable to the development of wellness programs and the successful execution of these programs by their participants. Prevention programs tend to fail in the long term because they are often too complicated and try to accomplish too much with limited resources. The entire concept of wellness needs to be simplified. Let's examine another opportunity to successfully apply a business model to a population-based health problem. Fos and Fine (2005) argue that the

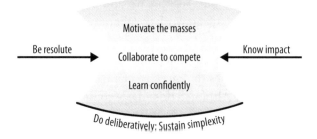

Figure 12.7   The Change Leader
Source: Fullan, 2011, p. 24.

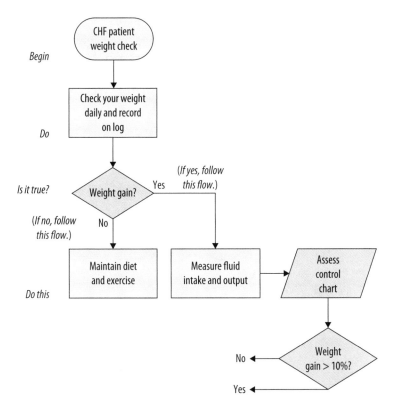

Figure 12.8 Example of a Flowchart Applied to a Health Problem
Source: Fos & Fine, 2005, p.191.

practice of creating flowcharts can easily be applied to health problems and managerial decision making.

Figure 12.8 displays a flowchart that is being used to assist individuals in following a weight reduction program. This is another example of a business tool that could be easily adapted to preventive health efforts both on an individual and a population basis. According to Fos and Fine (2005), flowcharts are extremely useful for describing a process along with identifying variation, which can then lead to correction of the variation and the building of a best process. The process of designing this tool can help program managers develop effective chronic disease prevention programs, and the tool itself can guide participants so that they can spot and respond to behavioral or outcome variations and stick with best processes or practices.

Figure 12.9 shows the **model for improvement**, another model from business that can be applied to the current epidemic of chronic diseases. This model employs a set of questions and the PDSA cycle originally discussed many years ago by W. Edwards Deming. As Healey and Zimmerman (2010) have pointed out, the **Deming cycle of PDSA (Plan, Do, Study, Act)** is a very appropriate model for use with health education and health

model for improvement
A model from business that focuses on outcomes and can be used to improve chronic disease management.

Deming cycle of PDSA (Plan, Do, Study, Act)
A management method used by businesses for the continuous improvement of quality.

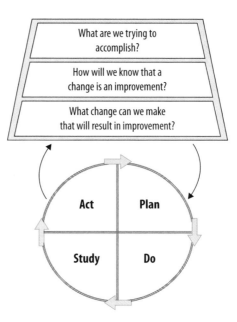

Figure 12.9 The Model for Improvement
Source: Provost & Murray, 2011, p. 4.

promotion efforts. Provost and Murray (2011), too, find that the PDSA cycle is widely applicable and easy to understand and utilize in numerous improvement efforts. Normally used in the improvement of business processes, it can be used to improve the results of many current initiatives for preventing the development of chronic diseases in the population. It can also be used with people who already have one or more chronic diseases. In the example later in this section, we will be designing a program to prevent the possible complications from chronic diseases.

In this model three fundamental questions form the basis for improvement:

- What are we trying to accomplish?
- How will we know that a change is an improvement?
- What changes can we make that will result in improvement? [Provost & Murray, 2011, p. 4].

It is not difficult to apply the PDSA cycle and attempt to answer these questions in the development of population-based chronic disease prevention and care programs. The following example of answering the questions uses the population-based problem of overweight and obesity.

What Are We Trying to Accomplish?

Provost and Murray (2011) argue that in order to improve a situation (such as the incidence of complications from overweight and obesity), all the important stakeholders need to agree on the reason for this effort. The best way to accomplish this critical component of the proposed program is to develop and agree upon an aim statement that is clear, concise, and results oriented. Here's a sample aim statement for our proposed overweight and obesity reduction program.

BOX 12.1. AIM STATEMENT

Community Weight Reduction Program

During the next year, the Wellness Task Force will reduce the average weight of the residents of County A by 20 percent.

Guidance: The focus for this weight reduction project will be health education programs for schools in the district on good nutrition and physical activity and a more advanced program for the workplaces in the county concerning appropriate weight and the value of physical activity.

How Will We Know That a Change Is an Improvement?

In order to keep community involvement high, there needs to be feedback that tells program managers whether or not the intervention is actually moving toward goal achievement. For example, measures of change in this project could be

- Percentage of children in the school district who are actively participating in the weight-loss program through improved nutrition and physical activity programs.

- Percentage of workplaces in the county that are actively participating in the weight-loss program through improved nutrition and physical activity programs.

What Change Can We Make That Will Result in Improvement?

According to Provost and Murray (2011), in many instances "the knowledge to support a specific change has existed for some time, but the conditions, resources, or inclination did not exist to make the change happen" (p. 7). This is the exact condition that we have been experiencing with the chronic disease epidemic in the United States.

For instance, Matthews et al. (2008) argue that Americans spend a large majority of their time in behaviors that are sedentary. The human body was not designed to be sedentary but is, rather, an amazing creation that thrives when physical activity becomes part of its daily routine. Lack of physical activity is contributing to our weight gain and subsequent development of chronic diseases. Increasing physical activity is a change that could drive prevention of these diseases or of their complications.

Another missing ingredient in chronic disease management that we have known about for some time is the way Medicare and most other insurers pay for care. Health care payment systems focus on activities performed by various providers rather than outcomes delivered by those providers. This focus on activities can result in enormous increases in health care costs, especially in the last several months of life when chronic diseases do the most damage but major interventions nevertheless often yield very poor outcomes. Having payment systems that focus more on outcomes is a change that might make real differences in the assistance people receive to manage their weight.

SUMMARY

Chronic diseases have become the leading cause of morbidity and mortality among the population and of cost escalation in health insurance premiums and health care costs in the United States over the last several years. This chronic disease epidemic has become the most serious medical threat to ever face the nation, and it is going to get worse until we as a nation decide to prevent it from growing. Reasons for this alarming increase in chronic diseases are the increase in high-risk health behaviors and a paradigm of medicine that concentrates on the cure rather than the prevention of disease.

Chronic diseases are responsible for over 75 percent of U.S. health care costs and are rapidly reducing the quality of life for a very large segment of the older population. These diseases can begin at a very early age, can continue to inflict damage in later life, and result in complications that cause pain, suffering, and quite often premature death.

We have not yet responded appropriately to the growing epidemic of chronic diseases and their complications, which is only going to get worse as the population continues to age. It is critical that all parts of the entire health care system work together with communities to develop a chronic disease plan of action to deal with these diseases and work on preventing the development of new cases in the future.

This collaborative approach to the chronic disease epidemic requires a new model for providers, insurers, and patients to follow. This new model can benefit from drawing on recent business models that have been successful in change management and program execution. Several business models that could be applied to health promotion programs were discussed in this chapter. The model for improvement was then applied to the problem of overweight and obesity, which is an underlying cause of numerous chronic diseases and their complications, not only in the United States but also around the world.

KEY TERMS

atherosclerosis	evidence-based system
body mass index (BMI)	hemorrhagic stroke
cancer	ischemic stroke
chronic care model	model for improvement
chronic disease	obesity
comorbidity	quarantining
Deming cycle of PDSA (Plan, Do, Study, Act)	self-management support
	stroke
diabetes	type 2 diabetes

DISCUSSION QUESTIONS

1. What are the major differences between communicable and chronic diseases?

2. What costs are associated with the chronic disease epidemic in the United States? Explain each of these costs.

3. How does the chronic care model differ from the way other diseases are handled by our health care delivery system?

4. How would you explain the use of the model for improvement in relation to the development and implementation of programs to prevent the development of chronic diseases or their complications?

REFERENCES

Agus, D. (2011). *The end of illness*. New York, NY: Free Press.

Akinci, F., Healey, B. J., & Coyne, J. (2003). Improving the health status of U.S. working adults with type 2 diabetes: A review. *Disease Management and Health Outcomes, 11*(8), 489–498.

American Diabetes Association. (2011). Diagnosis and classification of diabetes mellitus. *Diabetes Care, 34*(1), 562–569.

Bernstein, S. J. (2008). A new model for chronic-care delivery. *Frontiers of Health Services Management, 25*(2), 31–38.

Brown, D. (2012, May 7). Study predicts 42 percent of Americans will be obese in 2030. *Washington Post*. Retrieved from http://www.washingtonpost.com /national/health-science/study-predicts-42-percent-of-americans-will-be -obese-in-2030/2012/05/07/gIQAeaDL9T_story.html

Centers for Disease Control and Prevention. (2011). National diabetes fact sheet. Retrieved from http://www.cdc.gov/diabetes/pubs/general11.htm

Centers for Disease Control and Prevention. (2012a). Cancer prevention. Retrieved from http://www.cdc.gov/cancer/dcpc/prevention/index.htm

Centers for Disease Control and Prevention. (2012b). Heart disease and stroke deaths drop significantly for people with diabetes. Retrieved from http://www .cdc.gov/media/releases/2012/p0522_heart_disease.html

Centers for Disease Control and Prevention. (2012c). High-risk behaviors for skin cancer common among young adults. Retrieved from http://www.cdc.gov /media/releases/2012/p0510_skin_cancer.html

DeVol, R., & Bedroussian, A. (2007). *An unhealthy America: The economic burden of chronic disease*. Milken Institute. Retrieved from http://www.milkeninstitute .org/pdf/chronic_disease_report.pdf

Fos, P., & Fine, D. (2005). *Managerial epidemiology for health care organizations*. San Francisco, CA: Jossey-Bass.

Fuchs, V. R. (2009). Health reform: Getting the essentials right. *Health Affairs, 28*(2), 180–183.

Fullan, M. (2011). *Change leader: Learning to do what matters most*. San Francisco, CA: Jossey-Bass.

Gallo, C. (2011). *The innovation secrets of Steve Jobs: Insanely different principles for breakthrough success*. New York, NY: McGraw-Hill.

Glasgow, R. E., Orleans, C. T., & Wagner, E. H. (2001). Does the chronic care model serve also as a template for improving prevention? *Millbank Quarterly, 79*(4), 579–612.

Grady, D. (2012, April 29). Obesity-linked diabetes found harder to treat in children. *New York Times*, Editorial.

Graham, J. (2012, May 5). Obesity fight needs ambitious campaign, health leaders say. *USA Today*. Retrieved from http://usatoday30.usatoday.com/news /health/story/2012-05-05/childhood-obesity-tobacco/54745872/1

Harris, R. E. (2012). *Epidemiology of chronic disease: Global perspectives.* Burlington, MA: Jones & Bartlett Learning.

Healey, B. J., & Lesneski, C. D. (2011). *Transforming public health practice: Leadership and management essentials.* San Francisco, CA: Jossey-Bass.

Healey, B. J., & Zimmerman, R. S. (2010). *The new world of health promotion: New program development, implementation, and evaluation.* Sudbury, MA: Jones & Bartlett Learning.

Matthews, C. E., Chen, K. Y., Freedson, P. S., Buchowski, M. S., Beech, B. M., Pate, R. R., & Troiano, R. P. (2008). Amount of time spent in sedentary behaviors in the United States, 2003–2004. *American Journal of Epidemiology, 167*(7), 875–881.

McChesney, C., Covey, S., & Huling, J. (2012). *The 4 disciplines of execution.* New York, NY: Free Press.

Morewitz, S. J. (2006). *Chronic diseases and health care: New trends in diabetes, arthritis, osteoporosis, fibromyalgia, low back pain, cardiovascular disease, and cancer.* New York, NY: Springer.

Provost, L. P., & Murray, S. K. (2011). *The health care data guide: Learning from data for improvement.* San Francisco, CA: Jossey-Bass.

Remington, P. L., Brownson, R. C., & Wegner, M. V. (2010). *Chronic disease epidemiology and control* (3rd ed.). Washington, DC: American Public Health Association.

Schimpff, S. C. (2012). *The future of health care delivery: Why it must change and how it will affect you.* Washington, DC: Potomac Books.

Sultz, H. A., & Young, K. M. (2011). *Health care USA: Understanding its organization and delivery* (7th ed.). Sudbury, MA: Jones & Bartlett Learning.

Today Study Group. (2012). A clinical trial to maintain glycemic control in youth with type 2 diabetes. *New England Journal of Medicine, 366*(24), 2247–2256.

Turnock, B. (2009). *Public health: What it is and how it works* (4th ed.). Sudbury, MA: Jones & Bartlett Learning.

Wennberg, J. E., Fisher, E. S., Goodman, D. C., & Skinner, J. S. (2008). *Tracking the care of patients with severe chronic illness: The Dartmouth atlas of health care 2008.* Lebanon, NH: Dartmouth Institute for Health Policy and Clinical Practice.

Zook, C., & Allen, J. (2012). *Repeatability: Building enduring businesses for a world of constant change.* Boston, MA: Harvard Business Review Press.

CHAPTER 13

LEADERSHIP SOLUTIONS TO HEALTH CARE PROBLEMS

Bernard J. Healey

During a crisis the United States has in the past always been able to find leaders who come to the rescue and make things right. Unfortunately, with the massive change and resulting turmoil in our health care delivery system in recent years, there seems to be a shortage of real leadership to make quality health care equitable for all people.

One of the most difficult concepts for most individuals and institutions to understand and embrace is the need for constant change. Their argument is always that there is no need for change if, to their minds, everything is working well. In fact most people will use whatever personal and collective power they have to block change if it affects them in any way, owing to their fear of the unknown. They are incapable of seeing the opportunities that may result as a consequence of change. Health care organizations are no exception; they do not want to change.

Despite this reluctance to change there are numerous indications that the pace of change in our world is accelerating at a remarkable pace. There are many reasons for the escalation of change in our lives and businesses over the past twenty to thirty years, with improved communication being found at the top of the list of change process facilitators.

Understanding why change occurs is important, but not as important as gaining awareness of the fact that our individual and collective futures rely on how we accept change, adapt to change, and even play a part in creating change. It is no longer acceptable for individuals or businesses to simply react to change; instead they must become proactive in and be part of the creation of change. If an organization wants to remain relevant in

LEARNING OBJECTIVES

After reading this chapter you should be able to

- Describe the development of organizational conflict in health services delivery.

- Understand how leadership skills can help health care administrators meet the many challenges facing the U.S. health care industry.

- Identify ways in which the structure of a health care facility can block necessary change.

- Understand how creativity and innovation can develop in health care facilities.

the long term, it must actually seek out change and exploit that change for the opportunities it may offer. This is true for health care delivered by providers and received by consumers. The health care sector is ripe for change and the innovation in health care services that it may bring.

Serota (2013) argues that a major barrier to an improved system of health care in the United States is the fragmentation among the many players, resulting in a lack of coordination in care delivery. The Patient Protection and Affordable Care Act pays little attention to the financing of health care and virtually ignores the idea of designing financial incentives that would improve the delivery of health care services. However, health care reform should include financial incentives that are designed to allow cooperation between payers and providers of care to improve the quality of care and health outcomes. If we carefully craft these financial payments to improve health, rather than simply provide expensive and unnecessary services, we can eliminate a great deal of the current waste found in our health care delivery system. It is hard to understand why the designers of the Affordable Care Act ignored how and why we pay providers of health care services.

The United States has created a complex health care delivery system that is difficult for the average individual to understand. Perednia (2011) nevertheless argues that even though our health care system is extremely complex and dysfunctional, it can be understood if we spend some time dissecting the various incentives that guide its operation. In fact Christensen, Grossman, and Hwang (2009) state that the major problems facing the health care sector of our economy are not unique but are instead similar to the problems faced by many other large industries. At some point in their history, large industries that sell expensive products and services are transformed into making more affordable products and services, which then become available to more people. The agent of this transformation has been labeled **disruptive innovation**. Christensen and colleagues believe that this disruptive innovation is slowly presenting itself in all service industries, including education and health care delivery. This disruption will, over time, produce great change in the way business is done and services are delivered to patients who are evolving into consumers as they are becoming responsible for a larger portion of the costs. One of the most important components of this disruptive innovation is found in the concept of the **value-adding business process**. This process of adding value to the product or service offered to consumers requires a reduction in price or an increase in the quality of the final offering by the business.

The value-adding business process has been virtually missing in our health care organizations. In fact, for most health care facilities, adding value has usually been defined as adding more activities in order to increase the revenue stream for the health care provider. Unfortunately, many of

disruptive innovation
A new product or service that is capable of changing an existing market by improving convenience, access, and/or affordability.

value-adding business process
A new business process that increases the value of the current product or service.

these activities that add value for the provider offer little if any added value for the patient while at the same time increasing the cost of health care services and at times actually placing the patient in harm's way. A true value-added component would add real value as perceived by the customer.

Disruption is occurring in every business in the world, even health care delivery systems, whether they are private or government run. The U.S. health care delivery sector is also facing radical change, but who will lead that change? We need new leaders to repair our health service delivery system. In fact lack of leadership is probably the major reason that health care has had so little success in meeting recent challenges. Our health care sector is reluctantly moving to an understanding that bureaucratic organizations and poor leadership are the real cause of the system's failures in delivering quality health care services at a reasonable price.

In order for health care facilities to remain relevant they must develop and share a vision of the future that is acceptable to all their stakeholders. Although the final direction of an organization is the responsibility of its leaders, the change in direction must be a collaborative effort of the entire health care organization, including the consumers of its service.

Health Care Reform Beyond the ACA

The United States is in the process of the most dramatic health care reform it has ever experienced. The Affordable Care Act is the most important and controversial health legislation since the passage of Medicare and Medicaid in 1965. It seems as though we have been in a continuous state of health care reform with our efforts to reverse the fact that although we are spending more on health care delivery than every other country, we rank very low in health care outcomes compared to most other industrialized countries. Those who pay the health care bills keep asking for a change in reimbursement methods in order to improve our system of health care delivery.

Carroll, Chapman, Dodd, Hollister, and Harrington (2013) point out that health care costs are continuing to rise, and by the year 2020 these costs will total $4.6 trillion, representing almost 20 percent of our GDP. This cost escalation will occur despite the fact that the new health care reform law will have been fully implemented by 2020. The reforming health care sector is not only a result of new government laws and regulations but also represents a long overdue interest by consumers in health care services and how they are delivered to consumers and to their family members. This new interest in reform is a result of the patient of health care services being transformed into a consumer of health care services. This transformation was nudged along by more of the costs of health care being passed on to the consumers of these services in the form of higher deductibles and copayments. This is a critical turning point for the consumers of health care services, because changing their passive role to a more active voice in health care decisions is vital if we are going to reduce costs and improve the quality of health care services in our country.

According to Schimpff (2012) the purchasers of health care are demanding the same quality offered with the purchase of any other good or service. This means that they want a product or service that works, that is delivered on time by courteous employees who are responsive to their needs, and that is produced at an affordable price. The sad part is that many health care facilities are still not aware of the wave of consumerism that has hit health care services delivery. They are still living in their bureaucratic world, unaware of that their former patients have now become consumers with various competitors to choose from when purchasing health care products and services. Health care organizations must learn what the consumers of their services desire and then find out the best way to deliver these services at an affordable price. This represents an entirely new way of thinking for the managers of health care facilities.

Christensen et al. (2009) point out that disruptive innovation usually involves three elements: a technological enabler, a business model innovation, and a value network. In short a **technological enabler** allows the health care organization to take a solution to a problem and routinize it. A business model innovation allows a simplified solution to the problems associated with the costs and convenience of health care services delivery. The creation of a value network entails successful implementation of the disruptive economic models. Christensen et al. (2009) believe that since these elements of disruptive innovation have been successfully brought together in other large industries, they can also work their magic in health care services delivery.

technological enabler
New technology that contributes to radical change in a product or service.

Reengineering the Health Care Sector

Reform of the health care industry is occurring at a rapid rate that has never before been seen by this sector of our economy. This type of change cannot be managed but can, nevertheless, be led to its ultimate destination. Such leadership in the delivery of health care services will require a vision of a future delivery system of scarce health care services that cannot even be imagined today. In fact many health care administrators are requiring their facilities to reengineer their entire process of service delivery. According to Champy and Greenspun (2010), health care delivery is ready for redesign in an attempt to improve its quality, safety, and convenience that should ultimately result in a reduction in the cost of care.

The health care market has changed, and in some cases the consumer is dictating his or her demands to many providers and making choices almost as in any other market. This consumer choice and action in the health care decision-making process will become the normal way that health services are purchased. This will in turn force all health care providers to offer the consumers of health care quality services or those providers will no longer survive. The amount of health care information that is now available to consumers will allow health care delivery to function like any other market where the consumer is able to receive quality products and services at a reasonable price.

According to Jennings (2012) unless a business is constantly seeking radical change in its business practices, it will never be able to stay ahead of its competitors. As competitors increase their share of the market, those who missed the signal will begin losing share and eventually disappear. This is why individual and corporate reinvention is the new game being played and won by those who prepare and implement the change process on a daily basis in health services delivery. There are many parts of our current health care system that desperately need to be reinvented sooner rather than later. This reinvention, or reengineering, needs to begin with ending medical errors, eliminating wasteful testing and medical procedures, increasing efficiency and cost reduction, and then, finally, focusing on patient satisfaction. This is a great deal of change for an industry that has blocked change for years. To be successful in these lofty goals, health care needs strong leadership development. Leadership has to focus on consumer desires and how the health care system, through its employees, can deliver those services.

Understanding Power in the Health Care Sector

The health care sector of our economy represents an extremely large bureaucracy that has successfully blocked change for decades through the use of power mostly gained through legislation. The delivery of health care services in our country represents very big business that is controlled by very powerful interest groups. Tremendous power can be secured by constructing very large bureaucracies. A good example of a large bureaucracy in health care is found in the intermediaries who pay the health care bills for us. Goldhill (2013) argues that there are three large intermediaries that pay health care bills: private insurers, Medicare, and Medicaid. He calls them *surrogates* and points out that they have incentives in place that virtually guarantee the growth of the health care economy into the distant future. They have gained this surrogate status through **asymmetry of information**, defined as one party in an economic transaction having superior knowledge

asymmetry of information
A condition that exists when one party has more information than another party when making a decision.

of the product or service compared to the other party. In short we have abdicated from exercising our consumer purchasing power and given that power to the health care insurers. This power can be returned to consumers only if they demand its return and then also learn how to use the power.

These intermediaries are certainly one of the many special interest groups in health care services delivery who benefit from the growing expenditures in health care that we have witnessed since the 1960s. These interest groups have been successful in acquiring, developing, and using power in order to secure their enormous profits on a consistent basis over the last forty years. They are powerful enough to resist health care reform efforts and quite often turn any reform effort into a positive force for their own income stream. It is virtually impossible to improve the U.S. health care system without having a very good understanding of the role of power in that system.

Naim (2013) points out that concentrations of power are found in every field and have an important role in structuring relationships and interactions among individuals and organizations. Naim argues quite correctly that "power is the ability to direct or prevent the current or future actions of other groups and individuals" (p. 30). In order to regain consumer control over the U.S. health care system, we need a better understanding of where the power lies in our health care system and how to gain countervailing power to lead the system through positive change.

There is a great deal of evidence that the power of larger institutions in our country is diminishing, while power is accruing to smaller businesses that understand consumer wants and deliver them consistently. Consider how many large businesses are disappearing and being replaced by smaller start-ups. Examples include Blockbuster, Circuit City, and numerous airlines and financial institutions in recent years. In health care this loss of power can be seen in larger hospitals losing business to ambulatory care facilities. This power shift may help to improve the quality of services while lowering the price of delivering these services to consumers. This change cannot be managed, but strong leadership can seek out opportunities among the changes and exploit them. Now is the time for health care leaders and their followers to begin the long and challenging process of rebuilding the health care system so it can focus on better patient outcomes and efficient delivery of necessary patient services.

Changing the Health Care Environment

Everyone seems to agree that change in the health services sector of the U.S. economy is inevitable, even though the thought of change seems to terrify everyone and especially the providers of health care services. This is also a reason why there have been numerous efforts at health care reform over the last fifty years but very little change has resulted from them. In fact most of the reform efforts have actually increased the costs of health care services while having little if any effect on the quality of these services. Powerful interest groups have been blocking changes that do not increase their group profits or income. They do not want health care services to be like the markets that offer choice, quality, lower prices, and information to the consumer. The vast majority of providers in health care make their enormous profits year in and year out through consumer ignorance.

As discussed previously, there is a great deal of information asymmetry in health care. Goldhill (2013) points out that this difference in knowledge concerning a product or service makes it extremely difficult for the buyer to determine a product's true value and reasonable price at the time of the purchase. For instance, in an article called "Bitter Pill: Why Medical Bills Are Killing Us," Brill (2013) gives numerous examples of overpricing and wasteful purchases for hospitals that have occurred simply because there is no true transparency in health care billing practices.

The health care sector of our economy has been isolated from reality for a long time and it may also take a long time for acceptance of a normal market to occur. The market for health care services in the United States is very similar to the market for higher education in that it is not a real market of demanders and suppliers guided by a price system. The consumer or student takes what is offered and pays what the health care provider or the educational institution dictates. Also, the government provides grants and loans to some students, making them less sensitive to price increases, just as health insurance makes health care consumers less sensitive to the real costs of care. Fortunately, both education and health care services are experiencing disruptive innovation, which should eventually transform both these sectors of our economy for the better.

As stated previously, disruptive innovation usually results in an improved quality of product or service at a reduced price because of intense competition. But in order for disruptive innovation to work, the health care market must be freed from the power of special interest groups and Washington lobbyists. Fortunately, there is some evidence that power in health care is shifting from special interest groups back to the consumer. An example of this shift in power is found in the transparency provided by the use of electronic medical records that are open to the consumer. This recent development will not be enough in itself to unleash disruptive innovation in the health care sector, however. That will also require the development of leaders throughout health care facilities. These leaders will in turn have to empower their followers in a collaborative effort designed to improve health care quality and to deliver services efficiently in order to lower the cost of care.

Leadership Challenges

Rapid change in the business environment due mostly to technological growth and especially new communication technologies is ushering in widespread changes to the organizational structure and management of many industries. The new public availability of valuable information involving prices and quality of most products and services is driving these changes. This information can often change the nature and intensity of competition. It can turn industries upside down, forcing them to give consumers what they desire at a reduced cost. Those industries that fail to cater to the consumer are either absorbed by other companies or find themselves out of business. The health care sector of our economy is facing the same rapidly changing environment, creating challenges for leaders who deliver health care services.

The Need for Trust

There are thousands of books about leadership, with most claiming that a certain skill or attribute will help you to become a better leader. In the changing health care environment, leaders must be able to welcome and use innovation and creativity and to gain the trust of employees. Without trust in the leader and the organization, employees will not have the courage to take the risks that are necessary to improve the health care sector. As Horsager (2009) points out, "trust has become the world's most precious resource" (p. 2). He goes on to explain that a low level of trust in an organization results in reduced productivity, escalating costs, and reduced loyalty toward the leader and the business. Trust is a prerequisite for employees when they are attempting to be innovative in the delivery of products and services in a competitive environment.

Trust can be thought of as the magic potion that allows teams of health care professionals to collaborate to produce good patient outcomes at an affordable price. In order for teams to work together and concentrate on providing excellent service to their customers, they must trust each other and also respect and trust their leader. Without trust the entire process of health services delivery falls apart, hurting the patients first and slowly bringing down the entire organization. According to Burchell and Robin (2011), building trust in the organization reduces employee turnover and improves the workflow. Trust should also bring the followers and the leader together in successful attempts to add real value for their patients. Moreover, according to Horsager (2009), trust is a critical component of long-term organizational success and thus a necessary competency for anyone in a leadership position.

Leaders Who Are Trustworthy

- *Tell the truth as they understand it.* They don't shade or position the truth to benefit themselves: they are honest.

- *Do what they say they will do.* They keep their commitments. When they can't, they're clear and honest about what's changed.

- *Keep confidences.* They're rigorous about discretion; if they say they'll keep something private, they will.

- *Speak and act for the greater good.* Their words and actions are consonant and support the success of the enterprise.

- *Are capable and get results.* They have the skills and experience to do the job before them, and they do it [Andersen, 2012, p. 156].

This is a comprehensive list of the characteristics of a leader who is trustworthy and who can create a trusting environment that in turn helps the organization to simplify the work process, improve efficiency, and encourage innovation. This is important when the health care leader is trying to change the norms within the health care facility and encourage employees to be creative without the fear associated with failure. A good leader creates an environment that not only accepts change but also looks for change in order to create new opportunities.

One of the best ways to learn how to be a leader is by undertaking a complete analysis of any failure. Health care leaders need to be willing to encourage followers to try new ways of doing things. According to Weinzimmer and McConoughey (2013), many leaders learn the most from a trial-and-error process. These authors argue that mistakes are a large part of the pursuit of healthy risk taking by employees because they help people to reflect on new ways of approaching problems and turning them into potential opportunities. In other words, employees need to be allowed to fail in order to grow in their roles, including leadership roles. Obviously, any organization would like to limit the number of failures, but the most successful businesses encourage innovation and so they accept and encourage a certain amount of risk taking. As they do this, they also demonstrate trust.

Focusing on Outcomes

A growing number of health policymakers are arguing that health care providers should be paid for outcomes rather than for activities. In other words, we should place providers at risk of nonpayment for services that are not successful in the achievement of predetermined outcomes. We need to stop paying for activities that have not been shown to achieve good health but instead usually result in the waste of scarce health care resources. This certainly makes sense because many activities produced in health care today have very little, if any, value. For example, Brawley (2011) points out that the protein-specific antigen (PSA) test for prostate cancer is not only often a waste of time and money but in many situations it is also a dangerous test that can lead to unnecessary and harmful treatment. Brawley also argues that many transplants do not increase life expectancy, while costing a great deal of money and in many cases decreasing the quality of life. Additionally, many back surgeries, which cost a great deal of time and money, have poor results. Successful outcomes can be identified by the fact that they achieve predetermined goals of care. It may be difficult to determine which goals are the most important in any health care purchase, but it seems likely that consumers are looking for good health as their most sought-after outcome. Indeed the health care system should consider the prevention of illness and disease to be its primary desired outcome. Unfortunately, our current system of health care does not allocate many resources to prevention but does spend a great deal of money and time attempting to cure incurable chronic diseases and their various complications. Because health care providers make money only when people are sick, they make treatment more important than prevention of disease.

It will be up to the leaders of health care organizations to convince the payers of the health care bills that prevention activities, including health education, deserve reimbursement equal to or higher than that received by providers who bill for activities with little value. Halvorson (2009) points out that of the 18,000 billing codes for health care services, there are no codes for better outcomes. Our system of payment for health care does not incentivize prevention or the care oversight that a primary care physician responsible for the overall health of a patient might provide. In this role the primary care physician would monitor the various treatments and medications suggested by referrals to specialists. The only ones who benefit from all the wasteful testing and medical procedures performed currently are the people and organizations who supply these services and who have been given the power to create their own demand.

It is important for health care consumers and payers to examine the link between a predetermined outcome and the intervention that was performed by the health care provider. There are several outcomes that can be measured including whether or not the patient got better, the diagnosis was correct, the treatment was accurate, or the patient was harmed by a test or medical procedure. Was the health care provided appropriate, and was the technical aspect of care provided skillfully?

Preventing Disease

The primary reason for health care reform efforts over the last several decades has been to ensure access to health care services for the entire population of our country. The reason for this emphasis has been the mistaken belief that access to health insurance will guarantee good health for Americans. However, in order to remain healthy we need to remain free of illness and disease. Health insurance helps in our effort to remain well, but for effectiveness, health behaviors trump insurance coverage every time. Any health reform effort should be focused on the prevention of high-risk health behaviors that cause poor health.

The prevention of disease has always been discussed as a major goal of our health care system, but it has still not become a major goal in practice. The United States spends less than 3 percent of its entire health care budget on disease prevention activities. This means that over 97 percent of our almost $3 trillion annual health care expenditure is spent on attempting to cure disease. Given that most of the diseases that occur in the United States today are chronic diseases that are incurable, this is a waste of time and money. The only way to curtail this waste is to prevent chronic diseases before they start and go on to produce complications that lead to poor health and in many cases are life threatening.

Because money is made in health care only when individuals become ill, little attention and few resources are devoted to keeping individuals free of illness and disease. It is a sad commentary that wellness is not a profit center for health care providers but illness is. Even though the majority of health care organizations are classified as nonprofit, they are still very interested in making money. It is only through health care leadership that appropriate attention will ever be paid to the most important purpose of health care organizations and that is to keep individuals healthy. As these chapters have demonstrated over and over, achieving that purpose means changing poor health behaviors. One way to start this change is to have health programs that begin in elementary school, continue in the workplace, and are constantly reinforced by physicians.

Getting Control of Cost Increases

The cost of providing health care to Americans has been increasing at a rate higher than the rate of inflation for the last fifty years. This has occurred despite efforts by the third-party payers to contain costs through various reform efforts. These cost increases are no longer sustainable for those who are paying them: health care consumers, employers, and the government. Although health care costs have seen some stabilization (due in part to the recession in 2008 and 2009), most health policy experts predict an upward trend in costs to continue into the foreseeable future. These cost increases have surpassed not only the inflation rate but also the growth of the gross domestic product (GDP) and wage increases on an annual basis almost every year since the 1970s. Such price increases also mean that the productivity of the health care sector has been falling.

With the cost of health care expected to surpass 20 percent of GDP in the next few years something will have to change or the health care system is going to bankrupt the country. As mentioned earlier in this chapter, the ability of the providers of care to control pricing is most likely a direct result of information asymmetry, which places the individual purchaser and recipient of health care services at a great disadvantage.

The seller of health care services is usually a physician, who has a superior knowledge of medicine compared to the patient (consumer), who is usually not well versed in illness care. The health care consumer has never been allowed to be a knowledgeable participant in the medical care decision-making process. It has just been assumed that health care providers would always act in the best interest of the less knowledgeable patient. In the past patients simply ceded their decision-making authority regarding medical testing and procedures, hospitalizations, and all other medical decisions to their physician. The physician has thus been allowed to literally create his or her own demand. The answer to this possible conflict of interest is to make patients more knowledgeable in the expectation that this will make them active consumers of medical care and better able to participate in personal medical decisions. The most effective way to increase the health knowledge of patients is to increase the availability of medical information. For example, public health agencies can distribute medical knowledge to the media who will then make it available to the entire population.

Empowering Health Care Employees

The solutions to the problems found in health care delivery are not going to come from government or health care administrators but from those who work in health care delivery on a daily basis. These employees know best what is wrong with health care and also have suggestions about how to fix these problems. The most successful health care facilities in our country have one thing in common: they allow their employees the freedom and decision-making authority to solve problems as they are presented. This requires a team of collaborative employees empowered with the goal of improving service delivery for their patients.

Unfortunately, most health care organizations have a **bureaucratic structure**, with the power to make decisions residing at the top of the

bureaucratic structure
Power resides at the top of the organization and decisions are made by those in power.

hierarchy. This structure has failed in many ways, and the nation is not receiving good health outcomes despite the huge amount of money spent on health care every year. Health care facilities require collaboration among leaders, managers, and staff in order to achieve successful health outcomes for their patients. When leaders realize that they must involve their employees in decision making, better outcomes occur. This is why empowerment of staff members should be mandatory for all leaders and, in today's turbulent health care environment, especially for health care leaders.

Changing the Organizational Structure

The structure of an organization is a critical component in the way it makes decisions. In order to achieve maximum efficiency as the organization grows in size, many organizations institute the components of a bureaucratic organization, including rules, regulations, and a top-down command-and-control structure. This type of structure does not foster creativity and innovation, but it does work well when competition is limited or, as in some cases, nonexistent. In the long term most successful organizations change to a more decentralized structure, freeing their employees to be more creative in their approach to serving the needs of their customers. This decentralized approach needs to be adopted in health care organizations that are facing rapid change, a more demanding and a better-informed customer, and a need to control the cost escalation of health care services.

This change in organizational structure will not be easy because it will result in a great deal of organizational conflict. The bureaucracy will attempt to block conflict by issuing rules and regulations that employees must follow, virtually eliminating creativity. It is much wiser for a leader to not only allow and encourage conflict but also to manage conflict occurrence as the norm in the organizational culture.

Allowing Innovation in Health Care

Christensen et al. (2009) point out that health care has been frozen in a model of service delivery that is controlled by two major players: hospital managers and physicians. These players block change, innovation, and creativity through the scale of their operations and the power of their decision-making abilities. This service delivery model remains intact owing to their abundance of resources and their political base that has been secured by paid lobbyists. Change is simply not welcome in this industry because it is threatening to the bureaucratic model of health care created over a hundred years ago. This model does not represent what the consumer desires today. In fact the lack of innovation in the business model that controls the delivery of health care services today is probably the most important reason why health care costs continue to rise year after year.

Major industries and organizations require creativity and innovation in order to survive and grow. Wilkins and Carolin (2013) argue that the development and introduction of new products and services is the lifeblood of a successful organization. It is virtually impossible for an organization to remain relevant if it is not constantly changing the products and services that it produces in response to the pressure of competition and the desires of the consumer. Yet even conventional methods of fostering creativity and innovation have not found their way onto the radar of many health care service providers. Health care organizations have not received enough pressure from their competitors to spur innovation, and this allows them to continue to escalate costs.

Nussbaum (2013) argues that there is nothing rare about creativity; it can happen anywhere with any person who learns how to cultivate it. He points out that creativity is actually a result of an uncertain environment, where creative employees are allowed to excel as they react to unknown opportunities. Many health care organizations are now facing both short- and long-term challenges that are capable of ending their survival in this ever-changing industry. These organizations need leaders who will foster the development of creative staff who in turn will respond with innovation to multiple challenges.

Whitacre and Cauley (2013) argue that managers are not caretakers of an organization. They are instead the ones who are responsible for the success or failure of the business, and excuses for failing are of no value to anyone. When things are not working well, the manager is expected to step into the problem and make the appropriate corrections to make things work again. Hamel (2012) points out that one of the most important functions of the manager is to foster creativity and innovation in employees in the organization. This can be accomplished by allowing bold thinking by all employees, without fear of failure. Hamel argues that there is no shortage of human creativity but there is a lack of pro-innovation processes. This is why we need more farsighted leaders and fewer micromanagers. We also need health care leaders who are capable of instilling trust in their employees so that these workers feel able to produce services that respond to customer needs.

In many large industries this desire for innovation has taken the form of disruptive innovation and has radically changed the way products and services are being developed and delivered to demanding consumers. It has taken a long time but a combination of **creative destruction** and disruptive innovation has arrived in the majority of health care organizations in our country. As discussed in Chapter Six, creative destruction is a concept that was first described by the economist Joseph Schumpeter. This type of destruction usually results in radical innovation

creative destruction

The destruction of an old product or service in order to create a new product or service that is better.

that in turn produces major transformations. Creative destruction is the result of entrepreneurs seeking profits who produce a disruptive force that creates increased wealth even as previous vehicles of economic growth are destroyed. The creative destruction in health care will involve the breakdown of the bureaucratic structure, the elimination of an archaic system of reimbursement for health services, and the end of labeling those who seek health care as patients rather than consumers. Disruptive innovation, in contrast, involves the emergence of continuous innovation in order to improve the services for the new active consumer of health care services. There is a very large role to be played by public health departments in this educational initiative. There is evidence of successful dissemination of medical information to consumers in the fact that most consumers are questioning their doctor, asking for second opinions, and in some cases not accepting their physician's advice. Topol (2011) argues that the delivery of health care services in our country is very slowly bending to the desires of many to creatively destroy the old ways of doing business in order to build a better health care system that will focus on efficiency and the production of quality health services for our entire population.

It stands to reason that if we creatively destroy most of our current health care delivery system, we must replace it with alternative ways to deliver much needed health care services to an aging population. Disruptive innovation is the guiding force that replaces complicated and expensive products and services of health care with streamlined and cheaper procedures. Parts of the current health care system must be destroyed and then reconfigured in a way that offers positive outcomes at a price we can afford.

How Leaders Can Meet These Challenges

The bureaucratic system guiding health care delivery has allowed health care quality to diminish and costs to rise every year for the last several decades. These quality and cost issues have occurred despite a great deal of attention from health care managers to containing costs over the last few decades. These cost increases and the diminished quality of health care services are not sustainable for our businesses, people, and economy for the long term. In the past thirty years the federal government, one of the largest payers of health care bills, has focused a great deal of attention on reforming the system of health care delivery. The end of bureaucracy in health care organizations does not mean an end to management in health care services delivery. We will always need management in health care because we will always require efficiency. However, it has become increasingly clear that our system of health care delivery requires a complete reorganization of the way these services are delivered to the consumers of health care. The only way to meet and survive the many challenges is through the development of leadership skills in every person who works for the health care organization.

According to Rubino, Esparza, and Chassiakos (2014), managers spend the bulk of their time looking internally, with a major concentration on organizational processes. Leaders, in contrast, attempt to influence followers and spend their time monitoring external forces. This improves the leader's ability to predict changing environmental trends and to assist his or her followers in dealing with impending change. However, the leader can influence others only if these individuals allow themselves to be influenced. They are more likely to be willing to do this when they have respect for the leader and trust in him or her to do the right thing, for both the organization and the individuals who work for the organization.

In order for health care leaders to be successful in goal accomplishment, they will have to rely on their empowered staff to become creative in their approach to the delivery of health care services to customers in a transparent environment. This, in turn, will require the development of a positive culture in which employees can work in a collaborative manner to deliver appropriate and quality services to what will be very demanding customers. To be successful, health care organizations should be taking an outcome-oriented approach, supplemented with attention to the amenities that can and should be part of excellent health care.

The improvement of health care services is obviously a very difficult challenge that will require trial and error by both those in charge and those who follow. Harford (2011) argues that this trial-and-error process will most likely result in some failures, and this is why health care organizations must learn to adapt. His advice for successful adaptation is to experience three essential steps along the way: "to try new things, with the expectation that some will fail; to make failure survivable, because it will be common; and to make sure that you know when you've failed" (p. 36). The key here is to attempt to keep the failures to a minimum but also to learn from them. Failure can be a powerful tool in the process of leadership development. The development of leadership skills takes years, a great deal of experimentation, and a tolerance for some mistakes in the process.

This advice to help leaders and followers to successfully adapt to the changing health care environment sounds simple enough, but there are numerous barriers to successful implementation of the entire process. The greatest barrier will be overcome when the organization develops the ability to admit failure in the delivery of efficient and effective health services. Then leaders and followers can look at other potential solutions. In order to make this happen in health care, we need two things: leadership must emerge and followers must become aligned with the leadership.

Leaders and followers who are capable of becoming future leaders must face and eventually find solutions to very difficult challenges.

According to Andersen (2012) leaders require special characteristics if they are to gain followers who will support them in their current task or vision. These characteristics include being "farsighted, passionate, courageous, wise, generous and trustworthy" (p. 8). The most important characteristic the health care leader can exhibit is the ability to take a farsighted approach to confronting challenges. The leader needs to provide an honest vision of where he or she wants to take the health care organization in the long term. In order to get the followers on board in fulfilling this vision, the leader needs to be able to explain why it is the correct vision to follow at this point in time. In order to gain the trust of followers, a leader must be confident not only in the vision but in the method chosen to accomplish this vision.

Andersen (2012) points out that individuals are attracted to leaders who provide a farsighted approach to challenges and who see potential solutions for these challenges that will involve the followers.

Leaders Who Are Farsighted . . .

- See possible futures that are good for the enterprise
- Articulate their vision in a compelling and inclusive way
- Model their vision
- See past obstacles
- Invite others to participate in their vision [Andersen, 2012, p. 25].

These five important behaviors act like guideposts that point to a possible solution to the challenges faced by the health care industry. For example, individuals in positions of power need an articulated long-term vision and the ability to model this vision for their followers. These individuals need to be aware of obstacles in the way to achieving their vision and then work past the obstacles.

According to Kouzes and Posner (2010), the ability to imagine a future and then attract followers to share that future is one of the most important competencies of successful leaders. These leaders have the ability not only to see a future but also to convince others that this future is a real possibility. In fact Kouzes and Posner (2010) also discovered in their research that being forward looking is second only to being honest as the most admired aspect of leaders. It seems that followers desire leaders who have a strong vision of where they want to take their followers in the long run. These desired leaders are also honest with their followers about just how difficult it is to achieve the vision but are charismatic enough to gain followers' acceptance in their attempt to beat the odds.

There is no question that an important factor in the ability to lead an organization is the accuracy of the vision put forth by the leader. Reynolds (2013), in her book *Prescription for Lasting Success: Leadership Strategies to Diagnose Problems and Transform Your Organization*, argues that in order to build a dynamic organization the leader needs to apply the 4 P's model—Purpose, Passion, Planning, People—and also have the ability to Persevere. This model can be used to improve the way each health care facility diagnoses its problems and develops a plan to correct them. Reynolds, a physician, argues that health care facilities need to make a diagnosis of their major problems from the outside in and then deal with the real problems, not the symptoms of these problems.

Leaders are responsible for getting things done through their people; that is, through the professionals who actually deliver the care to the patient or consumer. Spiegelman and Berrett (2013) point out that if organizations do not treat their employees properly they shouldn't expect these employees to treat customers any better. In their book *Patients Come Second: Leading Change by Changing the Way You Lead,* these authors point out that if health care organizations treat their employees with respect these employees will, in turn, most likely do the same with patients, creating a culture of excellent service. This is the same philosophy that has been followed by a large number of businesses in the private for-profit sector of our economy. The former CEO for Southwest Airlines, Herb Kelleher, practiced this philosophy, resulting in a profit for his company in every year of his tenure.

SUMMARY

The health care sector of the American economy is undergoing tremendous change initiated by government reform and consumer demand for greater control over medical decisions. This changing health care environment is producing tremendous challenges, making it ripe for creativity and innovation in the way health services are delivered to over 300 million Americans.

The health care industry has been facing reform issues from the payers for health care services for the last few decades. There were several attempts back then at defining the problems and implementing solutions with the health care delivery system, with each attempt at reform actually making the problems worse. The Affordable Care Act of 2010 is the government's latest attempt at making our health care delivery system provide care to most Americans, but it does nothing about reforming the failing payment system. Although this latest attempt at health care reform may solve the access problem, it will not make the cost of care sustainable and will most likely accomplish little in terms of improving health outcomes. The starting point for a successful attempt at meeting the remaining challenges will be changing from a bureaucratically managed approach to a decentralized structure relying on leaders and empowering followers to implement innovative approaches.

There are numerous challenges facing our health care organizations over the next several years. A successful resolution will require creativity and innovation in turning these problems into real opportunities, producing motivation for those who seek problem solutions. This will require the emergence of effective leaders, the empowerment of followers, and the elimination of the special interest group power base that has created the challenges and has been successful up to this point in blocking solutions to those challenges. These leaders need well-developed communication skills along with the ability to gain the trust of followers. This ability to build trust is central to shaping an organization that seeks to welcome change and successfully exploit opportunities. This can only be achieved in a culture where mistakes are allowed to be made. These leaders will also need to be able to present members of the health care organization with a vision that the members believe they can attain, so they will work together to achieve goals that are important to all members of the organization and the community it serves.

KEY TERMS

asymmetry of information	disruptive innovation
bureaucratic structure	technological enabler
creative destruction	value-adding business process

DISCUSSION QUESTIONS

1. How will the reforming health care industry deal with disruptive innovation over the next few years? Be specific.

2. What are several of the important leadership challenges that will be faced by the U.S. health care delivery system over the next few years? Explain them in some detail.

3. How will the new health care legislation affect many health care organizations in our country?

4. How can the 4 P's approach be used to improve the efficiency and effectiveness of health care facilities?

REFERENCES

Andersen, E. (2012). *Leading so people will follow*. San Francisco, CA: Jossey-Bass.

Brawley, O. (2011). *How we do harm: A doctor breaks ranks about being sick in America*. New York, NY: St. Martin's Press.

Brill, S. (2013, April 4). Bitter pill: Why medical bills are killing us. *Time*. Retrieved from http://time.com/198/bitter-pill-why-medical-bills-are-killing-us

Burchell, M., & Robin, J. (2011). *The great workplace: How to build it, how to keep it, and why it matters*. San Francisco, CA: Jossey-Bass.

Carroll, L. E., Chapman, S. A., Dodd, C., Hollister, B., & Harrington, C. (2013). *Health policy: Crisis and reform* (6th ed.). Burlington, MA: Jones & Bartlett Learning.

Champy, J., & Greenspun, H. (2010). *Reengineering healthcare: A manifesto for radically rethinking healthcare delivery*. Upper Saddle River, NJ: Pearson Education.

Christensen, C. M., Grossman, J. H., & Hwang, J. (2009). *Innovator's prescription: A disruptive solution for health care*. New York, NY: McGraw-Hill.

Goldhill, D. (2013). *Catastrophic care: How American health care killed my father—and how we can fix it*. New York, NY: Knopf.

Halvorson, G. C. (2009). *Health care will not reform itself*. New York, NY: CRC Press.

Hamel, G. (2012). *What matters now: How to win in a world of relentless change, ferocious competition, and unstoppable innovation*. San Francisco, CA: Jossey-Bass.

Harford, T. (2011). *Adapt: Why success always starts with failure*. New York, NY: Farrar, Straus and Giroux.

Horsager, D. (2009). *The trust edge: How top leaders gain faster results, deeper relationships, and a stronger bottom line*. New York, NY: Free Press.

Jennings, J. (2012). *The reinventors: How extraordinary companies pursue radical continuous change*. New York, NY: Penguin Group.

Kouzes, J. M., & Posner, B. Z. (2010). *The truth about leadership*. San Francisco, CA: Jossey-Bass.

Naim, M. (2013). *The end of power: From boardrooms to battlefields and churches to states, why being in charge isn't what it used to be*. New York, NY: Basic Books.

Nussbaum, B. (2013). *Creative intelligence: Harnessing the power to create, connect, and inspire.* New York, NY: HarperCollins.

Perednia, D. A. (2011). *Overhauling America's healthcare machine: Stop the bleeding and save trillions.* Upper Saddle River, NJ: FT Press.

Reynolds, S. F. (2013). *Prescription for lasting success: Leadership strategies to diagnose problems and transform your organization.* San Francisco, CA: Jossey-Bass.

Rubino, L., Esparza, S., & Chassiakos, Y. R. (2014). *New leadership for today's health care professionals: Concepts and cases.* Burlington, MA: Jones & Bartlett Learning.

Schimpff, S. C. (2012). *The future of health-care delivery: Why it must change and how it will affect you.* Washington, DC: Potomac Books.

Serota, S. P. (2013). Insurer-provider integration: Insurers and providers integrating toward a common cause. In *Futurescan 2013: Healthcare Trends and Implications 2013-2018.* Chicago, IL: Health Administration Press.

Spiegelman, P., & Berrett, B. (2013). *Patients come second: Leading change by changing the way you lead.* Austin, TX: Greenleaf Book Group.

Topol, E. (2011). *The creative destruction of medicine: How the digital revolution will create better health care.* New York, NY: Basic Books.

Weinzimmer, L. G., & McConoughey, J. (2013). *The wisdom of failure: How to learn the tough leadership lessons without paying the price.* San Francisco, CA: Jossey-Bass.

Whitacre, E., & Cauley, L. (2013). *American turnaround: Reinventing AT&T and GM and the way to do business.* New York, NY: Business Plus.

Wilkins, D., & Carolin, G. (2013). *Leadership pure and simple: How transformative leaders create winning organizations.* New York, NY: McGraw-Hill.

CHAPTER 14

INTEGRATING CLINICAL SERVICES AND COMMUNITY PREVENTION

The Community-Centered Health Home Model

Larry Cohen
Leslie Mikkelsen
Jeremy Cantor
Rea Pañares
Janani Srikantharajah
Erica Valdovinos

The United States has a singular opportunity to reenvision its national approach to health. The health and well-being of individuals depends on both quality, coordinated health care services and community conditions that support health and safety. A successful, equitable health system will fuse these two areas, merging efficient, accessible, and culturally appropriate care with comprehensive efforts to prevent illness and injury in the first place by improving community environments. This coordinated thrust will produce the most effective, sustainable, and affordable health solutions. As Senator Tom Harkin has stated, "America's healthcare system is in crisis precisely because we systematically neglect wellness and prevention."

The Patient Protection and Affordable Care Act (ACA) is seeding extensive innovation along each of these lines. In addition to expanding insurance coverage, the ACA elevates the notion of a *health home* (or *medical home*), making it a key element of health care. The legislation leaves room for further delineating this concept, which is typically characterized as a site for coordinating and integrating medical and community services for individual patient care. The ACA also makes a historic investment in prevention, reflecting the growing understanding that community factors have a fundamental influence on health and safety.

LEARNING OBJECTIVES

After reading this chapter you should be able to

- Describe the economic and health and safety arguments that support an increased focus on community prevention.

- Understand the rationale and opportunity for linking clinical care with efforts to address community conditions.

- Identify the core elements of a community-centered health home.

- Discuss examples of clinical institutions that have demonstrated the impact on patient health of establishing partnerships to improve community conditions.

Now is the time to create a unified vision. Integrating the concept of health homes with a community prevention perspective produces multiple benefits: it is cost effective; it reduces demand for resources and services; and it improves health, safety, and equity outcomes on both community-wide and individual levels. Community prevention means investing in policies and infrastructure that create and support safe, healthy community environments to prevent illness, injuries, and violence from occurring *in the first place*. Therefore this approach alleviates the frustration of clinicians who feel powerless to change the social circumstances that shape the health of their patients. It provides a route through which medical professionals can apply their assets, expertise, and credibility to the challenge of creating environments that support health, equity, and safety.

The development of the **community-centered health home (CCHH)** framework, discussed in detail below, was initiated at the request of California's Community Clinics Initiative, which has a focus on community health centers (CHCs) (Cantor et al., 2011). This chapter lays out a coordinated set of CCHH practices that could be adopted by a range of health care institutions.

History of Clinical Services and Community Prevention Integration

The community-centered health home is intended to provide high-quality health care services, while also applying diagnostic and critical thinking skills to the underlying factors that shape patterns of injury and illness. By strategically engaging in efforts to improve community environments, CCHHs can improve the health and safety of their patient populations, improve health equity, and reduce the need for medical treatment. The CCHH model builds on a number of existing health care delivery models and practices (discussed in detail later and outlined in Figure 14.3), including the **patient-centered medical home** as defined by the Patient-Centered Primary Care Collaborative, and the **health home** (or *medical home*) as defined in the ACA. These models are not necessarily linear or sequential, as all are being advanced simultaneously and the concepts are evolving and expanding to include additional, complementary elements.

The community-centered health home approach builds on pioneering work on **community-oriented primary care (COPC)**. COPC, developed over a generation ago, made strong links between clinical practice and community action; the community-centered health home adds the sophistication and accumulated wisdom of prevention practice into a consistent approach that focuses efforts on policy and environmental change. Community-oriented primary care emerged in conjunction with

---

community-centered health home (CCHH)
A health care organization that actively participates in improving community factors (factors outside the health care system) that affect patient health.

patient-centered medical home
A primary care model that is patient-centered, comprehensive, team-based, coordinated, accessible, and focused on quality and safety.

health home
A team of health care professionals who provide whole-person care.

community-oriented primary care (COPC)
A primary care practice providing accessible, comprehensive, coordinated, continuous-over-time, and accountable health care services to a geographic or social community.

the development of community health centers. One example of this is the work of physician Jack Geiger in the 1960s.

In 1965, Jack Geiger opened one of the first community health centers in the United States, in Mound Bayou, Mississippi. The invention of the double-row cotton-picking machine had recently exacerbated poverty by replacing an entire population of sharecroppers. To assess the needs of the community, the Mississippi health center began by holding a series of meetings in homes, churches, and schools. As a result of these meetings, residents created ten community health associations, each with its own perspective and priorities. Some communities needed clean drinking water; others needed child care or elder care. The health center was seeing an enormous amount of malnutrition, stunted growth, and infection among infants and young children. Geiger and his colleagues linked hunger to acute poverty and linked poverty to the massive unemployment that had turned an entire population into squatters.

Geiger and his colleagues began writing prescriptions for food. Health center workers recruited local black-owned grocery stores to fill the prescriptions and reimbursed the stores out of the pharmacy budget. "Once we had the health center going, we started stocking food in the center pharmacy and distributing food—like drugs—to the people. A variety of officials got very nervous and said, 'You can't do that.' We said, 'Why not?' They said, 'It's a health center pharmacy, and it's supposed to carry drugs for the treatment of disease.' And we said, 'The last time we looked in the book, the specific therapy for malnutrition was food.'"

The health center then began urging people to start vegetable gardens and used a grant from a foundation to lease 600 acres of land to start the North Bolivar County Cooperative Farm. By pooling their labor to grow vegetables instead of cotton, members of a thousand families owned a share in the crops. In the first two years, tons of vegetables were grown. Health center workers also repaired housing, dug protected wells and sanitary privies, and later even started a bookstore focused on black history and culture. Reflecting on these efforts, Geiger stated, "You can do more than bail out these medical disasters after they have occurred, and go upstream from medical care to forge instruments of social change that will prevent such disasters from occurring in the first place. One of those disasters is the combination of racism and poverty" (Cohen, Chehimi, & Chavez, 2010, pp. 93–94).

Every step from traditional, segmented medical care toward a community-centered health home is an important improvement. As pioneering medical practitioners see it, the current emphasis on establishing medical homes is a tremendous step forward from the way the United States conducted health care for many decades, in which the focus was on treating sickness and injuries rather than promoting wellness and safety. The concept of the medical home is a seemingly simple one: all people should enter the medical system through a portal that manages their health holistically (comprehensive primary care, physical health, mental health, health education, etc.), treats them as individuals (with knowledge of their history, risk factors, concerns, and specific perspectives), and provides the highest-quality care efficiently (including both treatment and clinical prevention). In practice this requires a team approach, with smooth connections and communication between providers, staff who are comfortable coordinating care and collaborating with clients as partners, an electronic health records system that captures all relevant information and shares it with providers and patients, and a payment system that incentivizes efficient, collaborative work. Though the word *home* suggests a tangible place, in actuality the medical home is a set of practices that health care institutions can adopt to increase coordination between providers and provide comprehensive primary care (American Academy of Family Physicians, American Academy of Pediatrics, American College of Physicians, & American Osteopathic Association, 2007; Patient-Centered Primary Care Collaborative, 2013).

The ACA uses the term *health home* to describe a similar approach and set of core elements:

- Comprehensive care management
- Care coordination and health promotion
- Comprehensive transitional care from inpatient to other settings, including appropriate follow-up
- Support for patients, their families, and their authorized representatives
- Referral to community and social support services when needed
- Use of health information technology to link services, as feasible and appropriate

The ACA also provides funding that can support health home development, including $25 million in planning grants for states to develop health homes for Medicare and Medicaid enrollees with chronic conditions, a fund of $11 billion for community health center expansion, and $10 billion for the Center for Medicare & Medicaid Innovation to support health care delivery and payment reform.

The community-centered health home concept takes previous models a transformative step further by not only acknowledging that factors outside the health care system affect patient health outcomes but also actively participating in improving those factors. In addition to providing quality health care services, often to the most neglected and highest-need patients, community health centers are actively engaged in managing patients' disease through effective clinical prevention practices. Many are also equipped to refer patients, on an individual basis, to services in the community such as public health insurance options, legal services, and food stamps. These activities are critically important and reflect a commitment to a health care system that promotes health and well-being. The defining attribute of the CCHH is active involvement in community advocacy and change. In recent years more and more health care providers and institutions (particularly community health centers) have moved closer to this model, though still they remain a distinct, innovative minority. As institutions become focused on improving health at both the individual and population-wide level, they will work toward solutions that solve multiple problems simultaneously (e.g., improving neighborhood walkability would improve outcomes for diabetes, hypertension, and heart disease). Next, a hypothetical community-centered health home response to a spike in cases of lead poisoning serves as an example of the ways that a CCHH might engage in community change.

A young patient tests positive for elevated blood lead levels. Her pediatrician initiates appropriate clinical management protocols for treatment, including chelation—a necessary but risky and uncomfortable procedure to reduce the lead levels in her blood. As the diagnosis is entered into the community-centered health home's electronic records, it is instantly tracked alongside other lead-poisoning diagnoses in the community. In conducting the monthly data analysis, CCHH staff identify an increased number of cases among children in a certain neighborhood. The following week, at a monthly coordinating meeting held with a team including community health stakeholders, CCHH staff raise the issue with an affordable housing organization, the local health department, and a faith-based group. One of the community organizers recalls seeing children playing around a recently abandoned building. The team members work together to carry out a systematic response: the local health department tests the soil and structures at the site to establish the presence of lead; the housing organization works with the property owner to ensure that sources of lead are removed, as required by law; and CCHH staff and a community organizing group communicate with patients and families in the neighborhood about the risk. If lead poisoning continues to be a problem, clinic staff might engage in advocacy efforts to support stricter regulations and enforcement around lead exposures in housing. Even as the CCHH provides clinical treatment, its role in eliminating onsite lead reduces the risk of the young girl absorbing more lead and reduces the number of children who enter the clinic with lead poisoning in the first place.

Importance of Community Prevention

Community prevention is integral to effective health reform. It reduces the burden on the health system by reducing rates of preventable injury and illness and better aligning resources to address the factors that shape health and safety outcomes (Cohen et al., 2010, p. 4). Prevention can substantially diminish health inequities by focusing attention on unhealthy policies and inequitable resource distribution and improving community environments. Researchers have consistently concluded that the factors that have the greatest impact on health—the environments in which we live, work, and play and our behaviors (in part affected by those environments)—are outside the factors addressed by health care practices (Adler & Newman, 2002; Blum, 1980; Lee & Paxman, 1997). According to the best available estimates, environmental conditions, social circumstances, and behavioral choices that could be addressed through prevention have by far the greatest influence on determining health (Figure 14.1) (Institute for Alternative Futures, 2012). As primary health contacts and authorities, medical professionals and institutions have significant opportunities to play a far greater role in advancing the health of the populations they serve through community prevention efforts that address behaviors and environments.

Clinicians are typically trained and incentivized to engage only once a patient presents with symptoms. In general the linkage between clinical service and the community is thought of in terms of how health services can be provided in the community (e.g., vaccinations in schools) and how to engage needed community services to advance patient treatment (e.g., transit to get someone to the health center.) In a commentary in the *San Francisco Chronicle*, physician Laura Gottlieb described her experiences with patients and community factors: "I diagnosed 'abdominal pain' when the real problem was hunger; I confused social issues with medical problems in other patients too. I mislabeled the hopelessness of long-term unemployment as depression and the poverty that causes

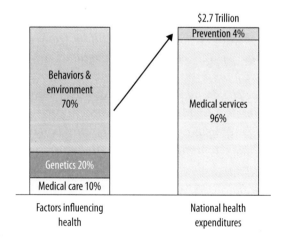

Figure 14.1 Discrepancy Between Health Determinants and Health Spending, 2012
Source: Bipartisan Policy Center, 2012.

patients to miss pills or appointments as noncompliance. In one older patient, I mistook the inability to read for dementia. My medical training had not prepared me for this ambush of social circumstance. Real-life obstacles had an enormous impact on my patients' lives, but because I had neither the skills nor the resources for treating them, I ignored the social context of disease altogether" (Gottlieb, 2010).

Additionally, our health system separates people into discrete categories, according to whether they are healthy, at-risk, or already ill or injured. Compartmentalizing is useful at times, but it can prevent us from seeing that health status is dynamic, constantly responding to the interplay with treatment and the environment. A better approach categorizes people when that's helpful for triage or delivering medical services but also considers the entire population in order to focus on environmental improvements that benefit all. As professor of clinical psychology George Albee put it, "no mass disorder afflicting mankind is ever brought under control or eliminated by attempts at treating the individual" (Albee, 1983, p. 24). For example, understanding the community conditions that produce and exacerbate type 2 diabetes helps inform an effective treatment plan. Actualizing the treatment plan will depend not only on individual medication and behavioral recommendations but also on making neighborhood improvements that facilitate access to healthy foods and safe places for physical activity. These environmental changes are important for preventing diabetes, for delaying and reducing its onset and extent, and for minimizing its impact for those who are already severely affected.

Prevention has a proven track record of saving lives. Since 1900, the average lifespan of people in the United States has increased by more than thirty years; twenty-five years of this gain are attributable to advances in public health, including the antitobacco policy, improved nutrition and sanitation, and safer workplaces (Bunker, Frazier, & Mosteller, 1994). Community prevention creates comprehensive changes that make health and safety the norm. Familiar examples include eliminating lead-based products; raising the minimum drinking age; and requiring the use of seatbelts, child car seats, and protective helmets.

Prevention also saves money. California's tobacco control program saved $86 billion in personal health care costs in its first fifteen years, while the state spent only $1.8 billion on the program, a fifty to one return on investment (Lightwood, Dinno, & Glantz, 2008). Every dollar invested in increasing the use of child safety seats has been demonstrated to return over $40 in reduced health care and social costs (Children's Safety Network, 2005). Recent analysis shows that in the United States investing $10 per person per year in proven community initiatives to increase physical activity, improve nutrition, and prevent tobacco use could produce a fivefold return in five years (Prevention Institute, Trust for America's Health, Urban Institute, & New York Academy of Medicine, 2008). Starting in the fifth year, a $3 billion investment would result in a $16 billion net savings in annual health care costs. Investments in communities at highest risk of disease would likely result in even greater savings and would help reduce health inequities. Prevention also lowers indirect costs such as those from workers' compensation claims and lost productivity (Goetzel & Ozminkowski, 2008; Goetzel et al., 2007; Hemp, 2004). In addition, it reduces the demand for medical treatment, enabling the system to operate more efficiently.

People intuitively understand the value of prevention. Our health systems and institutions typically focus prevention efforts primarily on education and screenings. While these services are important, they have limited capacity to effect broad-based change on their own. Transforming health at the population level comes from shifting social norms and creating policies that anchor other efforts. Prevention Institute, a national nonprofit focused on preventing illness and injury and on fostering equity, has developed **taking two steps to prevention**, a systematic methodology for applying prevention that traces a pathway from the medical condition to the behaviors and exposures that led to it and then to the environmental conditions that are at the root of the behaviors and exposures (Figure 14.2). For example, a man has chest pains, and his doctor diagnoses severe heart disease. Treatment may be expensive and may come too late to prevent impaired quality of life. While developing an appropriate treatment plan, a CCHH clinician will also reflect on how the man developed heart disease in the first place. Perhaps he ate poorly and didn't exercise. Earlier intervention might have led to healthier choices. But is it just about choice? Maybe he works long hours in a stressful, sedentary job where it is easiest to eat unhealthy, prepared foods at his desk. Perhaps his neighborhood environment isn't any better, lacking healthy food options and safe places to be active. The CCHH provider recognizes that significant, long-term health benefits could result from community-level interventions, so she helps to launch coordinated efforts that support people's need for healthy food and physical activity.

taking two steps to prevention
A systematic methodology for applying prevention that traces a pathway from the medical condition to the behaviors and exposures that led to it and then to the environmental conditions that are at the root of the behaviors and exposures.

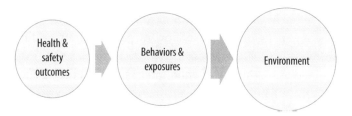

Figure 14.2 Taking Two Steps to Prevention
Source: Cohen et al., 2010, 43–45.

These changes benefit her patient as well as patients with other health concerns with related risk factors, such as diabetes and depression. They also help to protect the broader population from developing illness. They reduce or delay demand for costly medical services. The two steps to prevention framework offers a method to analyze what happens prior to the onset of illness and injury. This approach identifies the underlying factors that shape health and affect health equity to ensure that we are not only treating medical conditions but also reducing the likelihood they will occur in the first place. The first step to prevention is from disease or injury (e.g., type 2 diabetes, asthma) to exposures and behaviors that increase the risk for poor health (e.g., inadequate diet, limited physical activity, exposure to polluted air). The second step is to the environment (i.e., root factors and community conditions, such as lack of food outlets or the presence of polluting smokestacks) that shapes behaviors and leads to unhealthy exposures. Prevention Institute collaborated with a national expert panel to develop THRIVE (Toolkit for Health and Resilience in Vulnerable Environments), an evidence-based framework connecting health outcomes to community conditions, also known as community health factors. THRIVE's thirteen factors (displayed later in Exhibit 14.1) can guide thinking in the clinical context and with partners about the second step to prevention: getting specific about what elements in the community environment are shaping health, safety, and equity.

CHCs at the Center of Community Health

Community health centers are a particularly important venue for the initial implementation of the community-centered health home for a number of reasons. First, CHCs are philosophically committed to improving the health of communities and as a result are likely to be more inclined to try out innovative approaches that align with that commitment. Second, CHCs are especially dedicated to providing care to the most vulnerable populations (Health Resources and Services Administration, n.d.). Third, CHCs are closely connected to communities and thus are able to tailor their care to the context and demographics of the neighborhoods in which they are located. Many are already performing the services of a traditional health home or have gone a step further by linking individuals with non-health care services, such as SNAP, legal aid, or housing (Institute for Alternative Futures, 2012). Fourth and last, in the past decade CHCs, including community clinics, have seen their patient loads double (Gusmano, Fairbrother, & Park, 2002). Now, with the expanded coverage mandated by the ACA, much of the burden for providing services to 40 million individuals will fall to them (National Association of Community Health Centers, 2011). At the same time, CHCs are poised for expansion and innovation with $11 billion in ACA support for new construction, staff expansion and training, and updates to facilities and systems. By focusing on a CCHH approach, health centers can reduce the need for their services and make service delivery more manageable as well as improve patient outcomes. The role that CHCs play as a hub for community health and the current investment in innovation through the ACA means that CHCs are uniquely positioned to successfully implement the community-centered health home.

Elements of the Community-Centered Health Home

The skills needed to engage in community change efforts are closely aligned with the problem-solving skills providers currently employ to address individual health needs. It is a matter of applying these skills to communities. Specifically, with patients, practitioners follow a three-part process: collecting data (symptoms, vital signs, tests, etc.), diagnosing the problem, and undertaking a treatment plan. A CCHH functions in a parallel manner by developing capacity and expertise to follow a three-part process for addressing the health of the community; these parts are classified as *inquiry*, *analysis*, and *action*.

For example, CCHH staff might treat several seniors injured in falls, ask how they fell, and realize they live in the same housing development (inquiry). In discussion with community partners, CCHH staff discover most of the falls took place in a nearby park and that the pavement has been damaged by storms (analysis). In addition to treating the injuries, staff could contact the parks department or public works, join the neighborhood association in sponsoring an event highlighting the situation, write a letter to a local paper, and/or collect data from other patients on injuries sustained in the park in order to have a more robust analysis of the health impacts of conditions there (action). Inquiry, analysis, and action take time, just as individual treatment takes time, but the extra effort will be compensated by improvements in diagnosis and treatment success and the time saved from reducing patient load in the long run.

In order to simplify the next discussion, partnerships are described as progressively expanding from within the institution for inquiry to community representatives for analysis to the patient population and other institutions for action. In practice, depending on the context, those demarcations will likely be less discrete (patient representatives may participate in analysis, community partners may provide information for inquiry, etc.).

This three-part process is already being practiced by some community clinics. One example is St. John's Well Child and Family Center in Los Angeles.

Inquiry. When clinicians at St. John's noted a significant number of patients with conditions ranging from cockroaches in their ears to chronic lead poisoning, skin diseases, and insect and rodent bites, they inferred that many of the cases might be related to substandard housing conditions. The clinic incorporated into office visits a set of questions about patients' housing conditions and was able to collect not only standard health condition data (e.g., allergies, bites, severe rashes, gastrointestinal symptoms) but also housing condition information (e.g., presence of cockroaches, rats, or mice).

Analysis. St. John's clinic partnered with a local housing agency, a human rights organizing agency, and a tenant rights organization to form a collaborative to investigate substandard and slum housing in Los Angeles. The data that St. John's collected made the clinic an asset in the collaborative and helped the collaborative to gain partners.

Action. The collaborative developed and pursued a strategic plan to improve housing conditions in the area. The plan included community engagement, research, medical care and case management, home assessments, health education, litigation, and advocacy. The collaborative was able to get local administrative policies put in place and secured agreements from high-level leadership at local government agencies (LA City Attorney's Office and LA Department of Public Health) that led to improved landlord compliance with standard housing requirements.

The clinic now serves a surveillance role, reporting landlords who perpetuate substandard housing, and the community now has the infrastructure in place to ensure that landlords not in compliance are dealt the proper financial and legal consequences. Evaluation results show that residents' living conditions and health outcomes both improved as a result of collaborative efforts. For example, four out of every five residents who experienced anxiety related specifically to substandard housing conditions reported improved health outcomes. Additionally, of the 3,150 families living in the pilot project properties, over 90 percent experienced substantial improvements in their living conditions (Lowe & Haas, 2007).

Inquiry Elements

Given their constant contact with patients in the surrounding community, health centers and similar institutions are uniquely positioned to maintain a "finger on the pulse" of that community's health. In order to do this, they need to collect data that reflect community conditions, analyze existing data for community health implications, and capture clinician impressions and intuitions about underlying issues shaping prevalence of injuries and illnesses. The CCHH model in Figure 14.3 displays the elements that make up inquiry, analysis, and action and that are discussed next.

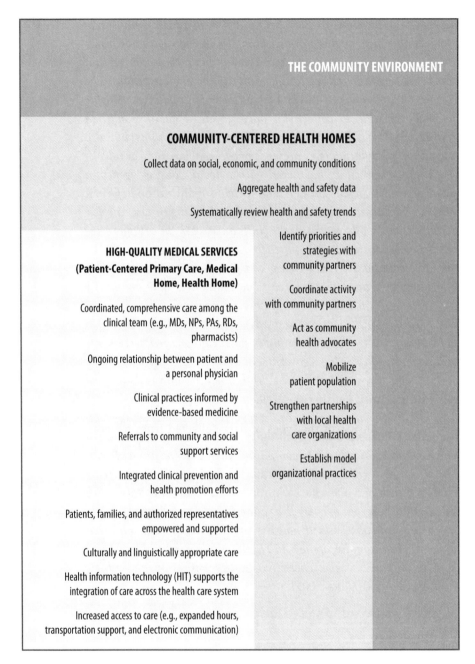

Figure 14.3   The CCHH Model: An Evolving Approach to Health

Source: Cantor et al., 2011, p. 8.

1. Collect Data on Social, Economic, and Community Conditions

Health centers already collect data on a host of patient demographics. CCHHs should use data collection to bring community conditions into the conversation about patient care within the institution. First, a set of questions on community, social, and economic conditions should be incorporated into the clinic's intake process (e.g., questions such as, How long does it take you to travel to a full service grocery store?, or, Do you feel safe walking or playing in your neighborhood?), and the resulting data incorporated into health records. A number of important issues need to be considered as this is implemented, including ensuring individual privacy; moving toward a consistent regional, state, and national approach so that information from multiple sites is comparable and analyzable in aggregate (see the section on metrics below); and striking a balance between using consistent questions and having the flexibility to modify the questions based on community health priorities. The latter issue may point toward a discrete menu of questions that is established at the national level and can be selected from to meet local considerations.

Second, prompts should be developed for use during clinical visits. These prompts should be contingent on diagnosis and be designed to take a very limited amount of time. For example, a clinician might see an adolescent with a trauma (e.g., a broken arm). Entering that diagnosis leads to prompts such as whether the injury was intentional or unintentional, whether unsafe neighborhood conditions were involved, and whether the patient is experiencing any symptoms of comorbidities (e.g., depression or anxiety).

Through this expansion of the types of data collected from patients, CCHH staff and their community partners will be positioned, in the analysis phase, to monitor trends and emerging issues in the patient population over time and geography and to create opportunities to explore the effectiveness of integrated community-oriented solutions and clinical interventions. With momentum building for the adoption of electronic health records and new resources available, health centers can use this opportunity to strengthen existing systems to fully capture each patient's, and eventually the community's, health profile.

2. Aggregate Health and Safety Data

In addition to implementing new types of data collection, health care organizations already collect a significant amount of information on diagnoses, test results, health history, and demographics. That information is potentially extremely important to analyze closely for trends and patterns of illness and injury that reflect health and safety outcomes across the community. In order to do that during the analysis part of this process, steps should be taken to aggregate and share patient health data at regular intervals. This could be done in the form of a monthly report that lists the most prevalent diagnoses from patient visits and flags any significant changes (either in the prevalence of a given condition or in the relative prevalence compared with other diagnoses).

Analysis Elements

Once health and safety information is collected, health centers can play a key role in helping to explore trends in patient health and safety and to link those trends with factors in the community in order to identify underlying problems and possible solutions. Essentially, the CCHH staff will analyze the data that the institution collects and then connect with community partners and collectively with those partners take the two steps to prevention described above (from health and safety outcomes to exposures and behaviors to the community environment). For example, if evidence from the CCHH and/or community partners shows increasing childhood obesity rates, the corresponding analysis might point to a dearth of accessible fresh foods or safe places to play. Existing research, resources, and tools, such as THRIVE (Exhibit 14.1), are available to support health centers in conducting an analysis. Universities and public health departments can also be ideal partners, both in supporting initial data analysis and also in monitoring and capturing successes. These partners can also help with aggregating data across regions and supporting longitudinal studies, comparative effectiveness research, and use of geographic mapping.

EXHIBIT 14.1. THRIVE COMMUNITY HEALTH FACTORS

Place

1. **What's Sold & How It's Promoted** is characterized by the availability and promotion of safe, healthy, affordable, culturally appropriate products and services (e.g., food, books and school supplies, sports equipment, arts and crafts supplies, and other recreational items) and the limited promotion and availability, or lack, of potentially harmful products and services (e.g., tobacco, firearms, alcohol, and other drugs).

2. **Look & Feel** is characterized by a well-maintained, appealing, clean, and culturally relevant visual and auditory environment.

3. **Parks & Open Space** is characterized by safe, clean, accessible parks; parks that appeal to interests and activities of all age groups; green space; outdoor space that is accessible to the community; natural/open space that is preserved through the planning process.

4. **Getting Around** is characterized by availability of safe, reliable, accessible, and affordable methods for moving people around. This includes public transit, walking, and biking.

5. **Housing** is characterized by the availability of safe and affordable housing to enable citizens from a wide range of economic levels and age groups to live within its boundaries.

6. **Air, Water, & Soil** is characterized by safe and non-toxic water, soil, indoor and outdoor air, and building materials. Community design should help conserve resources, minimize waste, and promote a healthy environment.

7. **Arts & Culture** is characterized by a variety of opportunities within the community for cultural and creative expression and participation through the arts.

Equitable Opportunity

8. **Racial Justice** is policies and organizational practices in the community that foster equitable opportunities and services for all. It is evident in positive relations between people of different races and ethnic backgrounds.

9. **Jobs & Local Ownership** is characterized by local ownership of assets, including homes and businesses, access to investment opportunities, job availability, and the ability to make a living wage.

10. **Education** is characterized by high-quality and available education and literacy development for all ages.

People

11. **Social Networks & Trust** is characterized by strong social ties among all people in the community—regardless of their role. These relationships are ideally built upon mutual obligations, opportunities to exchange information, and the ability to enforce standards and administer sanctions.

12. **Participation and Willingness to Act for the Common Good** is characterized by local leadership, involvement in community or social organizations, participation in the political process, and a willingness to intervene on behalf of the common good of the community.

13. **Norms/*Costumbres*** are characterized by community standards of behavior that suggest and define what the community sees as acceptable and unacceptable behavior.

Source: Cohen, Iton, Davis, & Rodriguez, 2009.

It is also critically important to be cognizant of existing community information and leadership, and to complement—rather than compete with—community prevention efforts. Analysis should not happen in a vacuum but rather as part of broader community efforts. The role of the CCHH will of course vary based on the visibility and capacity of community partners. In communities where advocacy networks, policy champions, and community prevention capacity are strong, the community health center may play a supportive, partnership, and facilitator role. In areas where leadership or community coalitions are lacking, the institution might need to play a more active role in community change. For example, the community health center might initiate and facilitate a local coalition if none exists or organize its patients to address specific health threats in the community.

3. Systematically Review Health and Safety Trends

The quantitative data gathered through the intake process and clinician prompts can provide vital insights into the major community health concerns. The quantitative data should be supplemented by qualitative information drawn from health care staff intuition and insight. To accomplish this, a venue should be established for review and discussion of the information gathered through the inquiry elements described above to be shared with community partners. This could happen as part of an existing problem-solving staff meeting or during grand rounds, or as a separate discussion. The goal of this review would be to identify underlying, community-level factors that might be shaping health and safety outcomes (Figure 14.4). These factors might come directly from the data collected (e.g., a large number of patients report that they don't feel safe walking in their neighborhood) or from clinician insight (e.g., "one of my patients told me they feel stressed going to school because of bullying. I wonder if that is a widespread factor in the mental health issues we're seeing."). Atul Gawande, a physician and journalist for *The New Yorker*, observed an effective process for systematic review of health and safety trends at the Special Care Center, a primary care clinic in Atlantic City, New Jersey. A CCHH builds on this process focused on individual patients' needs to consider actions to improve the whole community.

> I got a glimpse of how unusual the clinic is when I sat in on the staff meeting it holds each morning to review the medical issues of the patients on the appointment books. There was, for starters, the very existence of the meeting. I had never seen this kind of daily huddle at a doctor's office, with clinicians popping open their laptops and pulling up their patient lists together. Then there was the particular mixture of people who squeezed around the conference table. As in many primary-care offices, the staff had two physicians and two nurse practitioners. But a full-time social worker and the front-desk receptionist joined in for the patient review, too. And, outnumbering them all, were eight full-time "health coaches" [Gawande, 2011].

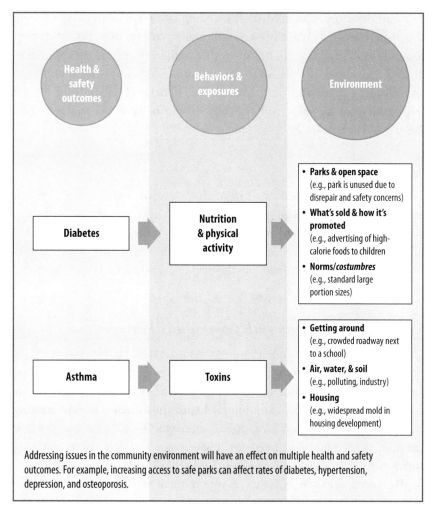

Figure 14.4   Two Steps in Practice: Identifying Community-Level Factors That Affect Health
Source: Cantor et al., 2011, p. 11.

4. Identify Priorities and Strategies with Community Partners

Working with partners outside the medical sector, through meaningful, ongoing relationships that go beyond resource referrals, will be central to the CCHH's ability to participate in community-level change. The CCHH will bring a tremendous amount of valuable community health data (described above). Other partners will bring important information about community perspectives, conditions, and priorities. This effort will likely require meeting at regular intervals, and engaging in communication and work in smaller groups between meetings. It is critical that there be a venue for sharing and discussion in order to identify potential actions to improve community health and safety. For example, after reviewing health data and priorities, and applying the taking two steps analysis, the CCHH and its partners may identify a need for a safe place for physical activity in a community. Then they can work together to figure out strategies to address the issue, given the realities of their community (e.g., joint-use agreements, rehabilitating an existing park, forming neighborhood walking clubs). Such community partnerships will typically extend beyond the analysis phase and play a key role in the action phase as well.

Action Elements

Given that medical professionals have a high level of credibility, clinical staff and health institutions can play critical roles in advancing broader systems change. This can happen in a number of ways, including engaging in or supporting targeted advocacy efforts and developing model organizational practices. Actions should build on the evidence and partnerships developed in the analysis phase.

5. Coordinate Activity with Community Partners

Effective community change requires a coordinated, comprehensive strategy, which in turn requires the capacity and engagement of multiple partners: some partners may have expertise in communicating with the media, others may be able to mobilize a broad constituency, and yet another may have expertise in crafting policy language. Building on the previous example of an identified need for a safe place for physical activity, the partners might identify a school facility that has recreational space but is largely closed after school hours. A subset of partners (e.g., the CCHH, the parks and recreation department, a youth service nonprofit, and a faith-based wellness program) could come together to work out and implement a plan to establish a joint-use agreement with the school and to have a sustainable approach to maintenance, operations, programming, and costs (including liability). Partnerships with organizations other than health care groups are vital, given that many of the decisions that have the greatest impact on health are made in other sectors, such as transportation, housing, and agriculture. Such partnerships can be mutually beneficial, as identified health impacts can be very useful in arguing for or against a given policy or decision.

The Beaufort Jasper Hampton Comprehensive Health Services (BJHCHS) provides comprehensive medical and dental services in Ridgeland, South Carolina. Beginning in the 1970s, the clinic noted at least five to seven pediatric cases of soil-transmitted helminths (ascaris, hookworm, and whipworm) each week, and attributed this pattern to poor water sanitation in and around the children's homes. Clinic staff knew that the best way to treat and prevent helminths, and other diseases caused by poor water sanitation, was to first improve home sanitation. So the clinic developed partnerships with local community organizations. Together, they sought grants to install septic systems and led the installation of septic systems and portable bathrooms in people's homes. Physicians ordered wheelchair ramps for those patients who needed them, and the environmental team for the project built the ramps. At its peak, the program installed 100 to 200 septic systems each year. Now, partnered with United Way, the clinic currently constructs twenty to twenty-five septic units each year. The clinic's role in the community has expanded beyond alleviating unsafe water conditions to include rodent and parasite reduction and addressing other environmental conditions. Today, the clinic does not see any cases of soil-transmitted helminths disease in its patients (Institute for Alternative Futures, 2012).

6. Act as Community Health Advocates

Clinicians can leverage their credibility on health issues and their direct experience with the health of community members to act as extremely effective advocates for health and equity through change in community environments. They can support community-identified advocacy goals by providing "expert" opinion in the form of testimony at hearings, interviews with the media, or talking directly with policymakers. There is a proud and effective history of such work—from physician-led campaigns resulting in car seat laws and thus reduced injuries to medical professionals' advocacy in support of tobacco control strategies and thus reduced lung cancer rates. As with the other steps in the analysis and action phases, this activity will be most effective when coordinated with partners and existing efforts. In particular, trusted allies can minimize the work and logistics involved in advocacy by creating opportunities for clinicians to engage.

Clinic staff at the East Boston Neighborhood Health Center, which serves the East Boston, Chelsea, Winthrop, and Revere communities of Massachusetts, became concerned with the number of children being identified as overweight in the clinic. Recognizing that many of their patients did not have a safe outdoor space to play, and that afterschool activities were inaccessible for many families, the clinic initiated its innovative Let's Get Movin' program. Through Let's Get Movin', the clinic provides community residents with a breadth of initiatives that support physical activity and healthy eating. In collaboration with Urban Youth Sports, a program of the nearby Northeastern University, the clinic offers afterschool programs at neighborhood schools and other community locations, with fun and structured physical activities and sports for children as well as nutrition education. The program was featured on the Discovery Health Channel, where physicians, nutritionists, and physical activity experts spoke about Let's Get Movin'. Gaining momentum through its work and the media, the clinic brought a farmers' market to East Boston, because it recognized that food access is key to healthy eating. The clinic also arranged for the purchase and distribution of farm shares in order to provide community members with fresh produce. Let's Get Movin' has supported other changes in the community; for example, it has worked with local stores in the neighborhood to get them to offer more healthy foods and has collaborated with local government through a Complete Streets grant to improve walking paths (East Boston Neighborhood Health Center, 2014).

7. Mobilize Patient Populations

Patients everywhere are directly affected by their community conditions. Thus the CCHH has a natural role in encouraging civic engagement and mobilizing its patient population in changing the local conditions. Engagement activities can range from providing voter registration at the health center to connecting patients to advocacy efforts that relate to their health concerns to identifying spokespeople who have authentic voices on community issues to bringing together and training groups of patients to take action on a priority issue. CCHHs should identify or hire staff who will be responsible for community engagement and incorporating community members' perspectives into institutional decision making and community prevention efforts. *Promotoras* (Hispanic or Latino community health workers) and other community health workers associated with the CCHH can play a strong role in mobilizing the patient population. Engaging patients—and their families—in community change is an important strategy: family-led campaigns, on such issues as changes in DUI laws, have made significant improvements to health and safety. Engaging patients in advocacy also leads to patient empowerment and indirect health improvements. As Makani Themba-Nixon, executive director of the Praxis Project, writes, "the act of organizing a community to engage in [a] policy initiative can increase social networks and reduce isolation and alienation, which can be as effective in reducing problems as the policy itself" (Cohen et al., 2010, p. 138).

8. Strengthen Partnerships with Local Health Care Organizations

Partnerships among the health care facilities in a community are a valuable step toward emphasizing community-wide health improvement goals. By working together, different health care facilities develop shared responsibility for the entire community beyond the individual patients that they serve. Community change efforts will inevitably affect the patient populations of multiple institutions. Many local and regional consortiums of community clinics already exist and can be used for this purpose. In other cases these consortiums may need to be convened. These relationships can support numerous activities of the CCHH: sharing data to gain a more complete picture of health issues and trends in the region, setting shared priorities, sharing promising practices and challenges, bringing key (non-health care) partners to the table, and advocating with one voice for mutual interests. Forming these consortiums can facilitate and incentivize the adoption of the same health information technology with the same questions, the same health goals, and the same capacity-building training across health care institutions. When many of the infrastructure components of the CCHH and other regional health centers are consistent across these organizations, there will be a stronger regional movement for community health.

9. Establish Model Organizational Practices

In many communities health institutions are the most visible authorities on health. Given that position, these institutions have a responsibility to ensure that their policies and practices promote health and safety. By enacting model policies, CCHHs can influence other community institutions and help set community norms. Examples of model policies include

- Policies that promote equity by eliminating institutional discrimination, ensuring the cultural competency of CCHH staff, and ensuring workforce diversity.

- Policies that ensure healthy foods and beverages are available and promoted in CCHH cafeterias, vending machines, coffee carts, and other concessions.

- Policies that encourage physical activity through CCHH building design (e.g., open, inviting stairways), meeting practices (e.g., walking meetings), and incentives for employees to travel to work by active means.

- Policies that favor serving locally and regionally grown healthy foods in the CCHH.

- Policies and practices in CCHH facilities that support the initiation and continuation of breast-feeding (e.g., baby-friendly hospitals).

Capacities Needed for Effective Implementation

Successful implementation of the nine inquiry, analysis, and action elements just described will depend in part on having certain capacities in place. In order to fully engage in the process of inquiry, analysis, and action, health centers and their partners should invest in strengthening certain internal capacities and resources. Some of these components may already be in place but would benefit from a more targeted focus on community prevention and community change.

1. Staff Training and Continuing Education

In order to achieve the goals of a CCHH, staff will need a firm understanding of the ways in which factors outside the clinical setting shape health, as well as information and tools that will enable them to play an active role in addressing those factors. One promising strategy for achieving these needs is a training process that might begin with a **community prevention readiness assessment**. This exercise would include an analysis of the CCHH's activity, current capacities, and staff needs. The focus of the training can then be based on the assessment findings. Training units might address such topics as understanding community prevention, community prevention strategy development for health centers, engaging in collaborative and intersectoral partnerships, and clinicians as community health advocates. Trainings should draw on existing research, promising practices, case studies, and existing resources.

community prevention readiness assessment
An assessment of a health care organization's capacities to engage in CCHH activities.

Clinics may want to explore existing requirements for ongoing professional development (such as continuing medical education) as an avenue for incorporating community prevention into continuing education. Incentivizing participation in trainings on community health and prevention—alongside existing courses on clinical prevention—elevates the importance of having a focus on the social determinants of health and developing skills in such areas as community engagement and advocacy.

2. A Dedicated and Diverse Team

Because community prevention is based on a multisector vision and approach to health, health centers will benefit from diverse staffing that takes into account the right mix of staff capacities and skills for each community. CCHH team members will include both clinical (e.g., physicians, nurses, and physician's assistants) and nonclinical (e.g., social workers and promotoras) staff, who communicate seamlessly and have a clear understanding of each other's roles and objectives. In addition to clinical duties, some staff will be responsible for tasks such as patient engagement, community prevention advocacy, participation in community partnerships and coalitions, and internal strategic planning to maintain an emphasis on community prevention in the clinic.

Moreover, staff will need to be equipped to understand the patient population and community (in terms of culture, language, history, and other demographics) and be able to respond to a wide variety of health and safety challenges. For example, an aging population has different needs than a population with a large percentage of children under five. Health conditions related to inadequate housing require a different set of clinical and community responses than health conditions related to unsafe streets. In some cases legal strategies will be necessary in order to achieve actions that improve health, in others an awareness of local policy or the latest clinical preventive service recommendations or transportation guidelines may be most useful.

Ideally, the CCHH will establish a dedicated, paid position to manage the implementation of the CCHH model and link the clinical and community components of the clinic's activities. The CCHH manager will be instrumental in transitioning to the CCHH model and maintaining the vision over time. Support from executive leaders, boards of directors, and advisory boards will also be critical in implementing necessary systems and operational changes.

3. Innovative Leadership

A fully functioning CCHH may require a shift from the institutional activities, culture, norms, and values that currently exist. As with any shift in thinking or operations, effective and innovative leadership is needed to implement and sustain these changes over time. These changes might create challenges for staff (new roles and skills will be required), clients (a new relationship with the staff), and stakeholders such as funders and partners. This change will be possible only if leadership is in place that is able to communicate direction clearly and engagingly, predict challenges, and create the sorts of systems and processes necessary to incrementally create change. This leadership will need to come from executive staff as well as members of the board of directors who have the skills and experience necessary to provide ongoing guidance and direction for the CCHH. These leaders will benefit from the shared learning that will occur when they are part of a network of CCHH executives (aligned with the networks discussed below).

Overarching Systems Change Recommendations

Community health centers are part of an integrated, complex health care system. Virtually every facet of their operation is influenced by external factors. Regulatory, funding, and training mechanisms can all be used to incentivize and support change within health institutions. In this section, five key areas for innovation at the systems level are discussed. In each case the issues raised are extremely complex, and the dialogue is far from comprehensive; the intent is to identify the venues for change and to lay out directions for additional exploration and strategy development.

Structure Health Care Payment Systems to Support Community Prevention Activity

Physicians, nurses, and other clinical providers are by definition concerned with the health of their clients, but current reimbursement systems limit the tools that providers have to protect and improve health (Chernew, Mechanic, Landon, & Safran, 2011; Lorber, 2011). Widespread adoption and promulgation of the CCHH model will require resources and incentives aligned with community health activity. Various options need to be explored. One option is to expand current reimbursements to support CCHH activities such as coordinating with public health departments and local leaders or to create incentives based on health and safety outcomes. In theory capitation payment systems could create a focus on keeping patients healthy (and thus lower costs), but such systems have been critiqued for their potential to incentivize systematic denial of care. Therefore other models under consideration would tie payments to achieving specific health and safety outcomes. If incentives were tied to health and safety outcomes, that would intrinsically elevate the role and importance of prevention and would motivate all health providers to think in terms of the most effective, and cost-effective, ways to maintain health.

There are a number of challenges. For example, insurers likely see only a fraction of the population as their responsibility and only for the relatively short period of time that the average individual stays with a health plan. As a result, *bundling* investment in community prevention from multiple sources will probably be necessary. Additionally, different communities start from different baselines in terms of the factors that shape health, so resources will need to be allocated based on need in order to ensure equitable outcomes.

Align Data and Measurement Across Sectors

In order to build the evidence base and to support the sort of funding changes discussed above, evaluation metrics are needed that assess clinics' success at both building capacity and engaging in community-level prevention. Creating a standard set of metrics to measure CCHHs will enable clear evaluation, the sharing of successful methods, and the ability to compare the effectiveness of clinical and nonclinical responses. It will also require defining concrete goals, thus helping to guide implementation. Additionally, metrics should be designed with sensitivity to the distinct conditions and challenges present in each community so that health equity is a fundamental consideration. The National Committee for Quality Assurance has undertaken a similar process to define the metrics for a patient-centered medical home by inviting the input of key stakeholders for the initial set of metrics (Lorber, 2011). A study released in 2011 by the Institute of Medicine (*For the Public's Health: The Role of Measurement in Action and Accountability*) makes the case for consistent measurement.

Standardizing metrics, along with the questions and information entered into the electronic health records, would ensure that health centers could compare data and that other institutions such as health departments and universities could use the data for research. A national convening of informed clinical and community prevention stakeholders would be instrumental in fine-tuning electronic health record practices and implementing these records to effectively collect expanded information.

Strengthen and Utilize Networks

As the approaches presented in this chapter are implemented, taking advantage of opportunities to share learning and collectively address challenges will be critical. Individual health centers will develop innovative approaches depending on their capacity and the specific needs of their respective communities, and sharing these approaches is central to the refinement and advancement of the CCHH concept. In addition to sharing promising approaches, collective discussion and problem solving around shared challenges and capacity-building training should be emphasized. Existing associations and forums that bring institutions and/or providers together can be used for this peer-networking and problem-solving purpose. In some cases, new learning networks may be necessary. Additionally, networks and associations can strategize and advocate for changes to local, state, and federal policy that would support the successful function of CCHHs. Examples of the sorts of issues that networks might weigh in on include changes to reimbursement systems, updates to the federally qualified health center guidelines, and the design of health information exchanges. Generating professional and political leverage will be critical to broad implementation of CCHHs.

Train Health Professionals to Work in CCHHs

Professional training programs for clinicians, such as medical school and nursing school programs, should be augmented to adequately prepare future health professionals to support community prevention efforts. Community prevention elements should be incorporated into the curriculum (e.g., the relationship between health outcomes and community conditions, and the role of the clinician as effective health advocate) and residency programs. A number of models exist both for classroom and hands-on learning (Cohen et al., 2010). What is needed is a commitment to develop and implement the most effective approaches.

The training curriculum should recognize that health centers across the country have differing needs and capacities and are located in diverse communities. Resource or technical assistance providers should be established to provide directed training and consultation responsive to the particular needs and issues of the community that the CCHH serves. Specialized training that targets and builds the capacity of health center leadership and boards of directors will likely be necessary. This sort of training could be delivered on a regional basis as a building block for a network of executives.

Professional societies and other national organizations with community prevention expertise have a role to play in preparing clinicians. In order to incentivize future health professionals to become more engaged in community prevention, programs such as the National Health Service Corps could be expanded to include a track for clinicians placed in positions with an explicit focus on addressing community conditions in underserved communities.

Identify Resources and Opportunities

Private foundations and community benefits programs have supported a number of clinics that have established the infrastructure and capacity to engage in community-level change. Philanthropy has the opportunity to support implementation of CCHHs and elevate learnings and promising practices as models. Funders can also encourage other grantees to engage substantively with the CCHH in their communities. Further, due to their unique understanding of community assets and needs, funders can play an important role in facilitating effective implementation.

The ACA includes funding streams that are aligned with CCHH principles and could be leveraged to spur implementation. The Center for Medicare and Medicaid Innovation reflects these concepts in its mission to improve quality of care, coordination of care, and community health and will be issuing proposals to support these outcomes. At the same time, Community Transformation Grant (CTG) funds will be awarded to communities to improve their environments to support healthy eating, active living, safety, and reduced tobacco use. By aligning health center funding with other community initiatives such as CTG, CCHH funding streams could be enhanced. In addition to linking efforts across the U.S. Department of Health and Human Services, there are important opportunities to link with other federal agencies (such as the Departments of Transportation, Agriculture, and Housing) and initiatives devoted to improving community conditions (such as Sustainable Communities, the Healthy Food Financing Initiative, Choice Neighborhoods, and Promise

Neighborhoods). Targeting funds to CHCs that are prepared to work with community partners to leverage one or more of these resources could help achieve reductions in health care costs while improving health outcomes.

SUMMARY

Health care has traditionally been largely a private matter between patients and clinicians, taking place within the walls of an exam room. Many clinicians know that by the time a patient reaches their office, his or her health has already been irrevocably compromised by factors that they are ill-equipped to address. The nation's health institutions are left to contend with a growing burden of complex but preventable illness and injury. The evidence argues for a new approach to health care: one that integrates quality health care services with strategies to support people in living healthier lives. This shift necessitates engaging in efforts to reshape communities. Smedley and Syme (2001, p. 4) summarized the situation in an Institute of Medicine report on health promotion: "It is unreasonable to expect people to change their behavior when so many forces in the social, cultural, and physical environment conspire against such change."

The concept of the community-centered health home builds on years of work and innovative thinking, including pioneering work on community-oriented primary care. This chapter is intended to catalyze discussion and to express ideas under development. Currently, there are groundbreaking and effective practices linking quality health care services with actions focused on community environments, but they are largely isolated initiatives. There is an opportunity to refine and systematically advance the community-centered health home model to reach across the country to the communities most in need. Revamping health care along these lines is imperative and could dramatically reduce demand for health care while extending the length and quality of life nationwide.

KEY TERMS

community-centered health home
   (CCHH)

community-oriented primary care
   (COPC)

community prevention readiness
   assessment

health home

patient-centered medical home

taking two steps to prevention

DISCUSSION QUESTIONS

1. Thinking about the thirteen THRIVE community health factors, how could clinical institutions gather data about community environments as part of their standard procedures—in particular, patient intake?

2. What kinds of partnerships would be valuable for each step of the CCHH model (*inquiry, analysis,* and *action*)? Also, what resources would be helpful in each step, and who in the community or field of work could provide expertise to execute each step?

3. How might staffing at clinical institutions need to change in order to implement the CCHH model in their clinics? What sorts of positions and capacities might be necessary?

4. What are some potential benefits and consequences of moving toward reimbursing based on health outcomes and benchmarks, rather than delivery of services?

REFERENCES

Adler, N. E., & Newman, K. (2002). Socioeconomic disparities in health: Pathways and policies. *Health Affairs, 21*(2), 60–76.

Albee, G. W. (1983). Psychology, prevention, and the just society. *Journal of Primary Prevention, 4*, 5–40.

American Academy of Family Physicians, American Academy of Pediatrics, American College of Physicians, & American Osteopathic Association. (2007). *Joint principles of the patient centered medical home.* Retrieved from http://www.aafp.org/dam/AAFP/documents/practice_management/pcmh/initiatives/PCMHJoint.pdf

Bipartisan Policy Center. (2012). *Lots to lose: How America's health and obesity crisis threatens our economic future.* Retrieved from http://bipartisanpolicy.org/library/report/lots-lose-how-americas-health-and-obesity-crisis-threatens-our-economic-future

Blum, H. L. (1980). Social perspective on risk reduction. *Family & Community Health, 3*(1), 41–61.

Bunker, J. P., Frazier, H. S., & Mosteller, F. (1994). Improving health: Measuring effects of medical care. *Milbank Quarterly, 72*(2), 225–258.

Cantor, J., Cohen, L., Mikkelsen, L., Pañares, R., Srikantharajah, J., & Valdovinos, E. (2011). *Community-centered health homes: Bridging the gap between health services and community prevention.* Oakland, CA: Prevention Institute.

Chernew, M. E., Mechanic, R. E., Landon, B. E., & Safran, D. G. (2011). Private-payer innovation in Massachusetts: The "Alternative Quality Contract." *Health Affairs, 30*(1), 51–61.

Children's Safety Network. (2005). *Child safety seats: How large are the benefits and who should pay?* Retrieved from http://www.childrenssafetynetwork.org

/sites/childrenssafetynetwork.org/files/child_safety_seats_childhood_injury
_cost_prevention.pdf

Cohen, L., Chehimi, S., & Chavez, V. (Eds.). (2010). *Prevention is primary: Strategies for community wellbeing*. San Francisco, CA: Jossey-Bass.

Cohen, L., Iton, A., Davis, R., & Rodriguez, S. (2009). *A time of opportunity: Local solutions to reduce inequities in health and safety*. Oakland, CA: Prevention Institute.

East Boston Neighborhood Health Center. (2014). *Let's Get Movin'*. Retrieved from http://www.ebnhc.org/en/strengthening-our-community/lets-get-movin /introduction.html

Gawande, A. (2011, January 24). The hot spotters. *The New Yorker*. Retrieved from http://www.newyorker.com/magazine/2011/01/24/the-hot-spotters

Goetzel, R. Z., & Ozminkowski, R. J. (2008). The health and cost benefits of work site health-promotion programs. *Annual Review of Public Health, 29*, 303–323.

Goetzel, R. Z., Shechter, D., Ozminkowski, R. J., Marmet, P. F., Tabrizi, M. J., & Roemer E. C. (2007). Promising practices in employer health and productivity management efforts: Findings from a benchmarking study. *Journal of Occupational and Environmental Medicine, 49*(2), 111–130.

Gottlieb, L. (2010, August 23). Funding healthy society helps cure health care. *San Francisco Chronicle*. Retrieved from http://www.sfgate.com/opinion/open forum/article/Funding-healthy-society-helps-cure-health-care-3177542.php

Gusmano, M., Fairbrother, G., & Park, H. (2002). Exploring the limits of the safety net: Community health centers and care for the uninsured. *Health Affairs, 21*(6), 188–194.

Health Resources and Services Administration. (n.d.). What is a health center? Retrieved from http://bphc.hrsa.gov/about

Hemp, P. (2004, October). Presenteeism: At work—but out of it. *Harvard Business Review*, 49–58.

Institute for Alternative Futures. (2012). Case study: Beaufort-Jasper-Hampton Comprehensive Health Services. In *Community health centers: Leveraging the social determinants of health*. Retrieved from http://www.altfutures.org /pubs/leveragingSDH/IAF-BJHCHS-CaseStudy.pdf

Institute of Medicine. (2011). *For the public's health: The role of measurement in action and accountability*. Washington, DC: National Academies Press.

Lee, P., & Paxman, D. (1997). Reinventing public health. *Annual Review of Public Health, 18*, 1–35.

Lightwood, J. M., Dinno, A., & Glantz, S. A. (2008). Effect of the California tobacco control programme on personal health care expenditures. *PLoS Medicine, 5*(8), e178. doi: 10.1371/journal.pmed.0050178

Lorber, D. (2011). Summary of private-payer innovation in Massachusetts: The "alternative quality contract." Retrieved from http://www.commonwealth fund.org/publications/in-the-literature/2011/jan/private-payer-innovation -in-ma

Lowe, A., & Haas, G. (Eds.). (2007). *The shame of the city: Slum housing and the critical threat to the health of L.A. children and families.* Retrieved from http://www.wellchild.org/SHAMEOFTHECITY.pdf

National Association of Community Health Centers. (2011). *Expanding health centers under health care reform: Doubling patient capacity and bringing down costs.* Retrieved from http://www.nachc.com/client/documents/HCR _New_Patients_Final.pdf

Patient-Centered Primary Care Collaborative. (2013). Defining the medical care home. Retrieved from http://www.pcpcc.org/about/medical-home

Prevention Institute, Trust for America's Health, Urban Institute, & New York Academy of Medicine. (2008). *Prevention for a healthier America.* Retrieved from www.preventioninstitute.org/component/jlibrary/article/id-75/127.html

Smedley, B. D., & Syme, L. S. (Eds.). (2001). *Promoting health: Intervention strategies from social and behavioral research.* Washington, DC: National Academies Press.

CHAPTER 15

A LOOK INTO THE FUTURE

Bernard J. Healey

Up until this point this book has focused on various components of the U.S. health care industry as they are currently structured, making recommendations on how they can be changed in order to improve the health of the population. It has also looked at the historical development of the major sectors of the health care industry, along with their role in delivering health care to consumers. This chapter will examine the future of health care delivery in the United States as a result of the various ongoing health care reforms that will alter the way that we deliver and receive health care.

Goodman (2012) argues that health care is a complex system that is so complicated that every individual sees only a small part of that system, making it very difficult for anyone to understand all the working parts. Over the years special interest groups (frequently with the aid of professional lobbyists) have manipulated health legislation so that it favors those special interests. Our current system of health care delivery is clearly in danger of bankrupting our country, and it does not seem that even the new health care reform efforts can save it. The newest health reform legislation, the Patient Protection and Affordable Care Act (ACA), does very little to change the way health care is financed, although it does succeed in increasing access for millions of the uninsured. This law also ignores the waste and fraud in health care delivery that is only going to increase with more people receiving their health insurance from the government. The ACA does encourage some preventive care but does very little to help educate the population about high-risk health behaviors that quite often result in the development of chronic diseases and complications from these diseases as people age.

LEARNING OBJECTIVES

After reading this chapter you should be able to

- Identify the major challenges found in the U.S. health care delivery system.

- Understand how health policy is formulated and implemented in the United States.

- Understand the value of health education programs in the prevention of chronic diseases.

- Discuss the reasons why the U.S. system of health care delivery needs to be reengineered.

- Explain how the reorganization of physician practices will change health care delivery.

The entrenched powers of special interest groups have long worked to prevent necessary change from occurring in the U.S. health care system. Quite often they stop change from occurring by citing the quality of health care as their reason when in reality they are protecting their own power, influence, and income. Fortunately, the debate surrounding the Affordable Care Act has helped millions of Americans better understand the current health care problems and potential solutions. These better-informed citizens and current or future consumers of health care services are now asking questions and becoming active rather than passive consumers of health care services. Power is shifting from special interest groups to the more informed and concerned consumer.

The American health care system exists in a capitalist system that utilizes markets and a pricing system, along with a decision-making process that relies heavily on profits and incentives, in order to function properly. Once we understand that health care delivery has become one of the largest businesses in the United States, we can begin to understand why many of its problems go unsolved. Fixing the problems facing our health care delivery system will result in fewer profits for special interest groups. These powerful groups have designed a health care system that meets their need for power, influence, and profits but does very little to increase quality and efficiency in delivering the necessary health services to the population.

The health care system pays little attention and devotes few resources to the prevention of disease because there is little profit to be made from healthy people. Health care organizations keep their power, prestige, and profits when people become ill and then spend a great deal of money trying to become well again. However, this system is now being confronted by numerous major challenges that can no longer be ignored by those responsible for health care delivery in our country.

Major Challenges Facing Health Care Delivery

There are numerous short-term and long-term health challenges facing the United States as it confronts an unsustainable escalation in the costs associated with funding the health care sector of the economy. It helps us to better understand the challenges and concentrate on better solutions when we realize that rising costs in health care are only symptoms of much larger problems. The challenges discussed in this section will require innovative approaches developed by the individuals who currently produce and consume health services. It is ironic that although these solutions are not going to come from government, they will not be able to happen without the help of government. Unfortunately, many of the challenges have actually been caused by government intervention in the health care sector. These challenges comprise physician shortages, lack of health care quality, the chronic disease epidemic, the high cost of pharmaceuticals, medical errors and medical malpractice, and fraud and waste.

Physician Shortages

U.S. legislators have attempted to deal with the escalating costs of health care delivery by opting to cut the salaries of those who make up the most important component of health care delivery, the physicians. Our country is currently experiencing a shortage of primary care physicians that could very easily become a shortage of medical specialists as well if we continue to cut their reimbursement rates. A side effect of reducing physician reimbursement is that many physicians are refusing to accept Medicaid recipients because the government reimbursement rate is too low. Making matters worse is the fact that the ACA will add millions of individuals to the Medicaid program, but the physician shortage may deny them access. They will have insurance coverage but not necessarily providers of health care (Lowrey & Pear, 2012).

The Association of Medical Colleges is predicting a shortage of more than 62,000 physicians by the year 2015. As a result, health economists predict that the price of health care will escalate at a much greater rate than we have previously seen or wait time for appointments will increase or both. Providing incentives to medical students who choose to work in primary care can reverse this shortage of primary care physicians. There also needs to be a commitment to legislation designed to free physicians from redundant paperwork and to allow physician extenders to perform more of the less skilled duties of physicians. The new health care law is actually replacing price rationing in health care with time rationing. As millions of Americans are added to the insured rolls because of the ACA, people will find it more difficult to get a physician appointment because of the shortages of providers. This shortage will result from increased demand for health services while the number of physicians diminishes.

Lack of Health Care Quality

Another concern of health policy experts is the lack of quality in the health care being supplied to consumers. This poor quality has been demonstrated by comparing the United States to other countries on many key health indices, such as infant mortality rate, length of life, quality of life as people age, and number of medical errors and nosocomial infections. The starting point for quality improvement in health care delivery is the development of a definition of what improved quality means to consumers.

There is an old adage that tells us, "You get what you pay for." That statement seems to be true everywhere except when we are purchasing health care services. Our country spends twice as much as other industrialized countries with far lower returns for our money in terms of improved health indices. Perednia (2011) argues that a large portion of what we spend on health care is wasted on things like redundant paperwork and other administrative costs that do nothing to improve individual or population health. According to Langley et al. (2009), "Fundamental changes that result in improvement in quality include

- Altering how work or activity is done or the makeup of a product
- Producing visible, positive differences in results relative to historical norms
- Having a lasting impact" [p.16]

In order to enhance health care quality we must first determine what it is that requires improvement, develop a process for advancement, and then evaluate the success or failure of the process. We also need to offer the necessary incentives to improve the quality of health care services. These incentives can include paying physicians for performance, especially when the performance includes health education for the patient and his or her family members. As mentioned previously, health education that leads to prevention is the only way to deal effectively with chronic diseases and their complications because these diseases cannot be cured. One of the most important things a physician can do for his or her patients and our health care system is to help those patients prevent disease. This type of intervention needs to be looked at as a long-term investment.

The Chronic Disease Epidemic

The chronic disease epidemic is growing rapidly in our country. It is fueled in no small part by the rise in obesity and is considered by most physicians and public health officials as the greatest medical threat to confront our system of medical care. These diseases cannot be allowed to continue to increase in incidence and prevalence or our health care system is indeed doomed to failure because these chronic diseases cannot be cured and the costs of their complications continue to grow as our nation ages. According to Schimpff (2012) this epidemic offers the United States an opportunity to improve population health by focusing on personal behaviors that are detrimental to health. This will require our health care system to shift resources away from the cure of disease and toward prevention efforts such as health education. Health education efforts need to begin in elementary school and continue on into the workplace.

According to Ogden, Carroll, Kit, and Fiegal (2012), more than one-third of adults and almost 17 percent of youth were obese in 2009 and 2010. This epidemic of obesity is growing at a rapid pace among children aged two to nineteen, claiming 5 million girls and approximately 7 million boys. This escalation in obesity at such a young age is going to result in early onset of chronic diseases like type 2 diabetes, resulting in life-threatening complications in these individuals' prime of life during their working age. It is extremely important to understand that we as a nation cannot sit back and allow this epidemic to slowly consume our young and our old. We have to take action against this chronic disease epidemic now because we are running out of time.

Along with the obesity problem (Figure 15.1), physical inactivity among the population (Figure 15.2) is also responsible for premature death and disability in epidemic proportions. According to *The Nation's Health* (Curry, 2012), physical inactivity results in about one in ten deaths worldwide and causes up to 10 percent of four chronic diseases: coronary heart disease, type 2 diabetes, breast cancer, and colon cancer. The epidemic of

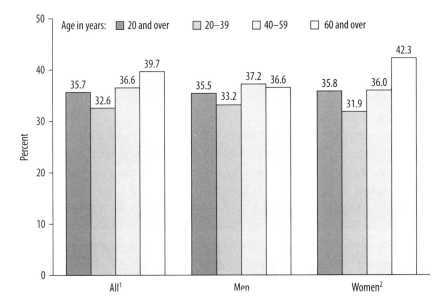

Figure 15.1 Prevalence of Obesity Among Adults Aged Twenty and over, by Sex and Age: United States, 2009–2010
Note: Estimates were age adjusted by the direct method to the 2000 U.S. Census population using the age groups 20–39, 40–59, and 60 and over.
[1] Significant increasing linear trend by age ($p < 0.01$).
[2] Significant increasing linear trend by age ($p < 0.001$).
Source: Ogden et al., 2012, fig. 1. Data from National Center for Health Statistics, National Health and Nutrition Examination Survey, 2009–2010.

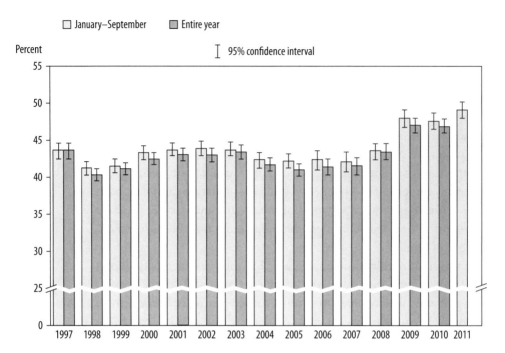

Figure 15.2 Percentage of Adults Aged Eighteen and over Who Met the 2008 Federal Physical Activity Guidelines for Aerobic Activity Through Leisure-Time Aerobic Activity: United States, 1997–September 2011

chronic diseases and their complications is going to continue growing and consuming increasing amounts of scarce resources unless we as a nation make the decision to prevent chronic diseases and their complications from occurring in the first place.

According to Marvassi and Stafford (2012), many modifiable risk factors for the development of chronic diseases are being ignored by the current U.S. medical care delivery system. These authors discuss Fries's **morbidity compression** model, which deals with the possibility of extending an individual's disease-free lifespan. Fries's model suggests that an individual's age at the onset of his or her first chronic infirmity can be postponed more readily than his or her age of death. If this is so, then the lifetime illness burden could be compressed into a shorter period of time nearer to the age of death. If we could postpone the complications from chronic diseases to a limited time period right before death, then we could reduce health care costs and improve the lives of patients at the same time. This change will require the reconnecting of medicine to public health departments and the use of primary care physicians.

morbidity compression

A reduction of the lifetime illness burden through postponing the onset of health complications from chronic diseases.

The High Cost of Pharmaceuticals

Pharmaceuticals are a for-profit component of the U.S. health care system; they cost approximately 10 percent of the more than $2 trillion a year spent on the health sector of our economy. The drug industry produces one of the highest profit levels on an annual basis of all American industries. In fact, until 2006, it was the most profitable industry in our country. It has since dropped to third place, but profit is still the ruler of the research agenda for the drug industry.

The pharmaceutical industry has developed solutions to many of the major threats to our health; it has discovered medicines that can mediate or cure many of the leading causes of disease. In order to increase research for new treatments for disease and because the drug industry reports that it costs between $800 million and $2 billion to bring each new drug to market, the FDA grants drug companies twenty-year patent protection for each new research discovery. This costs claim is refuted by Washington (2011), who cites a study completed by the U.S. government revealing that to bring a new drug to market takes only ten to twelve years at an average cost of only $359 million. Washington also points out that medical research has actually been harmed as pharmaceutical companies instruct their paid researchers to withhold damaging data from studies and hire ghostwriters to package their marketing messages as scientific studies.

The continuous increases in the prices of necessary drugs for treatment of medical conditions are not sustainable in the long term. At the same time, we desperately need continued research and development on new drugs to treat the leading causes of morbidity, mortality, and disability found in our country today. These innovations will come only from investment by government, academia, and pharmaceutical companies looking to make a profit. According to Christensen, Grossman, and Hwang (2009), the pharmaceutical industry is ripe for **disruptive innovation** and that process has already begun. As discussed in Chapter Thirteen, these authors argue that a disruptive innovation represents the application of a new set of values in the production process, with results that overtake the existing market. This type of innovation makes products or services less expensive and more accessible, allowing more consumers to enter and make purchases in the disrupted market. An innovation that is disruptive gives a whole new population of consumers at the bottom of a market access to a product or service that was historically accessible only to consumers with a lot of money or a lot of skill. To some extent, disruptive innovation in pharmaceuticals is a result of the pharmaceutical leaders attempting to

disruptive innovation
A new product or service that is capable of changing an existing market by improving convenience, access, and/or affordability

further increase their enormous profits by abandoning the least profitable of their activities. Disruptive firms are taking over these less profitable activities and turning them into value-added activities for the health care sector. This is allowing new entrants into the drug-producing industry, which was becoming monopolized by a few large firms. These hungry entrepreneurs may ultimately discover new cures for diseases that were previously unprofitable ventures for the large firms.

Medical Errors and Malpractice

Another major problem found in health care is the danger that patients face on a daily basis when they enter the health care system for assistance with their medical problems. Goodman (2012) points out that "as many as 187,000 patients die every year for some reason other than the medical condition that caused them to seek care. By another estimate, there are 6.1 million injuries caused by the healthcare system, including hospital-acquired infections that afflict one in every twenty hospital patients" (p. 95).

medical error
The failure of a planned action to be completed as intended or the use of a wrong plan to achieve an aim.

The United States is in the middle of a dangerous epidemic of medical errors, some of them arising from providing too much health care. Recall that the Institute of Medicine (IOM) (1999) defines a **medical error** as "the failure of a planned action to be completed as intended or the use of a wrong plan to achieve an aim." It seems that entering the medical care system, especially being admitted to a hospital, has become a potentially dangerous event. Brownlee (2007) points out that the most common medical error found in the delivery of medical care today is erroneous or inaccurate drug administration. These errors can be reduced only by better leadership along with empowered followers who are all working as a team to, first, discover why medical errors occur and, second, to rapidly move to prevent them from occurring in the future. This goal of reduced medical errors has been achieved by numerous health care facilities but has had its greatest success in the U.S. Department of Veterans Affairs (VA) hospitals. According to Longman (2012) the real cause of medical errors in health care facilities is the lack of a system designed to prevent these errors from ever occurring in the first place. Fortunately, the Veterans Health Administration (VHA), which runs the numerous VA hospitals for veterans, decided to do something about this epidemic of medical errors.

The starting point was the development of a way to gain full disclosure from all hospitals in the VA system regarding every single medical error. This was a very dangerous procedure to develop of course, because it meant that everyone, and especially the news media, would become a witness to medical errors among U.S. veterans. But it had to be done in order to gain an understanding of the volume of errors, their location, and their cause.

These error reports included operating on the wrong patient, operating on the wrong part of the body, medication errors, abuse, and even deaths during the delivery of medical care.

The next step involved discovering ways to prevent errors from happening. A checklist system was developed by the VHA, so that each medical procedure had a checklist that included all the necessary steps in the procedure. The VHA then began using the medical bracelet worn by each patient as an electronic storage system for information about the patient's prescribed drugs. A computer software program was written and used to record virtually every piece of medical information regarding every patient hospitalized in the VA hospital system. The VA became a shinning star in our nation's war on the epidemic of medical errors.

Fraud and Waste

The amount of fraud and waste in the U.S. health care delivery system has risen to historic levels and has become one of the most important challenges facing our nation. If our country were able to deal with this one area successfully, we could easily reverse the problem of escalating health care costs. A recent study conducted by the IOM (2013) found that the U.S. health care system wastes over $750 billion annually; that is enough money to fund Medicare and Medicaid into the distant future. According to the study report, this waste represents about thirty cents of every health care dollar, and immediate action to eliminate the waste is required.

The report identified six areas of waste: $210 billion in unnecessary services, $130 billion in inefficiency in the delivery of care, $190 billion in excess administration costs, $105 billion in inflated prices, $55 billion in prevention failures, and $75 billion in fraud. This report also offers a road map for finding the major areas of waste and fraud in our health care system, along with ten recommendations for ways to eliminate the waste and improve health care delivery for all. The most important recommendations are payment reforms that would reward quality, improved coordination of care, increased patient education, and better utilization of technology to aid in the improvement of clinical decision making.

An example of the seriousness of the fraud issue was brought to national attention by an investigation reported by the *New York Times*. According to Pear (2008), in the time period 2000 to 2007, Medicare paid 478,500 claims totaling $60 million to $92 million that were submitted by deceased physicians. As Hayes (2012) observes, the presence of large amounts of money has the ability to change individual and group behavior so that people participate in behavior they would usually avoid. Hayes also argues that reduced regulatory oversight and a culture of corruption are usually elements in successful attempts at fraud by both individuals and organizations. Fraud can also result from moral hazard. As discussed in Chapter Six, moral hazard refers to the perverse incentives that result when individuals are insulated from the costs associated with their actions. Many individuals involved in health care fraud seem to believe that they are just getting back what is owed them but not received because of government reductions in reimbursement.

An informative example of serious organizational fraud was investigated and reported by the *New York Times* in August 2012. The investigation centered on performing unnecessary cardiac work. It found that some cardiologists in Florida hospitals owned by HCA, the largest for-profit hospital chain in the United States, were unable to justify many of the procedures they were performing. In fact fully half of the cardiac catheterizations completed at Lawnwood Regional Medical Center in Fort Pierce, Florida, were performed on patients without significant heart disease (Abelson & Creswell, 2012).

Unfortunately, this type of fraud is widespread in health care, and up until now not a great deal has been done to eliminate fraud and abuse of our limited health care resources. To reduce fraud and waste in health care delivery we need to invest in the investigation of fraud and waste, set regulations, and prosecute offenders. We also need a rigorous evaluation of the costs and benefits associated with medical testing, procedures, and treatment of medical conditions. Better investigation and prosecution makes more sense than simply increasing premiums to make up for this illegal activity.

Accountable Care Organizations

accountable care organization (ACO)
A group of physicians and hospitals that share responsibility for the health and cost of care of a defined group of patients, with a goal of improving patient health while lowering cost of care.

The concept of the **accountable care organization (ACO)** was given birth in 2006 by Elliot Fisher, who was the director of the Center for Health Policy Research at Dartmouth Medical School. The ACO, which looks a lot like a health maintenance organization (HMO), is a health care organization designed to link payment and delivery of health care services to improved quality and cost reduction for a certain population. This new concept has gained traction among policy experts and is included in the new health care reform legislation. In an ACO various health care organizations, practices, and people—such as primary care physicians, specialists, hospitals, other providers, and payers—work together to provide and manage care. ACOs emphasize the alignment of incentives and accountability for providers across the continuum of care. Compared to HMOs, these new organizations will require greater use of information technology along with financial incentives in order to accomplish their goals.

On the one hand Starr (2011) points out that the ACO offers an attempt at experimentation that may lead to better ways to reduce the costs of health care delivery while improving the quality of health services. On the other hand Goodman (2012) is concerned that ACO incentives to providers may result in less care, which may actually harm the patient's health. Other possible problems with this care model are patients' limited choices of physicians and the possibility that patients may not see the same physician at each appointment.

According to Fisher et al. (2009), in order to improve the value of health care we need to deal with three barriers: "lack of accountability for the overall quality and cost of care and for decisions about local capacity; a payment system that rewards volume, growth, and intensity, regardless of value (and that penalizes providers who adopt cost-saving innovations); and the widespread belief—often in the face of relevant evidence to the contrary—that more medical care means better medical care" (p. 220). These barriers to the achievement of better value health care for the population are formidable, but they can be overcome with creativity and innovation in the delivery of health care.

To improve the quality of health care services, we need a primary care approach that uses a team model that coordinates medical care across time and various settings. For example, Shortell (2010) argues that the ACO model is particularly capable of serving the chronically ill cohort, where many patients have more than one chronic illness and are seen by multiple specialists. The goal for these patients should be to avoid the complications from their chronic diseases entirely. At the same time, Estes, Chapman, Dodd, Hollister, and Harrington (2013) observe that the current health care reform efforts are going to result in continuing power struggles between those who favor an approach of individual responsibility and those who see a role for government intervention in the workings of our health care system.

Areas of Future Concern

In addition to all these current concerns, there are areas of future concern that we should begin acting on soon as we move into the uncharted territory resulting from the various macro- and micro-forces involved in the reform of the American system of health care delivery. The remainder of this section discusses four of these major concerns: saving Medicare and Medicaid from bankruptcy, mitigating the effects of the ongoing consolidation of payers, developing strategies for more effective employment of physicians, and improving the process of developing health policy.

Saving Medicare and Medicaid

The Medicare and Medicaid entitlement programs need to be restructured and improved, and they also deserve immediate attention in this area instead of continuous criticism and funding cuts. There is no question that these government-financed programs are having serious financial difficulties due to increases in demand for health care services along with increased fraud and abuse in these programs. In fact both of these government health programs are predicted to go bankrupt in the very near future unless eligibility requirements are changed, costs are reduced, or taxes are raised on those paying the bill. We need a well-developed combination of these changes in order to shore up these government-financed health insurance efforts so they are available for the population in the future.

According to the Henry J. Kaiser Family Foundation (2012), the most discussed proposals for Medicare would transform it from a **defined benefit program**, in which beneficiaries are guaranteed coverage for a fixed set of benefits, to a defined contribution or **premium support program**, in which beneficiaries are guaranteed a fixed federal payment to help cover their health care expenses. Before any changes are made to these two important entitlement programs, health policy experts, including health economists, must clearly define the real problems in Medicare and Medicaid. There is an old saying that "a problem well defined is partially solved." This is where we need to have legitimate policy discussions absent the numerous lobbyists representing various groups that will be affected by making the necessary changes to these popular government programs. There are answers that can improve the financial position of these programs, but we have to eliminate the special interest groups from the legislative discussion, or we are never going to get at the real problems found in these programs.

Andes, Pauley, and Wilensky (2012) point out that Medicare is the largest purchaser of health services in the United States and its leverage is only going to increase with the aging of the baby boom generation. The payment structure of this government program is fee-for-service, which encourages much wasteful and expensive medicine. These authors recommend premium support for Medicare recipients, allowing them to shop around for their insurance coverage. This in itself should provide the necessary incentives for competition among insurance carriers. In addition, reduced restrictions and regulations for Medicare could foster innovations in the design of plans for the older population.

defined benefit program
A program that provides a fixed set of health care benefits.

premium support program
A program that provides a fixed federal payment to cover health care needs.

Mitigating the Consolidation of Payers

Goodman (2012) argues that health insurance is a secondary institution designed to be an adjunct to health care, not a substitute for it. The third-party payer was never envisioned as the entity that would make the decision of who receives health care and, more important, who does not receive this care. But that is exactly what has happened with our medical insurance. We have lost control of what is and what is not covered by the health insurance plans that we thought we owned. This problem is only going to get worse as the consolidation of health insurers continues, eliminating any type of valuable competition.

Ensuring Effective Employment of Physicians

Many members of the baby boomer generation remember their family physician as a solo practitioner whose medical office was quite often attached to his or her home. Their parents could call this family doctor at any time, and he or she would make a home visit or at least give them advice on what to do until they could make an office visit. This form of medical practice is long gone, and now many physicians are in group practices or have formed relationships with hospitals and health systems. Many of them have become full-time salaried employees of health care systems. This new physician is not always available, forcing many ill individuals to wait for long periods of time without care or in emergency rooms.

One thing that has not changed over the last fifty years is the fact that we still need the physician, who is still the most important player in the delivery of medical services. There is no question that people will always need physicians' medical expertise, but what no one needs is for these medical experts to waste their valuable time filling out redundant paperwork that is different for every health insurer.

Fabrizio (2011) categorizes the major concerns affecting physician employment as economic issues, personal issues, and competitive issues. The economic issues facing the most important players in our health care system are enormous. They start with a large student debt after they finish medical school, and that is followed by large costs to set up their medical practice and obtain malpractice insurance and by constant reductions in reimbursement from third-party payers, especially the government. Fabrizio (2011) points out that this leaves the physician few options about how to practice medicine. The only choices seem to be joining a medical group or becoming a salaried employee of a hospital or health care system.

The personal issues facing the physician today involve the desire to have a much different lifestyle from that experienced by older physicians who were solo practitioners running their own businesses. This new cohort of younger physicians places a greater value on having normal work hours, allowing them to spend more private time with their families. In order to accomplish this objective these physicians have opted to become salaried employees of a health care system, thus reducing their work hours. The economies of scale and professional office managers found in group practices and large health care systems cannot be matched by a solo practitioner, making the choice to be in group practice easier. All these factors are contributing to a reduction in the availability of physicians while the demand for these providers is escalating.

Improving the Process of Developing Health Policy

Health care legislation passed by the Congress and signed into law by the president is the major force shaping the U.S. health care system and its policies. According to Estes et al. (2013), when it comes to the division of scarce resources there is always great competition among special interest groups, usually resulting in political maneuvering to obtain the greatest share of these resources. The legislative processes surrounding health care policy in our country have become nothing more than a legitimated process for the redistribution of wealth guided by lobbyists representing special interest groups.

The process of health policy development, implementation, and evaluation is about to change. The stakes are too great for the health policy process to be under the control of lobbyists and special interest groups who are responsible for many of the perverse incentives that are currently found in our health care system. Over the years little attention has been paid to the process of developing health policy, especially at the state level. Therefore very little is known by the general public about the secondary economic effects of health policy. Understanding this is especially important when looking at the licensure process for health care professionals.

The process of developing health policy must become more transparent and involve more consumers in the discussion of what is and is not appropriate health policy. It has been said that all income for health care providers is determined by the legislative process, which in turn determines what various health care providers are allowed to do and not to do given their particular medical license. This usually results in increased income for the most powerful group in medicine, the physicians.

Miniter (2012) argues that a great deal of legislation created by the federal and state governments creates uncertainty that slows the process of risk taking that is so necessary for true innovation to be unleashed. Miniter points out that "if we seek to regulate future products and markets in advance, we'll impose rules that will almost certainly end up crushing innovation" (p. 110). We cannot let this interference with a functioning market continue in the health care sector of our economy.

Barlett and Steele (2012) observe that "Congress makes the rules when it enacts new laws and amends or rescinds others—and then votes on whether or not to provide the resources that determine whether the laws will be enforced" (p. 25). How laws are enacted is usually a result of the influence of individual legislators who are often guided by the information and support that they receive from those affected by the laws and their individual paid lobbyists. This is why it is so very important to look at all the possible secondary effects of proposed health legislation.

How to Meet These Challenges

These challenges are formidable, but they can be met and resolved by implementing some serious changes to the way we do business in health care today. Health care is one of the few remaining sectors of the U.S. economy that still use a bureaucratic organizational structure. Most businesses in the for-profit sector have realized that in order to continue to prosper, foster innovation, and retain talented workers, they need to change their strict bureaucratic method of management to a more organic structure where workers are encouraged to be creative and innovative and where trust can develop. This change in organizational design is slowly but surely making its way toward the health care sector. Some of the major changes that need to be made in the very near future in order to solve many of our health care problems include the expansion of health education, leadership replacing management, the encouragement of innovation by employees, and provision of the necessary incentives to make all these changes successful.

Houle and Fleece (2011) point out that at least part, if not all, of the current health care system is broken. The problem has become one of gaining agreement from the various stakeholders about what needs to be done to fix this broken system of health care delivery. There is indeed a paradigm shift coming in how we think about health care, how we deliver health care, and of course the economics of health care. These necessary changes in health care services delivery must occur sooner rather than later.

Invest in Health Education Programs

It seems obvious that the current focus in health care delivery of attempting to cure all diseases is not working. The major problems found in the current health care system—cost escalation, lack of access to care, and poor health levels among the population—would all go away if we remained healthy rather than becoming ill. In fact, as previously mentioned, the leading cause of morbidity and mortality in the United States is no longer curable communicable diseases but rather the incurable chronic diseases. This silent epidemic of chronic diseases cannot be treated but can be prevented if we as a nation are willing to invest sufficient resources in health education and health promotion programs designed to prevent people from acquiring these diseases in the first place.

Almost all the money spent on health care every year in this country is designated for finding disease and then curing the disease when found. The problem with this strategy is found in the fact that once one acquires a chronic disease there is no cure but only the management of the chronic disease in an attempt to prevent complications from it. Fortunately, there is another strategy that can be used to deal with the epidemic of chronic diseases. This strategy will take a long time to develop, implement, evaluate, and improve, but given time and resources it will work. Our health care system must move a large amount of resources from disease detection and attempted cure to health education and disease prevention. Health education is also a valuable strategy for the prevention of the complications that usually arise from having a chronic disease for a long period of time.

The idea of expanding health education and health promotion programs is not new. It has been a core function of public health departments for years. The problem has been that public health departments have never been allocated the necessary resources to make health education programs work. Why have health insurance providers not educated their members about the value of receiving health education and preventing chronic diseases from occurring in the first place? Doesn't it seem logical that if health insurance companies used their resources up front to prevent disease then they would not waste their resources attempting to cure the incurable chronic diseases later in life? The answer to these questions is found in the etiology of chronic diseases. These diseases take decades to develop and produce expensive medical complications. Because these complications usually occur in older individuals, these patients will most likely have moved into the Medicare system where they become the government's problem. There is simply no real monetary incentive for health insurance companies and employers to care much about keeping the population free from illness. Unfortunately, this attitude is costing the country as a whole enormous amounts of resources as the population grows older.

Barnes, Kroening-Roche, and Comfort (2012) point out that the new health law is requiring a strong primary care foundation for patient care. They also point out that the availability and use of patient-centered medical homes discussed in the previous chapter is growing across the United States; these medical homes are focused on promoting good health rather than just treating disease. They recognize that 40 percent of premature mortality is determined by individual health behavior and 15 percent by societal factors. Therefore, in order to improve the health of the population, more attention must be paid to preventing high-risk health behaviors like tobacco use, physical inactivity, and obesity. This will certainly result in health education becoming a vital part of primary care.

Engage in Leadership, Not Just Management

The most important skill necessary if we are to solve the many problems facing the health care industry and reform that industry is leadership. Without strong leadership from both formal and informal leaders in health care delivery, there will be little if any success. The current problems found in our health care system are far too large to be solved by management alone. The major challenges in health care today require vision and health care workers empowered to be creative and innovative in designing solutions. According to Hamel (2012) our large problems today demand radical new solutions, forcing organizations to change in ways that have no precedent. This is where our entire health care industry finds itself today. Change is coming so rapidly to health care organizations that current management processes are incapable of turning that change into opportunities for the organization.

Bureaucracies are designed to work slowly within rules and regulations, while changes in function or process meet with extreme resistance from those in control. Although bureaucratic structures are being rapidly replaced with decentralized management systems in most successful organizations, a few sectors in our economy, like health care, have retained a rigid bureaucratic structure. Health care management systems were never designed to deal with rapid change but rather to keep the organization running efficiently. This is especially true in bureaucratic organizations that are micromanaged by bureaucratic managers. These managers are not interested in the improvement of health care delivery, only in protecting their power and influence, which is found in their management position. Radical change brought about by innovation threatens their power base so they usually block change with their position power.

There is no magic bullet available to deal with the many challenges facing the health care sector of our economy. It requires creativity and innovation to turn the waste found in health services delivery today into efficient and productive changes designed to improve the health of our population at a price that we can all afford. Better management of the scarce health care resources is required, along with leaders who provide a vision and a plan to achieve that vision. Leaders must have a strategy to empower all staff in health care organizations to spend the majority of their time improving the quality of the services that they deliver every day. This is going to require the development of trust between the health care leader and those who actually deliver the services to the health care consumer. This process of building trust between leaders and followers begins when the leader of the health care organization recognizes that the most important resource found in the health care facility is the people providing the health services.

The enormous challenges faced by the restructuring health care sector require leaders with superb communication and conflict management skills, motivational expertise, and the ability to build and sustain a strong positive culture within the health care organization. These skills can help to release the innovative spirit throughout the organization, empowering all employees to improve service delivery on a daily basis. Just as the employee with innovation skills grows by using these skills, the leader grows by constantly using his or her leadership skills. With both the leader and the empowered employees growing in their positions, the health care facility should grow and prosper. The answers can be found in the people who work in all parts of the health care delivery system. These are the people who first recognize the problems and are also most likely to understand how to solve them.

Gross (2012) argues that it is not productive to use the enormity of the challenges that we face as an excuse for doing nothing. The most important attribute that we as a nation can bring to solving the challenges in health care is a desire to try new approaches and to adapt innovations to the way the business of health care services is conducted. This is where the vision of the leader, complemented by the talent of the empowered workers, comes into play.

O'Callaghan (2010) comments that in an organization facing a crisis, one of the most important things the leader can do is to gather numerous viewpoints on the causes of the problem and encourage a discussion of the various opportunities that are present for change. Jennings (2012) points out that all businesses must adapt to change or accept the fact that they are slowly going out of business. He finds that failing businesses usually waste valuable time blaming others for their failures rather than dealing with the root cause of their problem, their inability to respond rapidly to a changing environment. This is exactly what is happening in health care today. There needs to be radical change in the way health care is delivered, and we are all running out of time to address this change. Champy and Greenspun (2010) point out that many of the processes currently used in health care services delivery are in dire need of reengineering but have been ignored. If these health delivery processes were reorganized, they could maximize their quality, safety, and convenience while reducing costs of operation.

Leinwand and Mainardi (2011) argue that capable leaders are inspiring. They can provide leadership and empowerment to a group of creative individuals who understand why the organization has achieved success.

Vanourek and Vanourek (2012) point out that organizations that have developed a healthy culture have been able to achieve improved productivity, staff retention, increased profitability, and much better relationships with customers and suppliers. These authors use the Mayo Clinic as proof of this improved relationship and to illustrate the role of leadership in the daily improvement of the health of the organization's culture. The Mayo Clinic prides itself on its team approach to health care delivery. This is achieved through an emphasis on communication among all levels of the organization, along with collaboration among staff and patients on all medical decisions.

Create Innovations in Health Care Delivery

Florida (2011) states that creativity involves distinct habits of mind that are often stifled by the design of the organization. The great strength of a capitalist system is found in the entrepreneur who revolutionizes the pattern of production. All too often, as the organization grows because of a successful entrepreneur who has passion for the product or service and the confidence to take the risks associated with creativity, a bureaucratic system of management is installed to help with the growth process. Then, for efficiency and effectiveness within the growing organization, rules and regulations are instituted, which in turn all but eliminate the creativity of the organization. This is exactly what has happened to the health care sector of our economy.

The productivity of health care resources must be improved if we are going to be successful in dealing with the many challenges we face in the delivery of health care services. In order to improve health care resource productivity, we must be able to increase the availability of health care services at a lower price. This requires the development and implementation of innovations in health services delivery that are currently being blocked by bureaucratic organizations and the micromanagers that they employ. These innovations are also being blocked by powerful interest groups who resist changes that affect their members' income by supporting legislation that eliminates creativity and competition in the health care industry.

The way we receive medical care is in dire need of innovation. Consumers of health care services are demanding convenient, less expensive, quality health services that are delivered to them without their having to waste a large amount of their limited time filling out forms and waiting for care. According to Goodman (2012) this consumer demand has resulted in the growth of urgent care clinics and walk-in clinics. These innovations in health care delivery post their prices and usually offer excellent quality of care in a timely fashion. **Retail clinics** are a form of ambulatory care found in retail establishments like grocery stores, pharmacies, and many other types of stores. In a recent study Mehrotra and Lave (2012) found that the number of retail clinics is rapidly growing and these clinics are becoming a part of the U.S. health care delivery system. These authors have discovered a fourfold increase in retail clinic visits from 2007 to 2009. These clinics provide a desired service at a transparent and reasonable price. They offer after-hours availability, are usually conveniently located, and have short waiting times. The demand for retail clinics also reflects the increased demand for primary care because of the shortage of primary care physicians. The need for primary care will increase in the future as many of the uninsured become insured as a result of the Affordable Care Act now that it is being fully implemented.

Omachonu and Einspruch (2010) point out that information technology has become the most important component of innovation in health care. It has the ability to reduce the costs of health services delivery while improving the quality of care. Even though the federal government has put monetary incentives in place for providers of care to adopt technology in their practices and hospitals, the adoption rate of this technology is still moving at a frustratingly slow pace. This innovation is a critical requirement that must be fulfilled if we as a nation are ever going to deal with the challenges we face in health care, especially cost containment and quality improvement. We must first restructure the health care organization so that it encourages not only innovation but also disruptive innovation, which replaces older technologies with newer and value-added ideas.

Wagner (2012) argues that innovators require a skill set that includes curiosity, imagination, perseverance, critical thinking, a willingness to take risks, and the ability to accept failure. These skills are present in many individuals throughout health care organizations, no matter what their position or their formal education or training. The secret is to allow individuals with innovation skills to continue to develop their skills by using them. According to Chesbrough (2011) successful innovation efforts require changing the role of both the employee and the customer in the innovation process, thus empowering both groups.

The development of new products and services is the function of the entrepreneur who visualizes opportunities, pays the up-front costs associated with bringing the service or product to market, and ultimately takes all the market risks. The missing ingredient for success in innovation in health care delivery has been the entrepreneur. According to Miniter (2012) individuals with entrepreneurial skills are all around us and are well aware of the many opportunities that are present in the health care industry. Therefore the question that needs to be answered is, how can

retail c
Basic care
located i
other ret

we motivate these prospective health care entrepreneurs to channel their much needed skills toward solving the challenges currently faced by our health care industry?

Make Incentives Matter

Most incentives provided in the health care industry are dedicated to rewarding the players who have the most power and influence, but unfortunately these incentives do not improve the health of the population. Miniter (2012) points out that incentives matter in almost any attempt that is made to improve the chances of goal achievement. He offers the example of a **rent-seeking society**, where individuals and institutions spend a great deal of time attempting to increase their profits through politics rather than value creation. This rent seeking is evident in almost all the health care legislation that gets passed and implemented by our government. It is not proposed and ultimately turned into law by the people that it affects but rather it is a reflection of powerful health care providers and their lobbyists. They lobby government to pass legislation that hurts competitors while rewarding them with increased profits. This rent-seeking motive tends to reward nonproductive efforts and to discourage the very innovation required by our entire economy but especially the health care sector.

> **rent-seeking society**
> A society where individuals seeking profits put more emphasis on political influence than on creating value with innovations.

The current incentives in health care delivery encourage wasteful testing, unnecessary medical procedures, hospitalization when ambulatory care would work better, and often the unnecessary utilization of a hospital emergency room. These incentives must change or we are never going to get any semblance of the best way to deliver quality health care at a reasonable price. There's also a need to start providing incentives for preventive health care delivery that starts with health education in elementary school and continues right through the workplace. The only way to stop the epidemic of chronic diseases is to prevent high-risk behaviors from occurring in the first place. This will only happen once incentives are in place for the health care system and the nation as a whole to work together to prevent disease rather than attempt to cure disease after it has occurred. A very good example of an individual incentive would be a reduction in the insurance premium for various preventive health choices, such as participating in a company-sponsored wellness program. Miniter (2012) argues that the incentives found in a market provide individuals and companies with reasons necessary to choose productive activities, and so another example is found in the way we pay physicians for health care. The current method of payment is fee-for-service. The more activities produced by the physician, the larger the amount of money paid to the physician. The result of this incentive is a large number of activities, some of which are unnecessary. A better way to pay physicians would be for positive health outcomes.

SUMMARY

The American health care system is undergoing massive change, thanks to health care reform efforts that are producing many challenges and many opportunities for both providers and consumers of health care services. The cost escalation in health care is unsustainable and thus major changes in the health care delivery system are in order. Policymakers, providers of care, and consumers must make careful choices if the nation is to have better care at lower costs.

There are many challenges in health care delivery that require leadership rather than management for a solution. In order for leaders to come forth with a vision of innovation, we must first deal with the resistance to change among the special interest groups and the lobbyists who have been blocking any change by encouraging the development of poor health policy. It has been said that all income in health care is a direct result of health legislation. Unfortunately, our nation can no longer afford the rising price of health care service delivery.

The current health care delivery system in the United States provides incentives to waste scarce health care resources on unnecessary tests and medical procedures. Incentives need to be changed and redesigned to encourage preventive health care: first, through health education and, second, through the consumer becoming a more active participant in his or her health care decision making. If incentives are put in place that encourage health care providers to offer health education and preventive screening to their patients and discourage the use of unnecessary, wasteful, and sometimes dangerous testing and procedures, there will be a dramatic improvement in the health of the entire population.

KEY TERMS

accountable care organization (ACO)

defined benefit program

disruptive innovation

medical error

morbidity compression

premium support program

rent-seeking society

retail clinics

DISCUSSION QUESTIONS

1. What are some of the important challenges facing our health care system over the next several years? Explain the significance of each of these challenges.

2. What must be done, and why, in order to preserve Medicare and Medicaid for use by future generations?

3. What is an accountable care organization?

4. How can we deal with the current epidemic of chronic diseases facing our country?

REFERENCES

Abelson, R., & Creswell, J. (2012, August 6). Hospital chain inquiry cited unnecessary cardiac work. *New York Times*. Retrieved from http://www.nytimes.com/2012/08/07/business/hospital-chain-internal-reports-found-dubious-cardiac-work.html?_r=1&nl=todaysheadlines&emc=tha2_20120807&pagewanted=all.

Andes, J. P., Pauley, M. V., & Wilensky, G. R. (2012). Bending the cost curve through market-based incentives. *New England Journal of Medicine, 367*(10), 954–958.

Barlett, D. L., & Steele, J. B. (2012). *The betrayal of the American dream*. New York, NY: Public Affairs.

Barnes, K. A., Kroening-Roche, J. C., & Comfort, B. W. (2012). The developing vision of primary care. *New England Journal of Medicine, 367*(10), 891–893.

Brownlee, S. (2007). *Overtreated: Why too much medicine is making us sicker and poorer*. New York, NY: Bloomsbury USA.

Champy, J., & Greenspun, H. (2010). *Reengineering healthcare: A manifesto for radically rethinking healthcare delivery*. Upper Saddle River, NJ: Pearson Education.

Chesbrough, H. (2011). *Open services innovation: Rethinking your business to grow and compete in a new era*. Hoboken, NJ: Wiley.

Christensen, C. M., Grossman, J. H., & Hwang, J. (2009). *Innovator's prescription: A disruptive solution for health care*. New York, NY: McGraw-Hill.

Curry, D. (2012, September 1). Physical inactivity causes 1 in 10 deaths. *The Nation's Health*.

Estes, C. L., Chapman, S. A., Dodd, D., Hollister, B., & Harrington, C. (2013). *Health policy: Crisis and reform*. Burlington, MA: Jones & Bartlett Learning.

Fabrizio, N. A. (2011). Employing physicians: The future is now. In *Futurescan 2012: Healthcare trends and implications 2012-2017*. Chicago, IL: Health Administration Press.

Fisher, E. S., McClelland, M. B., Bertko, J., Lieberman, S. M., Lee, J. J., Lewis, J. L., & Skinner, J. S. (2009). Fostering accountable health care: Moving forward in Medicare. *Health Affairs, 28*(2), w219–w231.

Florida, R. (2011). *The rise of the creative class*. New York, NY: Basic Books.

Goodman, J. C. (2012). *Priceless: Curing the health care crisis*. Oakland, CA: The Independent Institute.

Gross, D. (2012). *The myth of American decline and the rise of the new economy: Better, stronger, faster*. New York, NY: Free Press.

Hamel, G. (2012). *What matters now: How to win in a world of relentless change, ferocious competition, and unstoppable innovation*. San Francisco, CA: Jossey-Bass.

Hayes, C. (2012). *Twilight of the elites: America after meritocracy*. New York, NY: Crown.

Henry J. Kaiser Family Foundation. (2012). *Comparison of Medicare premium support proposals*. Retrieved from http://kaiserfamilyfoundation.files.wordpress.com/2013/01/8284.pdf

Houle, D., & Fleece, J. (2011). *The new age: The future of health care in America*. Naperville, IL: Source Books.

Institute of Medicine. (1999). *To err is human: Building a safer health system*. Retrieved from http://www.nap.edu/openbook.php?record_id=9728.

Institute of Medicine. (2013). *Best care at lower cost: The path to continuously learning health care in America*. Washington, DC: National Academies Press.

Jennings, J. (2012). *The reinventors: How extraordinary companies pursue radical continuous change*. New York, NY: Penguin Group.

Langley, G. J., Moen, R. D., Nolan, K. M., Nolan, T. W., Norman, C. L., & Provost, L. P. (2009). *The improvement guide: A practical approach to enhancing organizational performance*. San Francisco, CA: Jossey-Bass.

Leinwand, P., & Mainardi, C. (2011). *The essential advantage: How to win with a capabilities-driven strategy*. Boston, MA: Harvard Business Review Press.

Longman, P. (2012). *Best care anywhere: Why VA health care would work better for everyone*. San Francisco, CA: Berrett-Koehler.

Lowrey, A., & Pear, R. (2012, July 28). Doctor shortage likely to worsen with health law. *New York Times*. Retrieved from http://www.nytimes.com/2012/07/29/health/policy/too-few-doctors-in-many-us-communities.html

Marvassi, F., & Stafford, R. S. (2012). From sick care to health care—reengineering prevention into the U.S. system. *New England Journal of Medicine, 367*(10), 889–893.

Mehrotra, A., & Lave, J. (2012). Visits to retail clinics grew fourfold from 2007 to 2009, although their share of overall outpatient visits remains low. *Health Affairs, 31*(9), 2123–2129.

Miniter, B. (2012). *The 4% solution: Unleashing the economic growth America needs.* New York, NY: Crown Business.

O'Callaghan, S. (2010). *Turnaround leadership: Making decisions, rebuilding trust and delivering results after a crisis.* Philadelphia, PA: Kogan Page.

Ogden, C. L., Carroll, M. D., Kit, B. K., & Fiegal, K. M. (2012, January). *Prevalence of obesity in the United States, 2009–2010* (Data Brief no. 82). Retrieved from http://www.cdc.gov/nchs/data/databriefs/db82.pdf

Omachonu, V. K., & Einspruch, N. G. (2010). Innovation in healthcare delivery systems: A conceptual framework. *The Innovation Journal: The Public Sector Innovation Journal, 15*(1), 1–20.

Pear, R. (2008, July 9). Report links dead doctors to payments by Medicare. *New York Times.* Retrieved from http://www.nytimes.com/2008/07/09/washington/09fraud.html.

Perednia, D. A. (2011). *Overhauling America's healthcare machine: Stop the bleeding and save trillions.* Upper Saddle River, NJ: FT Press.

Schimpff, S. C. (2012). *The future of health-care delivery: Why it must change and how it will affect you.* Washington, DC: Potomac Books.

Shortell, S. M. (2010). Challenges and opportunities for population health partnerships. *Preventing Chronic Disease, 7*(6), A114. Retrieved from http://www.cdc.gov/pcd/issues/2010/nov/10_0110.htm

Starr, P. (2011). *Remedy and reaction: The peculiar American struggle over health care reform.* New Haven, CT: Yale University Press.

Vanourek, B., & Vanourek, G. (2012). *Triple crown leadership: Building excellent, ethical, and enduring organizations.* New York, NY: McGraw-Hill.

Wagner, T. (2012). *Creating innovators: The making of young people who will change the world.* New York, NY: Simon & Schuster.

Washington, H. A. (2011). *Deadly monopolies.* New York, NY: Doubleday.

INNOVATION IN PHYSICIAN LEADERSHIP EDUCATION

Francis G. Belardi

The need for physician leadership education in the new millennium is underscored by the evolving complexity of the U.S. health care system. Traditionally, physician leaders were appointed to leadership positions based on their clinical reputation and personal interest in medical administration. Few of these physicians had formal training in leadership. Although some medical schools have begun to offer dual degrees like the MD-MBA to students interested in medical leadership, the number of U.S. physicians enrolled in this type of program is minimal and insufficient to meet the future leadership needs of the health care system.

Leadership Education at the Guthrie Clinic

The Guthrie Clinic is a 102-year-old, 270-physician, multispecialty group practice located in northeastern Pennsylvania. Prior to 2009, Guthrie did not sponsor a leadership program specifically for physician leaders, although Guthrie did sponsor leadership classes that were open to physicians as well as nonphysician administrative leaders. The annual leadership training requirement for physician leaders was minimal. A few physician leaders were sporadically enrolled in traditional, external MBA (master of business administration) and MMM (master of medical management) degree programs. In 2006, Guthrie underwent a significant change in its executive physician team, after which the team concluded that the current leadership education for the nearly sixty Guthrie physician leaders was inadequate. The decision was made to develop a physician-specific leadership curriculum within Guthrie in conjunction with an academic partner. There are three components to this physician leadership journey:

- An annual physician performance review for all Guthrie physicians to assess for leadership effectiveness and interest.

- A partnership between the Guthrie Clinic and King's College (located in Wilkes-Barre, Pennsylvania) to sponsor a physician leadership certificate program that would enable physicians to qualify for an MHA (master of health administration) degree. Since 2010, ten to fifteen physicians per year have enrolled in the curriculum, and to date, twenty-seven physicians at various levels of leadership in the Guthrie Clinic have been educated.

- A physician talent management program will begin in the near future.

The physician leadership certificate curriculum is composed of five master's degree courses. The program is offered annually and requires a physician commitment of ten months. The courses are web-based and physicians complete them from the privacy of their medical offices or from home. Each course generates three credits toward the MHA degree, and each course requires a midterm and a final examination as well as a term paper that is focused on a Guthrie-centric project pertinent to the course topic.

The current Guthrie Physician Leadership Certificate Program consists of the following courses:

- Healthcare Marketing
- Healthcare Law
- Human Resource Management
- Healthcare Financial Management
- Leadership and Executive Skills for the Physician

The curricular components were selected based on an assessment of the skills needed to provide appropriate physician leadership in positions from clinical section chiefs through board membership. The curriculum was designed to meet the requirements of King's MHA program as well. The Guthrie-King's program has generated significant interest among Guthrie physicians. The first class included the president of the Guthrie Clinic, several board members, and other physician leaders. By the end of 2012, 50 percent of Guthrie's physician leaders had completed the leadership certificate program.

An intramural physician leadership program has distinct advantages over external programs. Physicians are more likely to participate in a program that can be completed from their home base, minimizing time away from family and their professional practice. Guthrie's complete financial support for the certificate program tuition also makes that program an attractive alternative to external courses, which are significantly more expensive. Intramural programs also avoid the costs of transportation, lodging, and meals associated with traveling. Physicians have enjoyed the collegiality of joining practice partners in a Guthrie-centric program as well. Several projects developed through term papers have attained applicability within the Guthrie system.

Conclusion

The Guthrie Physician Leadership Certificate Program is still in the early stages, but results to date have been encouraging. The journey has been a process in evolution, beginning with physician annual performance reviews, continuing through the development of a physician leadership program with an academic institution, and finally, applying a physician talent management assessment process to appropriately evaluate each physician leader's knowledge and effectiveness before and after leadership education.

The future success of multispecialty group practices will depend on robust physician leadership and talent management programs. Guthrie currently seems well positioned to meet the physician leadership challenges facing the U.S. health care system.

DISCUSSION QUESTIONS

1. Why is leadership development so necessary for physicians as the health care industry responds to health care reform efforts?

2. What are the major components of the physician leadership development program offered to physicians employed by the Guthrie health care system?

3. How were the courses chosen for the Guthrie Physician Leadership Certificate Program?

4. What are the major advantages of an intramural physician leadership development program?

USING MARKETING TOOLS TO INCREASE EARLY REFERRALS OF CHILDREN WITH DEVELOPMENTAL AND BEHAVIORAL DISORDERS

Jeff Kile
Bernard J. Healey

A *developmental disability*, according to the Developmental Disabilities Assistance and Bill of Rights Act, is defined as a severe, chronic disability that originated at birth or during childhood, is expected to continue indefinitely, and substantially restricts the individual's functioning in several major life activities. According to Boyle, Decoufle, and Yeargin-Allsopp (1994), 17 percent of children in the United States have experienced a developmental disability causing a substantial impact on their health and learning ability. Boyle et al.'s research shows that developmental disabilities have a tremendous negative impact on children's health and educational functioning, and the impact can be different depending on the type of disability. Learning disabilities have been shown to have a profound effect on school performance.

Early diagnosis of and intervention with these disabilities can usually result in successful outcomes for the child. The key to this success is early referral of children to the services they require in order to reduce the effects of the disability. Head and Abbeduto (2007) point out that three goals need to be achieved when there is concern over development in children: diagnosis of the disability, intervention by medical providers, and evaluation of the progress of the intervention. However, because the participation rate of children in medical care for developmental disabilities is currently low, a concerted intervention is required to get children with these disabilities into treatment at an early age (Rosenberg, Zhang, & Robinson, 2008). This is not an easy task because awareness of the importance of early referral of these children is very limited in most communities. Thus there is a need for targeted educational programs for health care providers and parents (Sices, Feudtner, McLaughlin, Drotar, & Williams, 2004).

Early recognition of developmental disorders is a prerequisite to the improvement of outcomes and cost-effective care. It is known that less than half of affected children are identified before entering school. In most areas of the country, referrals to early intervention by parents and clinicians are made at a much lower rate for children under three years of age than they are for older children. Clearly, most referrals should be made well before the age of three for optimal intervention and outcome.

Using a PSA Program to Increase Awareness of Developmental Issues

The problem of a high prevalence of children residing in Luzerne County, Pennsylvania, with developmental and behavioral disabilities was identified by a local pediatric practice. These children with disabilities were not being referred for diagnosis and intervention by parents and medical care practices in northeastern Pennsylvania. A task force was organized to deal with the problem, and it was decided to utilize a marketing approach to increase the awareness of this problem among parents and other potential referral sources throughout the county. The marketing approach to solving this very serious health problem was launched in late 2007.

The marketing program was created and implemented by local pediatricians. Public service announcements (PSAs) were developed and disseminated in the local media, day-care centers, and other locations that support children's programs to communicate the need for increased awareness of potential childhood development problems, These PSAs were printed flyers containing information about the signs of behavioral and developmental problems that might be found in young children, along with a method of referral to appropriate medical care. The information from the PSAs was turned into a fact sheet that was used by local media, sports, and medical celebrities familiar to the targeted population to present the information. This promotional campaign also focused on making local physicians aware of the magnitude of this problem in Luzerne County. A secondary part of this campaign targeted whether or not a group of community volunteers could improve awareness and early referral of children less than three years of age to medical care. For this study, children's developmental and behavioral disabilities were defined as abnormalities involving speech, cognitive, fine motor, or gross motor development. The volunteers included pediatricians, family practice physicians, representatives from media outlets, and a number of community leaders from Luzerne County.

Table CS2.1   Preschool Referrals, July 1, 2005, to December 31, 2011

Fiscal/School Year (July 1-June 30)	Aggregate Count	Infant/Toddler Referred Students	Referred Students Other Than I/T Referrals	No. of Referred Students Diagnosed with Developmental Delay
2005–06	778	112	666	372
2006–07	782	105	677	392
2007–08	952	152	800	476
2008–09	980	171	809	490
2009–10	993	207	786	521
2010–11*	826*	100*	726	NA

Note: NA = Not available.
*For the time period July 1, 2010, to December 31, 2011.

This program has substantially increased referrals to early intervention programs, as shown in Table CS2.1. The number of infants and toddlers experiencing developmental and behavioral problems and referred to medical care has increased every year since 2006. This program continues to further develop this marketing approach to a community health problem and is expanding the program to neighboring counties.

Conclusion

The incidence of developmental and behavioral disabilities is much higher in Luzerne County than in most other counties in Pennsylvania. This problem motivated a community group to mobilize a task force of volunteers including physicians and community leaders to attempt to improve awareness of the problem and increase referrals of children with these disabilities to medical care, before they reach three years of age. The intervention was successful, and reports indicate that referrals to medical care for children with developmental disabilities have increased.

The success of this project has motivated the group of volunteers to consider the development of a website (to be hosted by a local college) to further increase awareness of this child health problem among a much larger percentage of the county population. The website will offer a pretest, followed by a ten-minute educational program about the signs and symptoms of developmental and behavioral disabilities, and then it will offer a posttest of knowledge gained from watching the program. This educational program will consist of a series of voice-narrated PowerPoint slides utilizing a local pediatrician who will discuss the signs and symptoms of these disabilities in children under the age of three and the need for early referral to medical care.

DISCUSSION QUESTIONS

1. What impact did a PSA have on identifying children with learning disabilities in this study?

2. How could this marketing approach be useful for other community health issues?

3. What other ways could be used to bring this developmental disabilities awareness program to more people?

REFERENCES

Boyle, C. A., Decoufle, P., & Yeargin-Allsopp, M. (1994). Prevalence and health impact of developmental disabilities in US children. *Pediatrics*, *93*(3), 399–403.

Head, L. S., & Abbeduto, L. (2007). Recognizing the role of parents in developmental outcomes: A systems approach to evaluating the child with developmental disabilities. *Mental Retardation and Developmental Disabilities Research Reviews*, *13*(4), 293–301.

Rosenberg, S. A., Zhang, D., & Robinson, C. C. (2008). Prevalence of developmental delays and participation in early intervention services for young children. *Pediatrics*, *121*(6), 1503–1509.

Sices, L., Feudtner, C., McLaughlin, J., Drotar, D., & Williams, M. (2004). How do primary care physicians manage children with possible developmental delays? A national survey with an experimental design. *Pediatrics*, *113*(2), 274–282.

FALL REDUCTION AT GEISINGER WYOMING VALLEY MEDICAL CENTER

"Above All, Do No Harm"

Daniel J. Amorino

The Hippocratic Oath is one of the most widely known tenets of a health care provider's code of conduct. The code requires a new health care provider to swear to uphold a number of professional ethical standards. One of the most popular phrases of the oath is "Above all, do no harm." In its groundbreaking report *To Err Is Human*, the Institute of Medicine (IOM) (1999) estimated that 98,000 patients die each year because of preventable medical harm. This death rate is equivalent to the death rate from three jumbo jets crashing every other day.

As a result of the sobering data brought to light by the IOM's 1999 report on medical errors, health care organizations have made reducing patient harm a key focus in quality improvement initiatives. Geisinger Wyoming Valley Medical Center (GWV) is one such organization that has undertaken a long and hard-fought journey to reduce patient harm. This case study focuses on GWV's efforts to reduce preventable harm by reducing fall rates.

Geisinger Health System and Geisinger Wyoming Valley

GWV is part of Geisinger Health System (GHS), a physician-led, integrated health care system that spans forty-four counties in Pennsylvania, serving over 2.6 million residents. As of the end of fiscal year 2011, GHS employed over 14,000 individuals, including over 1,300 doctors and advanced practitioners. In that same year the system had over 2.3 million outpatient visits and over 85,000 emergency room visits, and had total revenues of $2.7 billion (Geisinger Health System, 2011). Geisinger physician offices are strategically located in small and large towns and cities throughout the region, enabling patients to have close proximity to their providers.

In addition to nearly forty community practice sites, there are a number of hospitals, ambulatory surgery sites, and other Geisinger-affiliated programs or partnerships such as the Henry Hood Center for Health Research, Marworth Alcohol & Chemical Dependency Treatment Center, and the Life Flight® (air ambulance) program.

GWV has 243 licensed beds and features a state-of-the-art critical care building, the region's only freestanding heart hospital, a transplant and organ donation program, and various specialty programs in medicine and surgery. There are several nursing units with varying levels of acuity such as a labor and delivery unit, pediatrics unit, progressive care unit (PCU), intensive care unit (ICU), cardiac step-down unit, and several medical-surgical units.

Types of Preventable Harm in Hospitals

Some of the most common types of preventable errors in health care are hospital-acquired infections (HAIs). Some examples of typical HAIs are methicillin-resistant *Staphylococcus aureus* (MRSA), central line infections, ventilator-associated pneumonia (VAP), and urinary tract infections (UTIs). Another preventable error is medication error. More than 1 million serious medication errors occur every year in U.S. hospitals (Kuperman et al., 2007). *To Err Is Human* suggests that there are over 7,000 deaths per year from medication errors (Institute of Medicine, 1999). Two additional hospital-acquired conditions are wrong-site surgeries and objects being left in patients during surgery. Although it does not seem feasible that errors like these could happen, these serious and not-so-uncommon events do occur. Another preventable error and the focus of this case study is patient falls.

Falls are the leading cause of injury among adults sixty-five years old or older. In 2005, the total cost of falls in the entire U.S. health care system was $23.6 billion (Roudsari, Ebel, Corso, Molinari, & Koepsell, 2005). Estimates of costs for a fall in the hospital range from $4,000 to $37,000 (Inouye, Brown, & Tinetti, 2009; Rizzo et al., 1998; Wong et al., 2011). The caveat to the costs that hospitals incur to fix their mistakes is that as of October 1, 2008, the Centers for Medicare & Medicaid Services (CMS) will not reimburse costs for treating certain hospital-acquired (preventable) conditions. Falls in hospitals, along with several other hospital-acquired conditions, are among the original conditions Medicare will not cover the cost of treating due to their preventability (CMS, 2008).

Geisinger Quality Institute

The Geisinger Quality Institute (GQI) is a subdivision of the Division of Quality and Patient Safety within GHS. GQI employs full-time process improvement specialists, or coaches. These specialists travel throughout the entire Geisinger system. GQI specialists serve as coaches to facilitate improvement work that goes on in a clinical microsystem. A *clinical microsystem* in health care delivery is defined as a small group of people who work together on a regular basis to provide care to discrete subpopulations, including patients (Dartmouth Institute for Health Policy and Clinical Practice, 2012). GQI specialists embed themselves in a microsystem in order to address an issue or problem the group is facing. Their work is done methodically, through educational meetings and exercises using teaching tools. Groups learn quality improvement tools and apply these tools to the problems they are trying to address. The specialist also helps the microsystem implement several Plan, Do, Study, Act (PDSA) cycles in order to test potential solutions to the problems.

Fall Rates and Best Practices in Fall Reduction

A *fall rate* is calculated by taking the number of falls in a given area for a period of time and then dividing it into patient days or the number of days a patient is taking up a hospital bed in a given time period. Nationally, the median for fall rates is about three falls per 1,000 patient days (National Database of Nursing Quality Indicators [NDNQI], 2011). The Studer Group has done research into some of the best practices surrounding fall reduction. One Studer research study of the Sacred Heart Hospital in Pensacola, Florida, found that Sacred Heart Hospital was able to reduce fall rates by 33 percent by implementing effective hourly rounding (Studer Group, 2007). *Hourly rounding* is the process of a nurse or aide physically entering the room and assessing the patient for the 5 P's: Pain, Position, Potty, Placement, and P.O. (oral) fluids. Checking for the 5 P's is both visual and verbal. The nurse asks the patient proactive, direct questions about issues that the patient wouldn't necessarily think of if the nurse were to ask a general question such as, "Is there anything I can get for you?"

Another practice related to communication and fall reduction is the patient safety huddle (Institute for Healthcare Improvement, 2012). In general, nurses do not have an hour per shift to spend in an improvement meeting. A huddle is a five- to ten-minute meeting that all unit staff can attend in order to be educated about performance improvement initiatives. Huddles are ideal for testing various PDSA cycles. For example, the staff can try a PDSA cycle on one shift on one day and then have a huddle at the end of the shift to debrief. These huddles allow all staff to participate and be engaged in process improvement.

The use of pressure sensitive bed pad alarms has also helped to reduce falls. When the patient gets up from the bed pad for any reason, the alarm goes off, alerting staff that the patient is moving. Bed pad alarms have been around for at least twenty years, but these alarms are not always used consistently for patients who are at high risk for falls, due to lack of staff compliance, alarms getting lost, or financial constraints on the institution. The literature varies on the effectiveness of such alarms, but generally, the use of an alarm *in conjunction* with other monitoring processes has shown a modest reduction in falls (Donald, Pitt, Armstrong, & Shuttleworth, 2000; Healey, 1994; Sadler, 1993; Stevens & Olson, 2000).

As discussed in the next section, all these best practices were implemented along the way in GWV's journey to fall reduction. In addition, there were intangibles such as leadership and frontline staff accountability, daily monitoring, and increased knowledge that made a difference in driving fall reduction at GWV. GWV has brought about a tremendous change in fall rates. In relation to the rate in other medical-surgical units in teaching hospitals, GWV's fall rate went from being in the sixty-ninth percentile (4.54 falls per 1,000 patient days) in the fourth quarter of 2009 to being in the twenty-eighth percentile (2.33 falls per 1,000 patient days) in the fourth quarter of 2011 (National Database of Nursing Quality Indicators, 2011).

The Journey to Uphold the Oath

In the summer of 2004, The Joint Commission, the largest accrediting body for health care organizations in the United States, released its yearly patient safety goals for the following year. For 2005, the goal related to fall reduction was twofold:

- "Assess and periodically reassess each patient's risk for falling, including the potential risk associated with the patient's medication regimen, and take action to address any identified risks."
- "Implement a fall reduction program, including a transfer protocol, and evaluate the effectiveness of the program" (Geller & Guzman, 2005).

GWV had a fall prevention program in place for several years that addressed opportunities to reduce fall rates. This initiative came from best practices in fall reduction that had been publicized in nursing research and through other professional organizations, such as The Joint Commission and the Institute for Healthcare Improvement (IHI). GWV's Nursing Administration had also been active for some time in trying to reduce fall rates, but was never able to consistently reduce fall rates below the twenty-fifth percentile among NDNQI hospitals. Figure CS3.1 shows five years of data related to fall rates at GWV during this period.

It was not until the last quarter of 2011 and the first two quarters of 2012 that a significant reduction in fall rates began at GWV. The wake-up call came as the fall rate peaked at 5.46 falls per 1,000 patient days in June 2011. Nursing Administration felt a strong sense of urgency to reduce falls

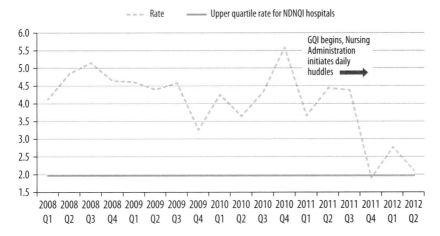

Figure CS3.1   GWV Fall Rates, 2008–2012

after the high rates were brought to the attention of the GHS board of directors. The board directed Nursing Administration to take the necessary steps to significantly reduce patient harm.

As a result of the board's call to action and recent consultations with the Studer Group, a health care consulting firm focused on operational, clinical, and financial outcomes, Nursing Administration took steps to home in on significantly reducing fall rates. Also during this time, GQI began working with the four units at GWV that had the highest fall rates in the hospital. The main focus initially was to look at safety rounds addressing the 5 P's. Observations by nurses and GQI showed that effective safety rounds were not being done reliably and consistently. For example, when a nurse entered a patient's room for rounding, it was not uncommon for the nurse or aide to ask, "How are you doing?" "Everything all right?" or "Can I get you anything?" This approach does not directly address the 5 P's.

A four-minute video focusing on the do's and don'ts for effective safety rounding was made, and all unit staff were shown the video and underwent a safety rounding seminar and certification conducted by Nursing Education. The seminar centered on how to ask direct questions related to the 5 P's. Questions such as "Are you in any pain?" "Can I help you to the bathroom?" "Do you need water?" "Are you comfortable in the position you are in?" and "Would you like to sit in the chair?" are the ones nurses need to ask patients. These direct questions address the areas that normally the patient is not thinking about unless he or she is asked directly. Effective questions are proactive; for example, informing the patient that he will be helped to the bathroom rather than asking if he needs to go to the bathroom.

Safety huddles are an important part of keeping patients safe. As mentioned previously, just about every quality improvement organization strongly encourages the use of huddles. In some GWV units, leaders decided that long team meetings were not engaging enough staff in improvement. So GQI led an effort to conduct safety huddles on each shift. Safety huddles were targeted at five minutes somewhere in the last half hour of the outgoing staff's shift. The huddles were always a *handoff* of knowledge from the outgoing to the incoming RN staff. Occasionally the aides would attend if they were not busy answering call bells or tending to other duties. The huddles, initially led by GQI staff, asked three questions:

1. Which patients are at risk for falls?

2. Why are these patients at risk for falls?

3. What is each patient's safety plan?

Most nurses acknowledged the benefit of taking time out of their busy routine to pause and focus solely on patients who were at risk. During the normal course of nursing reports, it may be mentioned that a patient is at risk, but the huddle focuses attention on all at-risk patients on the unit rather than just the ones the nurse is assigned to. The huddle can also be a great opportunity to discuss tests of changes or to relay important information to the entire group. Huddles are often times for a nurse manager, nurse leader, or charge nurse to recognize publicly the great work the staff is doing. The positive attitude that comes from this setting is powerful and can change the culture of a unit.

GQI then began to train the nursing leaders and charge nurses on the floor to conduct these huddles on their own. It is important to note that many times improvement initiatives start from the top (management) and come down, or they may even cut horizontally across the organization owing to the use of a consultative model like the GQI. However, the best and most effective way to achieve consistent improvement is by starting it from the ground up—among the nurses and staff working on the unit. If the frontline staff has bought into proposed changes that process improvement will bring about, they will personally make the necessary changes, ensure that others do so as well, and most important, guarantee that changes are sustained for time to come.

Nursing Administration support and accountability were integral to the success of this initiative. In June of 2011, Nursing Administration and the unit managers developed an action plan for immediate implementation. The plan covered the 5 P's, staffing, environmental rounds, change of shift procedures, bed alarms, safety huddles, and so forth. Another goal was to have weekly fall huddles among the unit managers and Nursing Administration. The chief nursing officer (CNO) and the vice president for nursing had been following the advice of the Studer Group to conduct weekly meetings or huddles that highlighted understanding challenges, transferring learning and best practices, rewarding and recognizing success, and holding leaders accountable for their results (Studer Group, 2007). However, after the meeting with the board, Nursing Administration began conducting daily five- to ten-minute huddles. Daily huddles created a sense of urgency throughout the entire organization to focus on fall reduction. As Margaret Hennelly-Bergin, the CNO at GWV, said about this initiative, "The key to improvement is to get the staff focused on one or two key things that will really lead to behavior change. We are asking our nursing staff to do a myriad of nursing tasks every day; they have so much on their minds. When they can direct their efforts on the one or two things related to fall prevention such as the 5 P's or safety huddles, it really helps to focus their attention on perfecting those particular tasks" (personal communication with the author, 2012).

The combination of using evidence-based practices more reliably and developing "cultural awareness" of fall prevention through leadership's communicating its heightened sense of urgency was the key determinant in enabling the great reduction in falls that has been sustained for nearly a year. In addition, the assistance that GQI offered as a third-party observer and facilitator was also essential to making the reduction in fall rates so successful. Other organizations should consider the use of a consultative model in which improvement specialists use a specific improvement methodology, such as PDSA, to help groups with important strategic initiatives. A third party's involvement can help groups to take an objective approach to improvement, as an outsider will have different perspectives and thoughts that can be very useful.

The overall reduction in falls was outstanding, and more specifically, the reduction in falls with injuries was also impressive (Figure CS3.2). It is

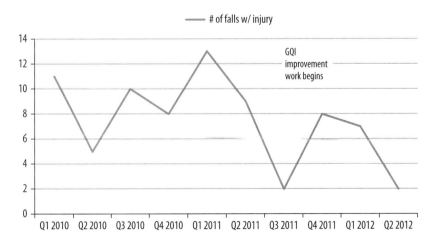

Figure CS3.2 GWV Reduction in Falls with Injuries over a Two-Year Period

estimated that by reducing falls with injuries, GQI helped GWV to avoid costs of over $375,000.

Conclusion

From its humble beginnings as a small hospital in rural Central Pennsylvania to its present status as one of the country's largest integrated health care systems, Geisinger has never forgotten its founder Abigail Geisinger's famous instruction that is now used as a slogan for the care that patients at Geisinger receive: "Make my hospital right; make it the best." Her prescript goes along nicely with the Hippocratic Oath that health care providers take when beginning their careers. No matter what the circumstances may be, we do the best we can do to make patients better off when they leave our care than they were before they entered it—to have them heal physically, mentally, emotionally, and even spiritually.

It is human nature to make mistakes, but in health care, mistakes can sometimes be fatal errors. The nursing staff at GWV make a commitment every day to reduce the errors that can be made when caring for patients at high risk for falls. In 2011 and 2012, GWV has reduced fall rates by over 35 percent. That change was not just chance. It came from the commitment of every nurse to change the way he or she practices clinical care. Through increased reliability in following and practicing evidenced-based guidelines, increased accountability for staff and management, greater emphasis on innovative thinking, and increased physical and educational resources, the nursing staff at GWV is journeying onward to uphold the oath and truly provide the best care.

DISCUSSION QUESTIONS

1. Think about the Hippocratic Oath and its charge to "do no harm". Besides falls, what are some other ways that harm occurs in the U.S. health care system?

2. If you were a manager on a unit that was experiencing high fall rates, what PDSA cycles would you test out to reduce those fall rates?

3. Why is it important to have executive leadership involvement when undertaking an improvement effort?

4. How would you compare and contrast the differences between (a) seeking help with an improvement effort from third parties (both internal and external consultants) and (b) making use of resources for improvement found in the unit or section that is experiencing a care gap?

REFERENCES

Centers for Medicare & Medicaid Services. (2008, July 31). Letter from Center for Medicaid and State Operations to state Medicaid directors (SMDL#08-004). Retrieved from http://www.cms.hhs.gov/SMDL/downloads/SMD073108.pdf

Dartmouth Institute for Health Policy and Clinical Practice. (2012). Resources within center. Retrieved from http://www.clinicalmicrosystem.org/about/background

Donald, I. P., Pitt, K., Armstrong, E., & Shuttleworth, H. (2000). Preventing falls on an elderly care rehabilitation ward. *Clinical Rehabilitation, 14*(2), 178–185.

Geisinger Health System. (2011). *Transforming health care.* Retrieved from http://www.geisinger.org/about/2011_AR_FINAL.pdf

Geller, K. H., & Guzman, J. L. (2005). JCAHO 2005 national patient safety goals. *Focus, 1,* 1–8.

Healey, F. (1994). Does flooring type affect risk of injury in older patients? *Nursing Times, 90,* 40–41.

Inouye, S. K., Brown, C. J., & Tinetti, M. E. (2009). Medicare nonpayment, hospital falls, and unintended consequences. *New England Journal of Medicine, 360*(23), 2390–2393.

Institute for Healthcare Improvement. (2012). Huddles. Retrieved from http://www.ihi.org/knowledge/Pages/Tools/Huddles.aspx

Institute of Medicine. (1999). *To err is human: Building a safer health system.* Washington, DC: National Academies Press.

Kuperman, G. J., Bobb, A., Payne, T. H., Avery, A. J., Gandhi, T. K., Burns, G., . . . Bates, D. W. (2007). Medication-related clinical decision support in computerized provider order entry systems: A review. *Journal of the American Medical Informatics Association, 14*(1), 29–40.

National Database of Nursing Quality Indicators. (2011, 4th quarter). Patient falls. In *2011 Quarterly Report: Staffing and Outcome Indicators.* Silver Spring, MD: American Nurses Association.

Rizzo, J. A., Friedkin, R., Williams, C. S., Nabors, J., Acampora, D., & Tinetti, M. E. (1998). Health care utilization and costs in a Medicare population by fall status. *Medical Care, 36*(8), 1174–1188.

Roudsari, B. S., Ebel, B. E., Corso, P. S., Molinari, N.-A., & Koepsell, T. D. (2005). The acute medical care costs of fall-related injuries among the U.S. older adults. *Injury, 36*(11), 1316–1322.

Sadler, C. (1993). Floored thinking. *Nursing Times, 89,* 20–21.

Stevens, J. A., & Olson, S. (2000). Reducing falls and resulting hip fractures among older women. *Morbidity and Mortality Weekly Report, 49*(RR-2), 1–12.

Studer Group. (2007). *Hourly rounding: Supplement.* Retrieved from http://www.mc.vanderbilt.edu/root/pdfs/nursing/hourly_rounding_supplement-studer_group.pdf

Wong, C. A., Recktenwald, A. J., Jones, M. L., Waterman, B. M., Bollini, M. L., & Dunagan, W. C. (2011). The cost of serious fall-related injuries at three Midwestern hospitals. *The Joint Commission Journal on Quality and Patient Safety, 37*(2), 81–87.

THE VA REINVENTS ITSELF

Joseph J. Marrone

The Veterans Health Administration (VHA) is the component of the U.S. Department of Veterans Affairs (VA) (sometimes referred to in short as the Veterans Administration) that implements the medical assistance program of the VA through the administration and operation of numerous VA medical centers. The VA has the most comprehensive system of assistance for veterans of any nation, developed or undeveloped, in the world. In 1776, the Continental Congress encouraged enlistment during the revolutionary war by providing pensions for soldiers who were disabled. Direct medical and hospital care were provided to veterans by individual states and communities. In 1811, the first medical facility for veterans was authorized by the federal government. During the nineteenth century, veterans' assistance was expanded to include benefits and pensions not only for veterans but also their widows and dependents.

When the United States entered World War I in 1917, a new system of benefits for veterans was rolled out. Included in these new programs were disability compensation, insurance for veterans and service persons, and vocational rehabilitation for the disabled. By 1920, the benefits were administered by three different government agencies: the Veterans Bureau, the Bureau of Pensions of the Interior Department, and the National Home for Disabled Volunteer Soldiers. The actual Department of Veterans Affairs (VA) was born in 1930 when Congress authorized the consolidation and coordination of government activities affecting war veterans. The three previous agencies were now combined into one.

The VA health care system has grown from 54 hospitals in 1930, to include 152 hospitals, 800 community-based outpatient clinics, 126 nursing home care units, and 35 domiciliary facilities. VA health care facilities provide a broad spectrum of medical, surgical, and rehabilitative care. The responsibilities and benefits programs of the Veterans Administration grew enormously during the following six decades. World War II resulted in not only a vast increase in the veteran population but also in a large number of new benefits enacted by Congress for veterans of the war. The World

War II GI Bill, signed into law on June 22, 1944, is said to have had more impact on the American way of life than any other law since the Homestead Act of 1862. The Veterans Administration was responsible for carrying out the law's key provisions: education and training; loan guaranty for homes, farms, or businesses; and unemployment pay. Further education assistance acts were passed for the benefit of veterans of the Korean conflict, the Vietnam War, Persian Gulf War, and the wars in Iraq and Afghanistan (U.S. Department of Veterans Affairs, n.d.).

During the past twenty years the VA has been blasted in the media and in political arenas for its medical treatment of veterans, many calling that treatment barbaric and cold. The VA took these comments and worked to change the opinions and to transform the quality of the health care. Today veterans and political pundits alike praise the VA for its use of electronic medical records, its focus on preventive care, and its outstanding results.

The Dark Years

One of the early examples of VA mismanagement is the Colonel Forbes debacle in 1923. Colonel Forbes was appointed to run the newly formed Veterans Bureau and to manage the building of new hospitals, staff them, and supply them. He went about doing this by taking kickbacks and selling off new supplies such as bed sheets and alcohol as army surplus. All the while the veterans coming home were not being treated because of shortages in the veterans' hospitals. These soldiers were exposed to all the hazards of World War I, such as mustard gas, only to return home and be treated poorly by the country they went to defend. Colonel Forbes is said to have swindled $200 million in 1923, or about $2.1 billion in today's dollars. He served time in Leavenworth for his mismanagement of taxpayer dollars, but his crime also had effects on health care services that created much mistrust in the Veterans Bureau. It was not until after World War II, when Omar Bradley was placed in the VA leadership role, that changes began to take hold.

In that role, Bradley was credited with working with deans of many medical schools, gaining their confidence and helping to turn the Veterans Administration around. The VA hospitals partnered with medical schools. The medical schools used the VA facilities as training hospitals for new internists, and in exchange, they raised the proficiency and abilities of the doctors serving at those hospitals. Bradley modernized and restructured an antiquated system, concentrating on the needs of the veterans rather than on political considerations.

Unfortunately, the high praise and good name of the Veterans Administration in that era did not last long. In the 1950s, the federal government began cutting the VA budget, leading to many layoffs and, again, poor service for the veterans. During this period many Korean War veterans could not get help at VA hospitals as they had difficulty proving they had service-related injuries. These issues continued into the Vietnam War era, where returning troops found the VA hospitals understaffed and in various states of disrepair.

The Beginning of Change

In the 1970s, a change was beginning to flow through the halls of the Veterans Administration. Everyone working in the VA saw a need for change, and some took it upon themselves to make it happen. One such person was Kenneth Dickie. Dickie began working on a project that was a secret from all but a few select people. What this new and innovative project started was an electronic medical records system for the Veterans Administration, a system now called VistA. VistA stands for Veterans Health Information System and Technology Architecture. The VistA system had a bottom-up design; that is, the initial users of the software contributed their input to its design and implementation as it was being written. VistA has transformed the way veterans' medical records are kept and reviewed. With the records electronically stored, the attending doctors and medical personnel can quickly and accurately call up the prescriptions for medications and the procedures prescribed for any patient at any time. VistA files also contain clinical data, such as patients' medical and health care utilization histories, demographics, diagnoses, and practitioner information. All patients treated at VA medical centers are included in the files, which are updated continuously at the point of care or as part of administrative processes. VistA has dramatically reduced medical errors at the VA while also improving diagnoses, quality of care, scientific understanding of the human body, and the development of medical protocols based on hard data about what drugs and procedures work best (Longman, 2012).

VistA has also helped to reduce costs for care by reducing duplicate tests and medications. VistA's support of email is another cost-saving feature that streamlines correspondence with patients. Instead of sending notifications to patients via a phone call or a mailed letter, a group of patients within the VistA database can be identified and contacted quickly with a single email. For example, information from drug manufacturers such as a drug recall can be sent out to all affected patients in the database at once.

Expanding upon its success with VistA, the VA is working with the Department of Defense to create one open source system and share the information across the two agencies. They would like to have an interacting, data-transferring system operational by 2017.

Putting Veterans' Health First

To reduce medication errors, the VA, along with the medical industry as a whole, has begun using a computerized system to dispense medications. Today, when dispensing a drug to a patient, an attending nurse uses a desktop computer to scan both the patient's ID bracelet, which has all the patient's pertinent information, and the medication prescribed to the patient. The computer cross-references the two scanned items and determines whether or not the specified medication is correct for that patient. This new technology reduces human error by the attending nurses or doctors. With this same system, medications can be checked for drug interactions and potential side affects.

A major shift came in 1997 when the VA agreed to begin documenting medical mistakes. This was no easy undertaking, as no one likes to admit blame, especially when it comes to something so serious. But taking this large risk and getting the doctors to agree made a wholesale change in the way VA health care worked. Knowing your mistakes makes it much easier to avoid them in the future. For example, with the VistA system, a surgeon can now scan a patient's wristband in order to check the procedure to be done and where on the patient's body it is to be done, thus avoiding wrong-site errors. Doctors have also begun marking the area or limb to be operated on with a pen. This is a very low-cost, simplistic answer to a difficult and possibly tragic problem. These new processes were made available simply by reporting errors, understanding them, and then finding ways to avoid them in the future.

In the past few years VA hospitals also have taken the lead in implementing patient-centered medical home (PCMH) care. Within this "home" for care, a physician, nurse practitioner, or physician's assistant; a registered nurse; a pharmacist; a social worker; and a psychologist work collaboratively to treat a patient. The result is improvements in access, chronic-disease management, and coordination between primary physicians and specialists.

The VA Answer for Everyone

In our current health care system doctors are paid a fee for service; the more patients they see, the more money they make. Under this same fee-for-service approach, when a doctor sends a patient to the hospital, he or she can charge that patient every time the doctor visits the patient in the hospital. Doctors can charge for each follow-up visit after tests or surgery. If a doctor or hospital were to institute a new program—for example, one that helps keep diabetics healthier—this would reduce visits to both the doctor and hospital. Under the current health care reimbursement system both the doctor and the hospital would lose money. They would lose money because there would be fewer patient visits and fewer payments from insurance companies. Currently, it is not sound business practice for the health care system to keep us healthy. Veterans Health Administration doctors are not paid on a fee-for-service basis, thus they have no interest in keeping a patient coming back for more and more care.

In a recent survey of patient satisfaction, the VA scored an 81 percent positive return. How many of us who use the traditional health care system can say that we are satisfied or happy with our service 81 percent of the time? Most people find their health care system cumbersome and cold. If the civilian health care industry would imitate VA practices, we would have a better all-around health care system for all people.

The VA's near-lifetime relationship with veterans gives it unique incentives and capabilities as an institution to maximize prevention, integration, and effective disease management. That long-term relationship is a function of the agency's scale; it would not exist to nearly the same extent if the VA served only a single city or region because it would be constantly losing patients who moved (Longman, 2012). Another benefit of the Veterans Administration is its sheer size and negotiating power. It is able to negotiate with drug companies and many other suppliers and that, by one estimate, results in savings of 48 percent on drugs and supplies (Blake, 2010).

Another important takeaway from the VA's transformation is its status as a mission-driven, nonprofit institution. As with all true HMOs, the VA's model of care minimizes overtreatment, if only because its doctors are on salary and thus lack financial incentives to perform unnecessary procedures. Also like all true HMOs, the VA operates within a fixed, or capitated, budget, as opposed to receiving fees for services, and this too minimizes overtreatment. But unlike many HMOs, the VA is not accountable to shareholders for maximizing profits, so it also lacks incentives to engage in *undertreatment* of patients (Longman, 2012).

Conclusion

The Department of Veterans Affairs has evolved from a chaotic and underserving agency to a well-designed organization focused on patient care. The reinvention of the VA began from the inside by people caring about what they do. The changes were not brought about by politicians and managerial people. Change came from the people working within the organization, a perfect example of bottom-up management as a success story and one to be followed. This case study has suggested many reasons why this model should and could be used to change the overall U.S. health care system and resolve the major health care issues facing our country today. The most apparent and obvious change would involve the fee-for-service method of payment for doctor's office visits and hospital care. This single change could save health care costs exponentially. There is support in the market place today for imitating the VA model, but so far nothing has been done to implement these changes. We continue to have exorbitant rises in our costs for health care with no end in sight. By using the VistA computer program across the country, the VA health system has been able to share records, reduce medical errors, and maintain continuity of care, thus reducing costs, while the rest of this country's health care system continues to work toward using electronic medical records in a piecemeal and uncoordinated fashion. Until the American health care industry adopts a universal working model such as VistA, we will continue to see exorbitant rises in health care. Only a coordinated effort by the entire industry can bring the cost of health care under control.

There are a few health care systems in the private sector that have a model similar to the VA's: the Cleveland Clinic, the Mayo Clinic, Intermountain Health Care, Geisinger Health System, and Kaiser Permanente. These health care systems are using innovative electronic health records and are developing and implementing innovative care models. However, overall, VA medical care is an excellent example of how it is the federal government that is leading on health care quality and cost.

DISCUSSION QUESTIONS

1. Recalling the way Colonel Forbes swindled $200 million from the government in 1923, would you think that kind of fraud would be caught more readily today, or could these things still happen? Explain your answer and give examples.

2. The VistA system was built using a bottom-up design. What does that mean, and what positive effects can it have when developing a software system like VistA?

3. What cost savings should result from using the email system incorporated into VistA to communicate with patients and providers?

4. VistA started the storing of electronic medical records. Now it is the standard being rolled out by the government. Do you think electronic health records are the correct way to improve coordination of care, or are there likely to be too many problems, including security risks, going forward?

REFERENCES

Blake, M. (2010, July–August). Dirty medicine. *Washington Monthly*, p. 1007.

Longman, P. (2012). *Best care anywhere: Why VA health care would work better for everyone.* San Francisco, CA: Barrett-Koehler.

U.S. Department of Veterans Affairs. (n.d.). History—VA history. Retrieved from http://www.va.gov/about_va/vahistory.asp